Nanomaterials

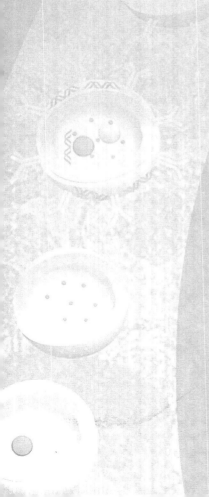

Nanomaterials
Science and Applications

edited by

Deborah Kane
Adam Micolich
Peter Roger

PAN STANFORD PUBLISHING

Published by

Pan Stanford Publishing Pte. Ltd.
Penthouse Level, Suntec Tower 3
8 Temasek Boulevard
Singapore 038988

Email: editorial@panstanford.com
Web: www.panstanford.com

British Library Cataloguing-in-Publication Data
A catalogue record for this book is available from the British Library.

Nanomaterials: Science and Applications

Copyright © 2016 Pan Stanford Publishing Pte. Ltd.

All rights reserved. This book, or parts thereof, may not be reproduced in any form or by any means, electronic or mechanical, including photocopying, recording or any information storage and retrieval system now known or to be invented, without written permission from the publisher.

For photocopying of material in this volume, please pay a copying fee through the Copyright Clearance Center, Inc., 222 Rosewood Drive, Danvers, MA 01923, USA. In this case permission to photocopy is not required from the publisher.

ISBN 978-981-4669-72-6 (Hardcover)
ISBN 978-981-4669-73-3 (eBook)

Printed in the USA

Contents

Preface xiii
Acknowledgments xix

1 **The Design and Testing of Multifunctional Nanoparticles for Drug Delivery Applications**   1
Tristan D. Clemons, Helena M. Viola, Michael J. House, Livia C. Hool, and K. Swaminathan Iyer
  1.1 Overview of Nanoparticles in Medicine   2
    1.1.1 Nanoparticles in Modern Medicine   2
      1.1.1.1 Nanoparticles for drug delivery   4
      1.1.1.2 Micelles, liposomes, and dendrimers for drug delivery applications   7
      1.1.1.3 Polymeric nanoparticles and nanocapsules as drug delivery vehicles   10
    1.1.2 Nanoparticle and Cell Interactions   11
      1.1.2.1 Nanoparticle endocytosis   14
      1.1.2.2 Strategies to enhance cellular internalization   16
    1.1.3 Multifunctional Nanoparticles   17
      1.1.3.1 Passive vs. targeted nanoparticles: Surface functionalities of multifunctional nanoparticles   19
      1.1.3.2 Multifunctional nanoparticles incorporating imaging functionalities   23
      1.1.3.3 Magnetic resonance imaging   27
      1.1.3.4 Magnetic resonance contrast agents   29
      1.1.3.5 Fluorescent probes for biological imaging   30
    1.1.4 Assessing Nanoparticle Toxicity   32

1.2 Multifunctional Poly(Glycidyl Methacrylate) Nanoparticles and Their Application in Cardiac Ischemia-Reperfusion Injuries 35
 1.2.1 Rationale and Design of PGMA Nanoparticles for Therapeutic Delivery 35
 1.2.2 Current Treatment of Cardiac Ischemia-Reperfusion Injuries 37
 1.2.3 PGMA Nanoparticle Characterization and Surface Peptide Loading 39
 1.2.4 A Comparison of Cellular Uptake and Biodistribution 42
 1.2.5 Nanoparticle and TAT-Mediated Delivery of the AID Peptide Reduces Damage Following Ischemia-Reperfusion Injury 45
 1.2.6 Conclusions and Future Work 47

2 Yolk–Shell-Structured Nanoparticles: Synthesis, Surface Functionalization, and Their Applications in Nanomedicine 61
Tianyu Yang, Jian Liu, and Michael J. Monteiro

2.1 Controllable Synthesis of Yolk–Shell-Structured Nanoparticles 62
 2.1.1 The Hard-Template Method 63
 2.1.2 The Soft-Template Assembly Method 67
2.2 Approaches to Composition Control 69
 2.2.1 Yolk–Shell-Structured Nanoparticles with an Inorganic Material Shell 69
  2.2.1.1 Silica-shell-based yolk–shell-structured nanoparticles 69
  2.2.1.2 Yolk–shell-structured nanoparticles with an organosilica shell 69
  2.2.1.3 Other inorganic-material-shell-based yolk–shell-structured nanoparticles 70
 2.2.2 Yolk–Shell-Structured Nanoparticles with a Polymer Shell 71
2.3 Control of Surface Properties in Silica-Based YSNs 72
 2.3.1 Modification of Silica-Based Nanoparticle Surface by Living Radical Polymerization Techniques 72

		2.3.1.1	Living radical polymerization techniques	73

		2.3.1.2	Graft-from methods	75
		2.3.1.3	Graft-to method	79
		2.3.1.4	Combined graft-to/graft-from method	79
	2.3.2	Silica Surface Modification via Silane Chemistry		80
2.4	YSNs for Biomedicine Applications			82
	2.4.1	YSNs for Chemotherepy		82
	2.4.2	YSNs for Gene/Protein Delivery		86
	2.4.3	YSNs for Photothermal Therapy		88
	2.4.4	YSNs for Bioimaging		88
	2.4.5	YSNs with Dual Functions for Bioimaging and Chemotherapy		90
	2.4.6	YSNs with Dual Function: Photothermal Therapy and Chemotherapy		91
	2.4.7	Multifunction YSNs: Multimodal Imaging, Photothermal Therapy, and Delivery to Therapeutic Site		93
2.5	Conclusion			95

3 Chemical and Biological Sensors Based on Microelectromechanical Systems — 107

Gino Putrino, Adrian Keating, Mariusz Martyniuk, Lorenzo Faraone, and John Dell

3.1	Microelectromechanical Systems for Chemical/Biological Sensing and Atomic Force Microscopy		108
	3.1.1	MEMS Chemical and Biological Sensors	108
		3.1.1.1 Static operation mode	109
		3.1.1.2 Dynamic operation mode	110
	3.1.2	MEMS Sensor Implementations	111
	3.1.3	Example: Palladium-Coated Cantilever Hydrogen Sensor	113
	3.1.4	Chapter Overview	114
3.2	Current Techniques for MEMS Position Readout and Their Limitations		115
	3.2.1	Optical Readout Techniques	115
	3.2.2	Electronic Readout Techniques	117

3.3	Integrated Gratings: A New Technique for Cantilever Readout	118
	3.3.1 Optical Modeling of the Structure	121
3.4	Integrated Grating Readout Technique Demonstration	126
	3.4.1 Device Fabrication	126
	3.4.2 Electrostatic Actuation	129
	3.4.3 Fabricated Microcantilevers	130
3.5	Grating Technique Noise and Limits of Detection Analysis	133
	3.5.1 Theoretical Noise Analysis	133
	3.5.1.1 Thermomechanical noise	135
	3.5.1.2 Shot noise	136
	3.5.1.3 Johnson noise	137
	3.5.1.4 Total noise	137
	3.5.2 Experimental Limits of Detection	138
3.6	Conclusions	140

4 Aluminum Gallium Nitride/Gallium Nitride Transistor-Based Biosensor   **147**

Anna Podolska, Gia Parish, and Brett Nener

4.1	Introduction to Aluminum Gallium Nitride/Gallium Nitride Transistor-Based Biosensors	148
4.2	Current Technological Challenges and Limitations	151
	4.2.1 Reference-Electrode-Free Operation	152
	4.2.2 Device Design, Fabrication, and Packaging	154
4.3	Investigation into Improved Biocompatibility	158
4.4	Drug Testing	162
	4.4.1 Sensing Human Coronary Artery Endothelial Cells	165
4.5	Conclusions	168

5 Understanding Melanin: A Nano-Based Material for the Future   **175**

A. B. Mostert, P. Meredith, B. J. Powell, I. R. Gentle, G. R. Hanson, and F. L. Pratt

5.1	Introduction	176
	5.1.1 Melanin, the Nanobioelectronic Material	176
	5.1.2 What Is Melanin?	179

5.2	The Basics of Melanin Charge Transport		181
	5.2.1 The Current Model: Amorphous Semiconductor		181
	5.2.2 Investigating Melanin Charge Transport		183
5.3	How Wet Is Melanin?		183
5.4	Determining the Hydration-Dependent Conductivity Data		185
	5.4.1 The Importance of Different Contact Geometries		185
	5.4.2 Photoconductivity Data		188
5.5	Muon Spin Resonance: Evidence for an Alternative Transport Model		190
	5.5.1 Introducing the Concepts behind Muon Spin Resonance		190
	5.5.2 μSR Relaxation Parameters		190
		5.5.2.1 μSR experiment	191
		5.5.2.2 μSR results	192
	5.5.3 The Origin of Charge Transport in Melanin: The Comproportionation Reaction		194
5.6	Melanin: The Potential Ionic-to-Electronic Transducing Material		196
5.7	Conclusions		197

6 Phase Transition in CdSe Quantum Dots and Deposition of CdSe Quantum Dots on Graphene Sheets — 203
Fehmida K. Kanodarwala and John A. Stride

6.1	Introduction: Colorful World of Quantum Dots	204
6.2	Phase Transition in CdSe Quantum Dots	209
6.3	Deposition of CdSe Quantum Dots on Graphene Sheets	218
6.4	Conclusion and Outlook	225

7 Design of Novel Nanostructured Photoanode Materials for Low-Cost and Efficient Dye-Sensitized Solar Cell Applications — 231
Yang Bai, Zhen Li, Rose Amal, and Lianzhou Wang

7.1	Introduction		232
7.2	How Does a Dye-Sensitized Solar Cell Work?		234
	7.2.1 Operating Principles		234
	7.2.2 Key Components		236

		7.2.2.1	Metal oxide photoanode	237
		7.2.2.2	Sensitizer for light absorption	238
		7.2.2.3	Electrolyte for electron transportation	242
		7.2.2.4	Counterelectrodes	244
	7.3	Characterization Techniques		245
		7.3.1	Photovoltaic Characteristic Measurements	245
		7.3.2	Electrochemical Methods	246
	7.4	Development of Nanostructured Photoanodes		248
		7.4.1	Mesoporous Nanoparticle Films	249
		7.4.2	Light-Scattering and LSPR Effects	252
		7.4.3	Higher-Order Nanostructures	256
	7.5	Stability and Commercial Development of DSSCs		263
	7.6	Our Recent Work on Design of Novel Nanostructured Photoanodes		264
		7.6.1	ZnO NW/TiO$_2$ NP Hybrid Photoanode	265
		7.6.2	Porous Titania NS/NP Hybrid Photoanode	268
	7.7	Conclusions and Outlook		270

8 Gas Transport Properties and Transport-Based Applications of Electrospun Nanofibers — **289**
Dahua Shou, Lin Ye, and Jintu Fan

	8.1	Introduction to Electrospun Nanofibers		290
		8.1.1	The Big World of Small Fibers	290
		8.1.2	What Is Electrospinning?	291
		8.1.3	What Affects Electrospun Nanofibers?	293
		8.1.4	Transport-Based Applications: Filters and Protective Clothing	295
		8.1.5	Limitations of Transport Modeling: Flow and Diffusion	296
	8.2	Filters and Protective Clothing		298
		8.2.1	Filters	298
			8.2.1.1 Evaluation of filtration performance	298
			8.2.1.2 Mechanisms of particle filtration	299
			8.2.1.3 Measurement of particle filtration	301
		8.2.2	Protective Clothing	304
			8.2.2.1 Good candidates for protective systems	304

		8.2.2.2	Measurement of diffusive and convective flow resistances	304

		8.2.2.2	Measurement of diffusive and convective flow resistances	304
		8.2.2.3	Breathable electrospun nanofibers	305
	8.2.3	A Call for Nanoscale Transport Models		307
8.3	Gas Flow in Nanofibrous Media			309
	8.3.1	Background of Gas Flow		309
	8.3.2	Present Model of Gas Flow		310
	8.3.3	What Can Be Found from the Flow Model?		314
8.4	Vapor Diffusion in Nanofibrous Media			315
	8.4.1	Background of Vapor Diffusion		315
	8.4.2	Present Model of Vapor Diffusion		317
	8.4.3	Experimental Measurement of Vapor Diffusivity		319
	8.4.4	What Can Be Obtained from the Diffusion Model?		321
8.5	Summary and Future Work			324
	8.5.1	Conclusive Summary		324
	8.5.2	Future Perspective		325

9 An Introduction to Blender 2.69 for Scientific Illustrations   335
Iwan Kelaiah

9.1	Setting Up Blender 2.69		336
	9.1.1	Getting the Latest Version of Blender	336
	9.1.2	Installing and Running Blender 2.69	337
	9.1.3	Setting Up User Preferences	337
9.2	User Interface		339
	9.2.1	Splitting Windows	341
	9.2.2	Customising Window Types	342
	9.2.3	Properties Window	343
9.3	Using Hotkeys in Blender		345
	9.3.1	Exercise: Orientation in 3D Space, Switching Orthogonal/Perspective View, and Rendering	345
	9.3.2	Exercise: Object Creation, Deletion, and Transformation	347
	9.3.3	Exercise: Object Editing, Transformation, and Rendering	348
9.4	3D Modeling		350
	9.4.1	Planning	351

	9.4.2	Creating a 3D Model of a Hepatitis B Virus	353
	9.4.3	Placing Objects in the Scene	354
9.5	Cycles, Light, and Materials		363
	9.5.1	Using Cycles Render	363
	9.5.2	Lighting and Background Color	364
	9.5.3	Shading	365
9.6	Render Setup and Saving Results		383
	9.6.1	Setting Render Size and Quality	384
	9.6.2	Saving Images	385
9.7	Conclusion		387

Index 391

Preface

This book reports up-to-the-minute research on nanoparticles for drug delivery and applications in nanomedicine, nanoelectronics and microelectromechanical systems (MEMS) for biosensors, melanin as a nano-based future material, nanostructured materials for solar cell applications, the world of quantum dots illustrated by CdSe, and gas transport and transport-based applications of electrospun nanofibers. The research was primarily undertaken within Australia and gives an excellent overview of topics in advanced nanomaterials and structures, and their applications. The reader also gets a tutorial introduction to the computer software used to generate the 3D illustrations that appear throughout the book.

This is the second book from a project developed and supported by the Australian Nanotechnology Network (ANN; formerly the Australian Research Council Nanotechnology Network). To quote from the ANN website [1]:

> The Nanotechnology field is one of the fastest growing areas of research and technology. The Australian Nanotechnology Network (ANN) is dedicated to substantially enhancing Australia's research outcomes in this important field by promoting effective collaborations, exposing researchers to alternative and complementary approaches from other fields, encouraging forums for postgraduate students and early career researchers, increasing nanotechnology infrastructure, enhancing awareness of existing infrastructure, and promoting international links.

One of the key aims of the research network is to support professional and research skill development in postgraduate research

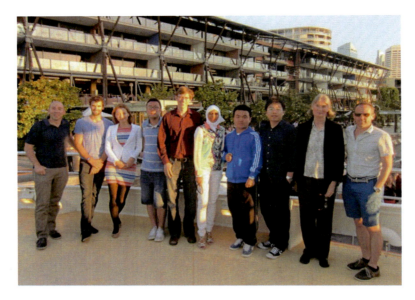

Figure 1 Participants in the book-writing workshop and two of the three editors. From left to right: Gino Putrino, Tristan Clemons, Anna Podolska, Tianyu Yang, Bernard Mostert, Fehmida, Kanodarwala, Dahua Shou, Yang Bai, Deb Kane, and Adam Micolich.

students and early career researchers. This book project was designed and implemented as an innovation in postgraduate/postdoctoral research skills and networking education. The program and process are described in some detail in the preface to the first book from the project [2]. Briefly, it involved workshopping the writing of the chapters within the community of first-named chapter authors and the editors at a book-writing workshop (see Fig. 1). The workshop supporting this book was held from December 4 to 10, 2013, at Macquarie University in Sydney, Australia [3]. Additional support and training on producing high-quality graphics to visualize the research work being reported in the chapters were undertaken. A guide to using Blender [4] for this purpose is included as Chapter 9 of this book, authored by Dr. Iwan Kelaiah. He trained and supported the workshop participants to use this application to produce figures for their individual book chapters. Some examples of the graphics produced appear on the cover and in Figs. 2–4.

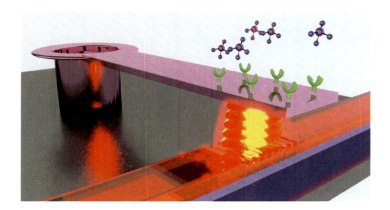

Figure 2

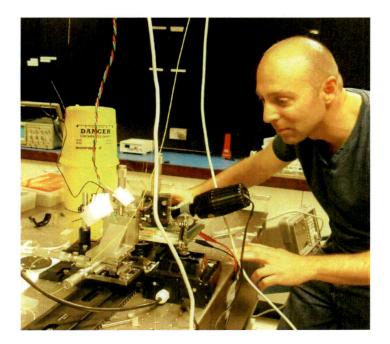

Figure 3

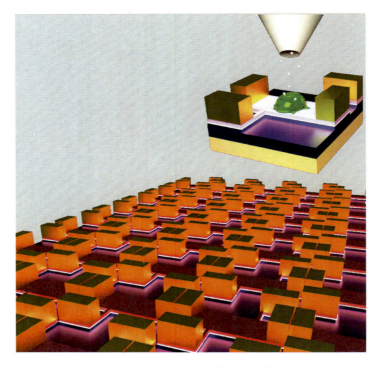

Figure 4 Schematic representation of an AlGaN/GaN sensor array; sensing live human cells for diagnosing diseases and developing new treatments.

Chapters 1 and 2 cover topics on nanoparticles for nanomedicine. Chapter 1 gives a review of nanoparticles developed for drug delivery and then discusses the development and characterization of a multifunctional poly(glycidyl methacrylate) (PGMA) nanoparticle system designed for therapeutic delivery. This system has been researched to deliver a therapeutic peptide for effective use in cardiac ischemia-reperfusion injury. The results have broad applicability beyond the treatment of this condition to a range of disease and injury sites that require rapid cellular delivery of a therapeutic agent. Chapter 2 reports on yolk–shell nanoparticles (YSNs), or "nanorattles," which have a distinct core–void–shell structure. These structures are being researched for delivery of therapeutics and for diagnostic purposes in nanomedicine. Different active medical agents can be delivered by YSNs. These include chemotherapeutic drug and gene delivery, molecular imaging by incorporating different magnetic and fluorescent contrast agents, and photothermal therapy by encapsulating various photoheat-converting agents. The safety and potential toxicity of these advanced nanoparticles are also discussed.

Chapters 3 and 4 report on biosensors that use nanotechnology in their device design and in the principle of sensing. In Chapter 3 the principle of a cantilever functionalized to absorb the molecule/nano-object to be sensed is incorporated into a MEMS device, which has an easy-to-view readout. In Chapter 4 top-down nanotechnology devices—AlGaN/GaN transistors—are engineered into a biosensor for living cells. The biocompatibility, sensitivity, and optimized operational design of these biosensors are discussed, and they emerge as having strong potential for further research.

Chapter 5 details advances in the understanding of the charge transport properties of melanin, an amorphous semiconductor. This is supporting the potential of melanin as a bioelectronic material for use in nanoscale devices where it can act as a transducer of ionic signals to electronic signals. The physical properties of melanin include bistable electrical switching, broadband optical absorbance, water-dependent conductivity, and potential protonic conduction, among others. The improving charge transport model is becoming a tool for nanodevice design and evaluation. In Chapter 6 the methods researched to synthesize, and verify, high-quality crystalline CdSe quantum dots are reported. Also, successful decoration of graphene nanosheets with these quantum dots represents an interesting nanocomposite material with potential for applications.

Applications in energy capture, conversion, and/or storage are among the applications for which nanotechnology and nanoscience research is generating the knowledge to meet future needs. Chapter 7 reviews dye-sensitized solar cells (DSSCs), the third generation of solar cells, which are being considered as a promising alternative to expensive conventional silicon-based photovoltaic devices. Original research on improving the dye uptake ability, efficient charge transfer, and enhanced light harvesting of DSSCs using novel nanostructured designs for the photoanode shows real promise for low-cost solar cells.

Chapter 8 introduces the applications of electrospun nanofibers in, for example, filtration, protective clothing, tissue engineering, thermal insulation, and fuel cells. Electrospun nanofibers have significant advantages for gas transport–based applications, but the physical basis of this has been poorly understood. New mechanistic models for the main transport phenomena at the nanoscale are detailed, thus advancing the in-depth understanding of the improved characteristics.

Deborah M. Kane
Adam P. Micolich
Peter Roger

References

1. http://www.ausnano.net: web page of the ANN.
2. Kane, D. M., Micolich, A. P., and Rabeau, J. R. (eds.). *Nanotechnology in Australia: Showcase of Early Career Research*, Pan Stanford, Singapore, 2011.
3. http://www.ausnano.net/content/bookwriting_project2: web page describing the 2013 ANN Book Writing Workshop and Project.
4. https://www.blender.org/; http://www.blender.org/download/.

Acknowledgments

This book would not have been possible without the support of the ANN. Professor Chennupati Jagadish, convenor of the network, is acknowledged, in particular, for his leadership in advancing activities that benefit postgraduate students and early career researchers. Professor Erich Weigold, chair of the network, and the management committee of the network are also thanked for their strong support. Ms. Liz Micallef, the network manager, is thanked for overseeing communications within the network and project support. Professor Clive Baldock, dean of science at Macquarie University, and Associate Professor Judith Dawes, head of the Department of Physics and Astronomy, are thanked for supporting the workshop by approving access to facilities and administrative support. Mr. Adam Joyce, professional officer, Department of Physics, Macquarie University, is thanked for providing professional support for the Maths and Physics Computing Laboratory, before and during the workshop. The staff at Dunmore Lang College made sure the participants and editors were well catered for during our stay there. Mr. Stanford Chong, director and publisher at Pan Stanford Publishing, is thanked for his enthusiastic support. Ms. Archana Ziradkar is thanked as the managing editor for the publication. The editors thank the participants for their strong engagement with, and enthusiasm for, this project.

Chapter 1

The Design and Testing of Multifunctional Nanoparticles for Drug Delivery Applications

Tristan D. Clemons,[a] Helena M. Viola,[b] Michael J. House,[c] Livia C. Hool,[b] and K. Swaminathan Iyer[a]

[a]*School of Chemistry and Biochemistry, University of Western Australia, 35 Stirling Highway, Crawley, WA 6009, Australia*
[b]*School of Anatomy, Physiology and Human Biology, University of Western Australia, 35 Stirling Highway, Crawley, WA 6009, Australia*
[c]*School of Physics, University of Western Australia, 35 Stirling Highway, Crawley, WA 6009, Australia*
Tristan.clemons@uwa.edu.au

Nanotechnology has the potential to revolutionize the medical profession by improving on traditional drug delivery methods and transforming how disease and injury are currently diagnosed, monitored, and treated. The effective delivery of small-molecule drugs, peptides, and proteins to a site of disease or injury has faced considerable barriers in the past. These include premature clearance from the body, off-site toxicity, and poor bioavailability or pharmacokinetics. Nanoparticles can be used to help improve these characteristics by aiding delivery of therapeutics that otherwise show little efficacy without assisted delivery. This chapter contains

---

Nanomaterials: Science and Applications
Edited by Deborah Kane, Adam Micolich, and Peter Roger
Copyright © 2016 Pan Stanford Publishing Pte. Ltd.
ISBN 978-981-4669-72-6 (Hardcover), 978-981-4669-73-3 (eBook)
www.panstanford.com

two separate yet highly related sections. The first section will provide a review and introduction to the field of nanoparticles developed for drug delivery. This introduction will cover a range of different nanoparticle formulations and their associated merits and pitfalls. The second portion will provide an insight into some of our research on the development and characterization of a multifunctional poly(glycidyl methacrylate) (PGMA) nanoparticle system designed for therapeutic delivery. Here we show this multifunctional nanoparticle system and its ability to effectively deliver a therapeutic peptide designed to modulate L-type calcium channel activity following cardiac ischemia-reperfusion injury. These results have broad applicability beyond the treatment of this injury into a range of disease and injury sites that require rapid cellular delivery of an appropriate therapeutic payload. This nanoparticle system provides sound proof-of-concept for peptide delivery ex vivo. With further testing it has the potential to change how we currently treat one of the major contributors to cardiac failure.

1.1 Overview of Nanoparticles in Medicine

1.1.1 Nanoparticles in Modern Medicine

Nanotechnology is characterized by the creation and use of engineered materials or devices that have at least one dimension in the range of 1–100 nm in size [1]. It exploits the physical and chemical properties of nanoparticles, which, as a result of their size, are remarkably different from both atomic species and bulk materials [2]. Since the properties depend on the dimensions of the nanostructure, reliable and continual changes can be achieved by changing the size of single particles. The best example of this is with quantum dots, where altering the size of the quantum dot particle can change the optical properties of the material (Fig. 1.1).

Not only is nanotechnology interesting from a synthetic approach, but this scale also mirrors that of many biological targets and systems. Many proteins, viruses, and important biological molecules are in the size range of 1–10 nm. As a result, structures that can be accurately designed on the nanometer scale have the ability

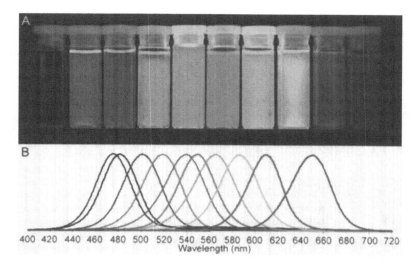

Figure 1.1 (A) Quantum dots possess unique photophysical properties, making them ideal for applications in biological imaging due to the ability to tune the emission color by altering the quantum dot size (particle size increasing from violet emitters on the left to red emitters on the far right). (B) Narrow emission spectra along with efficient light absorption throughout a wide spectrum of wavelengths make quantum dots suitable for a range of applications, especially in biological imaging. Reprinted from Ref. [5], Copyright (2009), with permission from Elsevier.

to interact on the cellular, subcellular, and molecular levels with unique specificity [1, 3]. This specificity can result in explicit interactions within cells and tissues without causing undesirable side effects [3]. A major field of nanotechnology research is the synthesis of nanoparticles for medical applications, including disease diagnosis, imaging, and most importantly treatment through the delivery of therapeutics. It is envisaged that the global market for nanotechnology-related applications in the medical field could increase to between US$70 and US$160 billion by the year 2015 [4].

Nanotechnology and nanoparticle drug delivery vehicles provide an exciting prospect for the delivery of therapeutics in the treatment of a range of diseases and injuries in comparison to current clinical methods [6, 7]. Nanoparticles in particular possess a range of advantages as drug delivery vehicles. These include drug protection from clearance and degradation, high levels of drug loading, the potential for multiple therapeutics to be delivered from the same entity, preferential drug release at target tissues, modifiable drug release kinetics, and, finally, ease of nanoparticle modification for the incorporation of imaging probes that target moieties and surface structure functionalities [8]. This review provides insight into some significant breakthroughs and also highlights some of the challenges still facing engineered nanoparticles designed for drug delivery applications. Following this introduction an application of our own nanoparticle system will be presented in its use as a peptide delivery vehicle in a relevant cardiac ischemia-reperfusion injury model.

1.1.1.1 Nanoparticles for drug delivery

In drug discovery it is easy to find a long list of drug candidates that, although possessing high potency, are unsuitable for clinical application due to poor solubility or poor circulation within the body. Often these candidates have been overlooked in preference for drugs possessing lower potency but better solubility and half-lives [4]. Nanotechnology has the potential to change this by rewriting the rules of drug discovery and improving drug characteristics that were previously seen as limiting or significant enough to warrant rejection [4]. Nanoparticle-based drug delivery systems have been developed to ultimately improve the efficiency of delivery and to reduce systemic toxicity of a wide range of therapeutics. The application of nanoparticles and nanocapsules for drug encapsulation has looked to build on this concept down to the nanoscale. The first generation of nanoparticles developed for drug delivery often only provided one function: drug coating and protection to enhance either drug solubility or circulation time. These nanoparticles are now currently being tested in clinical trials, with some gaining recent approval for clinical applications (Table 1.1) [9]. A wide variety of nanoparticle formulations have been used for drug delivery applications, including liposomes, dendrimers, microemulsions, micelles, solid lipid and polymer nanoparticles, and soluble polymers that have a therapeutic attached via biodegradable linkages (Fig. 1.2). Particles already approved for clinical use include those based on liposomes, biodegradable polymeric nanoparticles,

Table 1.1 Nontargeted nanoparticles that have been approved for clinical use or undergoing clinical trials [9]

Brand Name	Composition	Indication	Status
Liposome-based nanoparticle			
Doxil/Caelyx	PEGylated liposomal doxorubicin	Ovarian cancer, Kaposi's sarcoma	Approved
DaunoXome (Galen)	Liposomal daunorubicin	Kaposi's sarcoma	Approved
Myocet (Sopherion)	Non-PEGylated liposomal doxorubicin	Breast cancer	Approved
Micelle-based nanoparticle			
Genexol-PM	Paclitaxel-loaded PEG-PLA micelle	Breast cancer, lung cancer	Approved
NK911	Doxorubicin-loaded PEG-pAsp micelle	Various cancers	Phase 2
NK012	SN-38-loaded PEG-Pglu (SN-38) micelle	Breast cancer	Phase 2
NC-6004	Cisplatin-loaded PEG-Pglu micelle	Various cancers	Phase 1
SP1049C	Doxorubicin-loaded pluronic micelle	Gastric cancer	Phase 3
NK105	Paclitaxel-loaded PEG-PAA micelle	Breast cancer	Phase 3
Polymer–drug conjugate–based nanoparticle			
OPAXIO (Cell Therapeutics)	Paclitaxel combined with a polyglutamate polymer	Ovarian cancer	Phase 3
IT-101	Camptothecin conjugated to cyclodextrin-based polymer	Various cancers	Phase 1/2
HPMA-DOX (PK1)	Doxorubicin bound to HPMA	Lung cancer, breast cancer	Phase 2
HPMA-DOX-galactosamine (PK2)	Doxorubicin linked to HPMA bearing galactosamine	Hepatocellular carcinoma	Phase 1/2
CT-2106	Camptothecin poly-l-glutamate conjugate	Various cancers	Phase 1/2
Albumin-based nanoparticle			
Abraxane	Albumin-bound paclitaxel nanoparticles	Metastatic breast cancer	Approved

PLA, poly(l-lactide); pAsp, poly(l-aspartic acid); PEG, poly(ethylene glycol) Pglu, polyglutamate; PAA, poly(l-aspartate); HPMA, N-(2-hydroxypropyl)-methacrylamide-copolymer

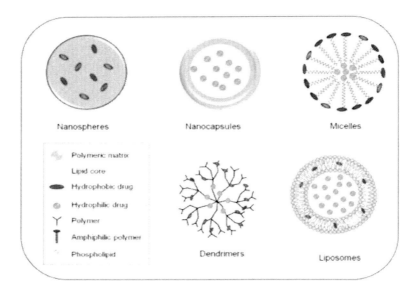

Figure 1.2 Schematic representation of some of the main classes of nanoparticle formulations currently being applied in drug delivery applications. Nanocapsules and nanospheres are some of the simplest drug delivery vehicles. Nanocapsules provide an internal cavity suitable for the loading of a drug of interest, whereas nanospheres usually provide drug protection through incorporation within the nanosphere structure. Both of these systems provide suitable platforms for drug release to the intended microenvironment, while offering drug protection from potentially harmful surroundings. Micelles are spherical structures produced from amphiphilic molecules such as detergents. In an aqueous environment the hydrophobic groups are internalized and will group together to form a tight spherical structure with the hydrophilic portion of the molecules on the outside. In a nonaqueous environment the reverse micelle structure will occur. Micelles have found application in the encapsulation of non-water-soluble drugs required for intravenous administration. Dendrimers are highly branched polymeric structures where the 3D branching about a central core can be well controlled. These branches can be easily functionalized to improve targeting or drug-loading characteristics. Liposomes are spherical vesicles comprising one or more lipid bilayers around a central aqueous core. Reprinted from Ref. [11], Copyright (2009), with permission from Elsevier.

and poly(ethylene glycol) (PEG) or protein-based nanoparticle drug conjugates (Table 1.1) [9, 10]. The following section will introduce these major classes of nanoparticles currently being investigated for drug delivery applications.

1.1.1.2 Micelles, liposomes, and dendrimers for drug delivery applications

Micellar nanoparticles consist of a hydrophobic core that is surrounded by amphiphilic block copolymers that have assembled around this hydrophobic core to produce a core/shell architecture in aqueous media [12, 13]. The hydrophobic core region of the micelle acts as a reservoir for hydrophobic drugs; the hydrophilic exterior of the micelle allows for nanoparticle stability in aqueous media [13]. Micelles have the ability to encapsulate a range of therapeutic cargoes, including hydrophobic drugs, oligonucleotides, proteins, and imaging agents with high loading levels (up to 30% w/w) [12, 14]. Micelle nanoparticles have shown great promise as delivery systems, with a number currently in phase 3 clinical trials (Table 1.1). Micelles can also be produced from stimuli-responsive block copolymers to allow disassembly in the presence of triggers such as pH, temperature, light, or ultrasound [15]. This allows for targeted release of the therapeutic payload held within the micelle structure.

A 2012 study by Lee et al. encapsulated the photosensitive Protoporphyrin IX (PpIX) within a pH-responsive micelle based on the block copolymer of PEG-poly(β-amino ester) (Fig. 1.3) [15]. The pH of the microenvironment surrounding tumor tissue is lower (pH 6.4–6.8) than that of normal tissue (pH 7.4) [16, 17]. This reduction in pH allows for protonation of the tertiary amines present in the amino ester, resulting in an increase in the hydrophilicity of the polymer [16]. This change results in rapid de-micellization in the regions surrounding the tumor tissue and leads to the release of the encapsulated photosensitizer PpIX. The strong fluorescent signal of PpIX allows its location, surrounding the tumor microenvironment, to be identified (Fig. 1.3B). Furthermore, when irradiated with the appropriate wavelength of light, PpIX produces cytotoxic singlet oxygen (photodynamic therapy), which in turn destroys nearby tumor cells (Fig. 1.3D).

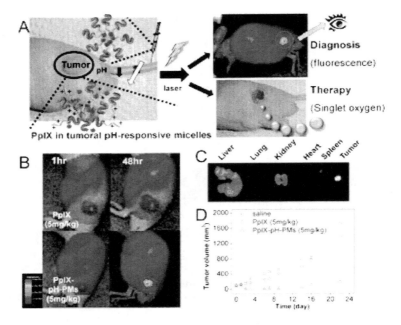

Figure 1.3 Polymeric micelles for optical imaging and photodynamic therapy. (A) Schematic illustration of PpIX-encapsulated pH-responsive polymeric micelles for tumor diagnosis and photodynamic therapy. (B) Fluorescence images after injection of PpIX-encapsulated pH-responsive polymeric micelles. (C) Ex vivo images of organs and tumors. (D) Tumor growth after injection and laser irradiation. Reproduced from Ref. [15], Copyright (2012), with permission of the Royal Society of Chemistry (http://pubs.rsc.org/en/content/articlelanding/2012/cs/c2cs15261d#!divAbstract).

Similar to micelles, liposomes are closed colloidal structures consisting of an aqueous core surrounded by a phospholipid bilayer, with their main application in the delivery of aqueous biomolecules and hydrophilic drugs [12]. Liposomes have the potential to entrap relatively large amounts of hydrophilic drugs within their aqueous core or between the lipid bilayer shell structure if the therapeutic is lipophilic [14]. A major advantage of liposomes is that they form spontaneously in solution and they essentially possess no inherent toxicity due to the presence of the components of liposomes throughout the body in all cell membranes [12]. Liposomes have had great success in the delivery of anthracycline-based chemotherapeutics, including doxorubicin and daunorubicin, for the treatment of metastatic breast cancer [18, 19], ovarian cancer [18], and AIDS-related Kaposi's sarcoma [20]. An interesting application of liposomes for drug delivery is the utilization of liposomes for the encapsulation and aerosol delivery of the vasoactive intestinal peptide (VIP) for the treatment of various lung diseases such as asthma and pulmonary hypertension. A study from 2008 by Hajos et al. found that encapsulation of the VIP within liposomes was successful in allowing the VIP to avoid enzymatic degradation once inhaled and deposited within the bronchi [21]. This study found that loading of the VIP within the liposomes for inhalation therapy improved the pharmacological and biological activity of the VIP treatment in comparison to the delivery of free VIP [21].

Dendrimers are not nanoparticles per se but more strictly defined as a polymeric macromolecule of nanometer dimensions composed of highly branched monomers that emerge radially from a central core, as shown in Fig. 1.2 [13]. Dendrimers can be biodegradable or nonbiodegradable structures. Natural polymers such as glycogen, and some proteoglycans consist of a dendrimer-like structure. However, for drug delivery, the synthetic polymer poly(amidoamine) (PAMAM) is the most extensively studied [13, 22]. PAMAM has been shown to be effective for the binding and subsequent delivery of cisplatin both in vitro and in vivo where it shows improved efficacy in comparison to cisplatin delivered without the dendrimer [23]. Properties that make dendrimers attractive for drug delivery applications include monodispersed size distributions, modifiable surface chemistry, multivalency, water solubility, and an internal cavity available for drug loading [22]. Due to the ease with which dendrimer surface chemistry can be modified, the addition of contrast agents, imaging probes, and targeting ligands can be coupled with a therapeutic for delivery. This combination of imaging and therapy has led to the production of dendrimer-based multifunctional drug delivery systems [22]. Dendrimers can be produced with low cytotoxicity. Surface decoration of the dendritic structure with PEG can prolong its circulation half-life. Although there is significant interest in dendrimers as drug delivery vehicles, few have translated into clinical trials. Vivagel® is the most promising candidate, currently in phase 2 clinical trials [24]. Vivagel® is an L-lysine dendrimer that contains a polyanionic outer surface, which exhibits antiviral activity against the sexually transmitted herpes simplex virus (HSV) and the human immunodeficiency virus (HIV) [24].

1.1.1.3 Polymeric nanoparticles and nanocapsules as drug delivery vehicles

Polymeric nanoparticles and nanocapsules are solid formulations ranging in size from 10 to 1000 nm in diameter and can be synthesized from natural or artificial polymers. Generally speaking, the major advantage of polymeric nanosystems over other nanodelivery systems is their inherent stability and structural rigidity [12]. These polymeric nanoparticles often incorporate the therapeutic to be delivered via drugs that are adsorbed, dissolved, entrapped, encapsulated, or covalently linked to the nanoparticle [25, 26]. The most commonly used synthetic materials for the synthesis of biodegradable polymeric nanoparticles are poly(lactic acid) (PLA), poly(D-L-glycolide) (PLG), or the copolymer of these synthetic polymers, poly(lactic-co-glyoclic acid) (PLGA). These are adopted due to their low toxicity, biodegradability, Food and Drug Administration (FDA) approval, and tissue compatibility [26, 27]. Biodegradable nanoparticles based on these aforementioned polymers have been used for the delivery of a range of therapeutics in vivo, for the treatment of cancers [28] and neurodegenerative disorders [29], and for the controlled release of contraceptive steroids and fertility control systems [30, 31].

Nanoparticles synthesized from naturally occurring polymers such as chitosan, albumin, and heparin have been popular choices for the delivery of oligonucleotides, proteins, and small-molecule drugs. Despite significant research in the use of polymers for nanoparticle drug delivery systems, only one, Abraxane, has been approved for clinical applications to date [32]. Abraxane is an albumin-based nanoparticle system developed for the delivery of paclitaxel, a proven chemotherapeutic agent to metastatic breast cancers [32]. Furthermore, Abraxane is currently undergoing clinical trials for delivery to a variety of other cancers, including non-small-cell lung cancer (phase II trial) [33] and advanced nonhematologic malignancies (phase 1 and pharmacokinetics trials) [34].

A number of approaches have been developed for the synthesis of polymeric nanoparticles, most of which involve the use of block copolymers consisting of polymer chains of differing solubilities. The more common techniques for polymeric nanoparticle formulations include layer-by-layer (LbL) approaches, nanoprecipitation (sometimes referred to as the solvent displacement method), emulsification, solvent evaporation methods, and the salting-out method. Further to these traditional methods, techniques that make use of microfluidics, supercritical technology, and the premix membrane emulsification method are increasingly favored due to their potential for producing highly monodispersed nanoparticles in high yields [27]. Usually, the choice of nanoparticle formulation method is dictated by the physicochemical properties of the drug, the polymer intended for encapsulation, and particle size requirements [8].

1.1.2 Nanoparticle and Cell Interactions

In addition to accurate synthesis and drug loading, another integral consideration for nanoparticles developed for drug delivery is how they interact with biological systems. For drugs with intracellular targets, often the cell membrane can loom as a formidable barrier. The concept of nanoparticles, which can be tailored to carry these drugs across the cell membrane and to relevant subcellular compartments, provides an attractive means to achieve improved pharmaceutical transport. Proof-of-concept studies in the 1970s have shown that submicron-sized liposomes [35], as well as synthetic polymer nanoparticles [36], were able to deliver and concentrate in cells therapeutics that previously were unable to do so on their own. The plasma membrane is the barrier that protects the cell against unwanted intruders such as pathogens, macromolecules, and even nanoparticles from entering the cell from the extracellular space [37]. It consists of a self-assembled bilayer of lipids where the hydrophobic interior of this layer is responsible for restricting the passage of water-soluble substances into the cell. Although the passage of small molecules, amino acids, and ions

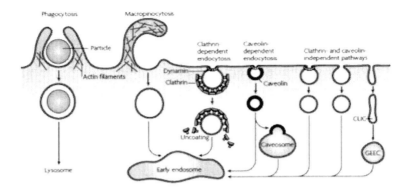

Figure 1.4 Pathways of entry into cells. Large particles can be internalized by phagocytosis, whereas fluid uptake occurs by macropinocytosis. Both processes appear to be triggered by and are dependent on actin-mediated remodeling of the plasma membrane at a large scale. Compared to the other endocytotic pathways, the size of the intracellular vesicles formed by phagocytosis and macropinocytosis is much larger. Numerous cargoes can be endocytosed by mechanisms that are independent of the coat protein clathrin and the fission GTPase, dynamin. Most internalized cargoes are delivered to the early endosome via vesicular (clathrin- or caveolin-coated vesicles) or tubular intermediates (known as clathrin- and dynamin-independent carriers [CLIC]) that are derived from the plasma membrane. Some pathways may first traffic to intermediate compartments, such as the caveosome or glycosyl phosphatidylinositol–anchored protein-enriched early endosomal compartments (GEEC), en route to the early endosome. Reprinted by permission from Macmillan Publishers Ltd: Nature Reviews Molecular Cell Biology (Ref. [43]), copyright (2007).

occurs through specialized membrane protein pumps and selected ion channels on the cell surface, the majority of nanoparticles must undergo some form of membrane interaction before the process of endocytosis can occur [38]. Endocytosis can occur through a range of mechanisms (Fig. 1.4) that can be broadly categorized into either phagocytosis (cell "eating" for solid particles) or nonphagocytic pathways (cell "drinking" processes) [38, 39]. With reference to nanoparticles, however, these classical references of cell eating and drinking are not as relevant due to the ability of solid nanoparticles to still be internalized through nonphagocytic pathways [40]. It is important to have an understanding of the relevant pathways of cell entry that could act on or affect nanoparticle uptake, as this will have direct effects on the drug physicochemical characteristics as well as the intracellular fate of the nanoparticle carrier and in turn its therapeutic cargo [40].

Phagocytosis for the internalization of macromolecules and indeed most nanoparticles occurs primarily in specialized cells known as phagocytes, which include macrophages, monocytes, neutrophils, astrocytes, and dendritic cells [41]. Phagocytosis can be described as a general three-step process. An important first step is recognition of the nanoparticle by opsonin proteins in the bloodstream to tag the nanoparticle for phagocytosis. Secondly, this signaling triggers the plasma membrane to form an invagination preparing for the nanoparticle to be internalized, and finally the plasma membrane will pinch off from the surrounding plasma membrane to engulf the nanoparticle, producing a discrete package bound by plasma membrane proteins within the cell (Fig. 1.4) [39, 42, 43]. The internalized vesicle, known as a phagosome, is trafficked within the cytoplasm until it becomes accessible to early endosomes. The phagosome then begins to acidify and matures, fusing with late endosomes and finally lysosomes to form a phagolysosome [41]. The speed with which this process occurs is highly dependent on the particle and its surface characteristics, but typically the process can take from minutes to hours [41].

Phagolysosomes become acidified due to the proton pump ATPase located in the membrane of the phagolysosome; the recruitment of an enzyme cocktail to aid in the degradation of the foreign body also occurs at this time [44]. Although a minimum size of 0.5 μm is often considered the limit for phagocytosis, previous studies have shown nanoparticles ranging from 250 nm to 3 μm in diameter can undergo in vitro phagocytosis [40]. Careful control of the nanoparticle surface coating and nanoparticle size can play important roles in producing nanoparticles that can avoid phagocytic uptake [45]. It is generally accepted however that the in vivo fate of nanoparticles is to be opsonized, that is, marked for phagocyte removal, and in turn phagocytosed with little discrimination for nanoparticle composition. This occurs unless the particles are very small in size, that is, less than 100 nm, or, more importantly, possess a specific hydrophilic coating such as PEG to aid in the avoidance of opsonin recognition [40].

Nonphagocytic pathways, normally referred to as pinocytosis, are not restricted to specialized cells and contain processes that are used by almost all cells for the internalization of fluids and solutes alike. Nonphagocytic uptake into cells can occur through four main mechanisms: clathrin-mediated endocytosis, caveolae-mediated endocytosis, micropinocytosis, and other clathrin- and caveolae-independent processes (Fig. 1.4) [40, 43]. Clathrin-mediated endocytosis, the most common mechanism for uptake, results in trafficking of cargoes into the lysosomal pathway for biodegradation [42]. Conversely, caveolae-mediated uptake has been shown to produce caveolar vesicles that do not contain a degradative enzymatic cocktail, and hence caveolae-dependent uptake is seen as a mechanism that, if targeted, could avoid trafficking of nanoparticles to the degradative lysosomal pathway [45]. A third process known as macropinocytosis is where actin-derived protrusions from the cell membrane can engulf cargoes, upon which the protrusions collapse to again fuse with the cell membrane. These macropinosome cavities containing their entrapped cargo will often fuse with lysosomes, which in turn acidify for the degradation of the payload [40]. By having a better understanding of the variety of internalization pathways by which nanoparticles can be internalized, a clearer understanding will be gained as to what kind of environment nanoparticles may be exposed to once they are internalized. This information is important, for example, when developing new nanoparticles with site-specific drug release capabilities or biodegradation qualities or if the nanoparticle vehicle is engineered with specific escape mechanisms to avoid degradation in endosomes [46, 47].

1.1.2.1 Nanoparticle endocytosis

Nanoparticle size, shape, and relative hardness can dictate which endocytosis pathway is activated and utilized for nanoparticle uptake. A study in 2004 by Rejman et al. investigated the internalization of uniform spherical polystyrene nanoparticles of differing sizes in murine melanoma cells (B16-F10) [45]. This study demonstrated that polystyrene spherical nanoparticles with diameters of 50 and 100 nm were rapidly internalized in less than 30 minutes by a clathrin-mediated pathway [45]. In comparison, larger nanoparticles (200 and 500 nm in diameter), also made from polystyrene, were internalized much more slowly (2–3 h) and exhibit an 8–10-fold decrease in internalization when compared to the smaller particles [45].

The shape of nanoparticles has also been recently investigated to see the role it plays on nanoparticle internalization. Gratton et al. in 2008 investigated the internalization of a series of nanoparticles in HeLa cells where the nanoparticles were fabricated to have differing aspect ratios [48]. High-aspect-ratio rod-shaped nanoparticles were internalized in HeLa cells at a greater rate than spherical nanoparticles of a similar internal volume, a phenomenon similar to that of the appreciable increase seen in the uptake of rod-shaped bacteria in nonphagocytic cell lines [48]. Even nanoparticle hardness can influence the interactions of nanoparticles with the cell membrane and in turn can have a direct influence over cell internalization. In 2009 a study by Banquy et al. investigated the internalization of similar particles of differing hardness, that is, Young's modulus [49]. This study found that 150 nm hydrogel nanoparticles with an intermediate Young's modulus (35 and 136 kPa) were internalized by a range of different mechanisms in macrophages, whereas softer nanoparticles (150 nm diameter hydrogel nanoparticles, 18 kPa) were preferentially internalized by macropinocytosis and stiffer nanoparticles (150 nm diameter hydrogel nanoparticles, 211 kPa) via clathrin-mediated endocytosis [49]. Further to this, these nanoparticles with intermediate hardness experienced approximately 67% higher internalization than softer nanoparticles and approximately 25% higher internalization in comparison to the harder nanoparticles [49].

It is evident that size, shape, and hardness can affect nanoparticle endocytosis, but another important characteristic is that of nanoparticle surface charge. The surface charge of nanoparticles plays an integral role in determining by which endocytosis pathway nanoparticles are internalized [39]. Positively charged nanoparticles are the most efficient at plasma membrane interactions and in turn internalization as they interact favorably with the negatively charged residues present on the cell surface [39]. Nonetheless, uptake of nanoparticles with negative surface charges has also been observed despite the unfavorable electrostatic interactions that occur between the nanoparticles and the negatively charged cell membrane [39, 50]. For example, a study in 2008 by Harush-Frenkel et al. investigating the internalization of cationic and anionic nanoparticles in epithelial Madin–Darby canine kidney cells found that cationic nanoparticles experienced rapid uptake, while the anionic nanoparticles, although at a slower rate, still experienced effective cellular internalization [50]. The majority of both nanoparticle formulations was targeted mainly to the clathrin-dependent endocytosis pathways, with a small proportion of both formulations experiencing macropinocytosis-dependent uptake [50]. Further studies from the same group investigated a similar effect in HeLa cells, where it was determined that the cationic nanoparticles once again experienced rapid clathrin-dependent uptake compared to the anionic nanoparticles, being internalized more slowly by a different endocytosis pathway [51].

1.1.2.2 Strategies to enhance cellular internalization

Poly(ethyleneimine) (PEI) is a synthetic polycation well known for its long history as a nonviral transfection agent. Studies have used PEI for intracellular delivery of a range of cargoes, including nanoparticles, proteins, and small-molecule drugs [52–55]. PEI is also suitable for the delivery of short interfering RNA (siRNA) and DNA due to the ability of this positively charged polymer to condense around oligonucleotides, thus enabling transfection of the anionic cell membrane [56–59]. PEI can promote and facilitate endosomal escape due to its strong buffering characteristics in what is referred to as the "proton sponge" effect [52, 53]. After endocytosis, the natural acidification within the endosome protonates PEI, inducing chloride ion influx, osmotic swelling, and destabilization of the vesicle, resulting in the nanoparticles being released into the cytoplasm [60, 61]. The major downfall associated with PEI as a nonviral vector is its inherent toxicity, which has been shown to scale with its molecular weight and transfection efficiency [53].

Another method other than cationic polymers that has had success in transfecting therapeutic cargoes and nanoparticles across cellular membranes is the incorporation of cell-penetrating peptides (CPPs). CPPs are short cationic peptide sequences that were first discovered by investigating the ability of the HIV *trans*-activator of transcription protein to penetrate cells and subsequently effectively deliver the HIV-1-specific genes [62]. There is a broad spectrum of CPPs available, with most consisting of fewer than 20 amino acids, the most common of these being the *trans*-activator of transcription (TAT), or, as it is more commonly known, the TAT peptide [37]. TAT is an 11-residue-long peptide taken from the protein transduction domain of the HIV-1 TAT protein; this domain is responsible for viral transfection [63]. The TAT peptide is rich in arginine and lysine residues, making it a highly positively charged, basic, and hydrophilic peptide suitable for attachment to the anionic cell membrane and in turn subsequent internalization [63]. The TAT peptide sequence has also been widely used to improve the cellular delivery of a plethora of molecular cargoes, from small-molecule drugs to large proteins and nanoparticles [64].

The exact mechanism for TAT transfection is still an area of debate and contradicting theories. However, most studies agree on the importance of direct contact between the TAT peptide and the negative residues on the cell surface as a preliminary requirement for successful transfection to occur [63–66]. Despite this agreement, TAT-mediated therapeutic delivery still has some major drawbacks yet to be fully addressed. These include the nonspecificity of the current TAT sequence, as well as the associated social stigma surrounding its use due to the origins of this sequence in the debilitating and currently incurable HIV infection [67]. Finally, and just as important, is the possible immunogenicity of the TAT delivery system. It has been speculated that TAT, especially through repeated dosing, could produce a significant immunogenic response, thus limiting its clinical applications, an issue yet to be examined further [62].

1.1.3 Multifunctional Nanoparticles

A major downside to the nanoparticles that are currently being investigated for clinical trials (Table 1.1) is their ability to perform

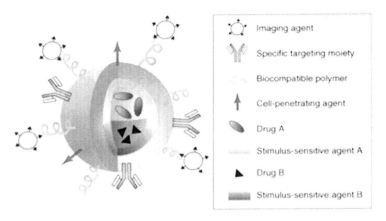

Figure 1.5 Multifunctional nanoparticles for drug delivery. Multifunctional nanocarriers can be developed to include and combine a range of functions. Some of these functions will include targeting agents (usually an antibody or a peptide), imaging agents (such as fluorescent dyes, quantum dots, or magnetic nanoparticles), a cell-penetrating agent to aid in cellular uptake (e.g., the polyArg peptide, TAT), a stimulus-sensitive element to aid in drug release (i.e., pH or a photosensitive polymer), and a stabilizing polymer to ensure biocompatibility (with the most common of these being PEG or PEG derivatives). The above functions combined within a solitary delivery vehicle along with one or multiple therapeutics provide exciting prospects for drug delivery technology. Development of novel strategies for controlled release of drugs as well as timed release will provide nanoparticles with the capability to deliver two or more therapeutic agents on differing time scales. Reprinted from Ref. [68], Copyright (2008), with permission from Elsevier.

only one primary role as delivery agents. More recent work has resulted in the production of multifunctional nanoparticles for drug delivery that aim to achieve combinations including imaging probes, high drug loading, modifiable drug release kinetics, drug release triggers, targeting ligands (such as antibodies, proteins, and peptides), and nanoparticle coatings to improve circulation times. Figure 1.5 provides a schematic of such a nanoparticle, conveying broadly the different aspects that scientists may look to incorporate into a multifunctional nanoparticle system [68]. Research in this field has resulted in a plethora of nanoparticle formulations and combinations of functions being presented within the literature.

A 2012 study by Zhou et al. describes an octafunctional nanoparticle suitable for the delivery of siRNA to tumors for RNA interference (RNAi) [69]. The octafunctional nanoparticle included (1) a biodegradable PLGA polymer matrix for controlled release; the core of the particle contained (2) siRNA for gene knockdown; (3) an agent to facilitate endosomal escape; (4) an agent to enhance siRNA potency, with the nanoparticle surface containing a range of functionalities, including (5) the attachment of a CPP; (6) a peptide to aid in endosomal escape; (7) a tumor homing peptide; and finally (8) PEGylation of the surface to improve circulation time [69]. It is important to realize, however, that the addition of extra functions results in increases in the cost and time associated with production and purification, as well as the complexity of the nanoparticle system. As a result, there is an ongoing battle in evaluating the benefits of added functionalities versus the extra cost of adding those functions in these multicomponent nanoparticle systems. The following sections will address some of the key considerations and functionalities currently being investigated in the application of multifunctional nanoparticles for drug delivery applications, paying special attention to some pivotal examples making use of these additions.

1.1.3.1 Passive vs. targeted nanoparticles: Surface functionalities of multifunctional nanoparticles

Probably the most significant effort, following on from first-generation nanoparticles for drug delivery, is that of nanoparticle targeting. Targeting can be achieved by two main avenues. The first is passive targeting, that is, nanoparticle targeting resulting from disease pathophysiology. The second is active targeting, where targeting ligands and moieties are added to the nanoparticles to produce preferential nanoparticle binding and at times cellular uptake in target tissue [70]. Nanoparticles produced for the treatment of malignant tumors and cancers can be considered to be targeting tumor tissue through a passive process known as the enhanced permeability and retention (EPR) effect (Fig. 1.6) [71]. This is an effect directly due to the leakiness of tumor vasculature combined with poor lymphatic drainage and the high fluid flow

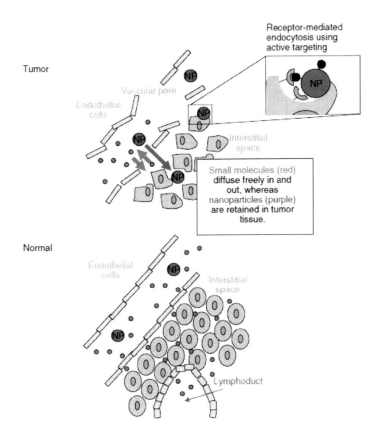

Figure 1.6 Schematic representation of nanoparticle active and passive targeting via the EPR effect. The schematic demonstrates the increased "leaky" vasculature consistent with the rich vascular network of a tumor in comparison to that of normal healthy tissue. Reprinted with permission from from Ref. [78]. Copyright © 2010, John Wiley & Sons, Inc.

often seen with many solid tumors [10]. Tumor vasculature enables nanoparticles to accumulate within tumor tissue without the addition of specific targeting moieties to the nanoparticle surface for tumor recognition [72]. Animal studies have shown that a 50-fold increase in nanoparticle accumulation can be achieved through this passive process when compared to healthy tissue [73]. Hence, to optimize uptake due to the passive process of the

EPR effect, an important characteristic of nanoparticle systems is to ensure long blood circulation times to avoid nanoparticle removal before accumulation can occur. Both nanoparticles and liposomes are known to be rapidly recognized and cleared from the blood by cells of the mononuclear phagocytic system (MPS), particularly macrophages present in the liver and spleen [74–77]. As alluded to earlier, nanoparticle removal by macrophages is initiated by interactions with the hydrophobic nanoparticle surface and plasma opsonin proteins, including immunoglobulins, albumin, and fibronectin, in a process known as opsonization [41, 70]. These plasma proteins are recognized by specific receptors on macrophages, which then phagocytose the nanoparticles (as discussed in detail in Section 1.3) [76, 77].

Studies have shown that through alteration of the nanoparticle surface with hydrophilic, flexible, and nonionic polymer chains, avoidance of macrophage removal or "stealth like" nanoparticles can be produced [79]. The coating of nanoparticle surfaces with PEG, a process sometimes referred to as PEGylation, has been extensively used in providing nanoparticles with a stealth-like coating [80]. The addition of neutrally charged hydrophilic polymer chains to the surface of a nanoparticle can provide a means for avoiding phagocytosis and recognition by macrophages. In turn this leads to longer circulation times [80, 81]. Improved circulation times enhance the EPR effect, as generally the longer the nanoparticle circulation time, the greater the EPR-induced nanoparticle accumulation experienced within tumor tissue [82]. Due to the large variability seen between tumors, it is difficult to assess the optimum nanoparticle surface charge and size of nanoparticles to best exploit the EPR effect. However, generally nanoparticles on the scale of 10–100 nm demonstrate the most effective uptake on tumors [83]. However, there are also reports that show nanoparticles of 400 nm penetrating tumors as a result of the EPR effect [71]. Passive targeting using nanoparticles via the EPR effect still face some challenges. The longer circulation times of drug-loaded nanoparticles can lead to adverse effects, as has been seen with DOXIL, which can cause severe hand-foot syndrome. Hand-foot syndrome causes redness, swelling, and pain on the palms of the hands and/or the soles of the feet similar to severe sunburn.

Sometimes blisters may also appear [84]. In addition to this, the tumor vasculature is highly dependent on tumor type and age, and hence the EPR effect is not suitable for all tumors or all tumor stages of development [85]. The heterogeneous nature of tumors emphasizes the need to identify and develop alternate targeting strategies to enhance the effectiveness of particle-based delivery systems and therapies [10, 85].

Active targeting of nanoparticles has the ability to further complement the EPR effect. Active targeting can be achieved through the addition of proteins, ligands, or antibodies to the nanoparticle surface to exploit receptors and other signaling molecules associated with diseased states. Targeted nanoparticles possess major advantages in drug delivery, such as the potential for lower dosing, reduced systemic toxicity, and the potential for the safe delivery of more potent therapeutics. These moieties with corresponding specific receptors in target tissue can greatly enhance specific cell uptake of a nanoparticle vehicle and its subsequent drug payload [9]. One example is a study conducted in 2011 by Poon et al. where the authors found folate targeted paclitaxel-loaded micelles resulted in a significant increase in tumor accumulation and retention when compared to nontargeted micelles [86]. There was a fourfold increase in the efficiency of paclitaxel when delivered in the targeted nanoparticle system, while also significantly reducing in vivo toxicity of the chemotherapeutic treatment [86]. Folate is an attractive targeting moiety for cancer with folate receptors, responsible for delivery of folic acid into cells, showing a 100- to 300-fold overexpression in a wide spectrum of cancer cells [87]. Furthermore, the application of active targeted nanoparticles for the treatment of cancer has an added advantage with regard to the treatment of small metastases (<100 mm^3), as these sites are poorly vascularized and do not evoke a significant EPR effect suitable for passive nanoparticle targeting [78].

However, despite the significant upside to nanoparticle targeting, both passive and active, there are still major problems to be overcome. This is further supported by the fact that currently only a handful of targeted formulations have made it into clinical trials, with none so far being clinically approved despite targeted nanoparticles being around for some decades now [9]. The added difficulty and time during synthesis required for the addition of ligands, the potential for off-target effects if the ligand–receptor pair is not highly specific, and also increased monetary expense are all valid reasons to question the balance of cost to benefits when discussing targeted nanoparticles.

Furthermore, the attachment of targeting moieties can compromise the stealth capabilities of the nanoparticles and in turn accelerate their clearance by the host through recognition by opsonin proteins [9, 88]. It has been shown that nontargeted liposomes can achieve comparable tumor accumulation to that of folic acid–conjugated liposomes as they benefit from higher circulation times and in turn a longer period of accumulation resulting from the EPR effect [88]. Hence, the addition of targeting moieties has the potential for producing very selective drug delivery vehicles. However, substantial consideration must be given to the choice of targeting ligand and in turn the estimated costs and benefits of its use in a given application.

1.1.3.2 Multifunctional nanoparticles incorporating imaging functionalities

Recent trends in multifunctional nanoparticles have endeavored to do more than improve pharmacokinetic properties of a therapeutic and/or increase blood circulation time and targeting. In addition, they look to include imaging agents within the nanoconstruct suitable for imaging in a clinical setting. The introduction of magnetic resonance imaging (MRI) contrast agents and fluorescent/optical imaging probes are two of the most common modifications that still have strong prevalence and applicability in the clinic. Further to these two, positron emission tomography (PET), computed tomography (CT), ultrasound, and single-photon emission computed tomography (SPECT) are all finding applications for nanoparticles developed for drug delivery. Figure 1.7 shows the characteristics of each of these imaging modalities currently used in the clinical field, displaying each mode's advantages along with its intrinsic limitations [15]. The ability to use imaging tools to follow a nanoparticle in vivo has great applications in drug delivery due to the ability to provide key information to help physicians make better

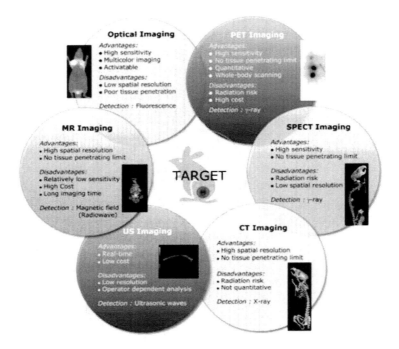

Figure 1.7 Characteristics of imaging modalities currently used for biomedical applications. Reproduced from Ref. [15], Copyright (2012), with permission of the Royal Society of Chemistry (http://pubs.rsc.org/en/content/articlelanding/2012/cs/c2cs15261d#!divAbstract).

informed decisions regarding drug dosage, timing of drug delivery, and drug choice, resulting in a powerful addition to personalized treatment strategies [9].

Furthermore, the integration of two or more imaging modalities, when chosen carefully, can allow for the advantages of one imaging mode to overlap with the disadvantages of another to produce an entity that is detectable and suitable for imaging across a range of length scales, instrumentations, time points, and resolutions. With this, nanoparticles have the potential to overcome a common conundrum of modality selection in clinical diagnostic imaging where the modalities with the highest sensitivities have relatively poor resolutions, while those that can achieve high resolution often have relatively poor sensitivity [89]. Another important consideration to the type of imaging modality is the relative amount or dose of imaging or contrast agent. For example, PET or fluorescent probes often only require low concentrations when compared to the doses required for MRI or CT imaging [15].

PET imaging is a technique that can potentially provide functional information about a disease with high sensitivity. This complements a technique such as MRI or CT, which both offer high-resolution images for anatomical information. A 2011 study by de Rosales et al. combining PET with MRI demonstrated these benefits. In this study a novel bifunctional chelator was designed to allow for radiolabeling of iron oxide nanoparticles with ^{64}Cu. In their study they demonstrated the ability for the bifunctional chelator to bind ^{64}Cu to Endorem®, a commercially available iron oxide MRI contrast agent, and demonstrated the PET/MRI capabilities of this nanoparticle conjugate in the detection of lymph nodes in vivo (Fig. 1.8) [90].

CT imaging is a very widely used imaging technique due to its affordable price, high spatial resolution, and unlimited depth. Accurate anatomical information can be determined with CT-generated reconstructed 3D images [15]. In CT imaging, X-rays are emitted from a focused source, which rotates around a subject placed in the center of the CT scanner. As X-rays pass through the subject, they are absorbed in inverse proportion to the density of the subject's tissue before being detected by detectors on the other side of the subject [91]. This information can then be used to produce high-resolution tomographic anatomical images by reconstruction through a series of back calculations [92]. One of the major downfalls of this technique, however, is its lack of soft tissue contrast, resulting in large amounts (gram quantities) of CT-compatible contrast agents, for example, iodine, often being required [91]. However, iodine has also been problematic as a CT contrast agent due to its rapid renal clearance, poor sensitivity, and issues surrounding its toxicity. The use of gold nanoparticles has overcome some of these problems due to their X-ray absorbing and fluorescent quenching characteristics. A recent study looking to combine CT and fluorescence imaging made use of gold nanoparticles conjugated with a Cy5.5 metalloproteinase (MMP)-sensitive peptide, which upon degradation produced a near-infrared fluorescent signal (Fig. 1.9A) [93]. In vivo accumulation

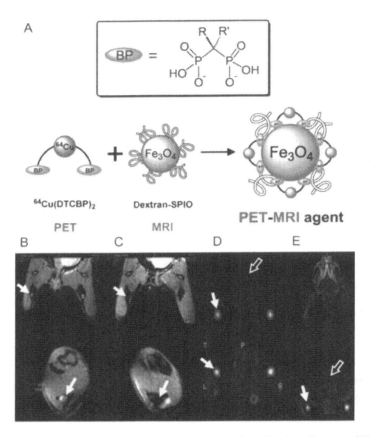

Figure 1.8 (A) Schematic representations of a bisphosphonate (BP; top) and the conjugation reaction between the BP-based PET tracer [64Cu(dtcbp)2] and the dextran-coated iron oxide nanoparticle MRI probe Endorem/Feridex (bottom). (B-E) In vivo PET-MRI studies with [64Cu(dtcbp)2]-Endorem in a mouse. (B, C) Coronal (top) and short-axis (bottom) MRI images of the lower abdominal area and upper hind legs, showing the popliteal lymph nodes (solid arrows) before (A) and after (B) footpad injection of [64Cu(dtcbp)2]-Endorem. (D) Coronal (top) and short-axis (bottom) NanoPET-CT images of the same mouse as in (C) showing the uptake of [64Cu(dtcbp)2]-Endorem in the popliteal (solid arrow) and iliac lymph nodes (hollow arrow). E) Whole-body NanoPET-CT images showing sole uptake of [64Cu(dtcbp)2]-Endorem in the popliteal and iliac lymph nodes. Reprinted with permission from from Ref. [90]. Copyright © 2011 John Wiley & Sons, Inc.

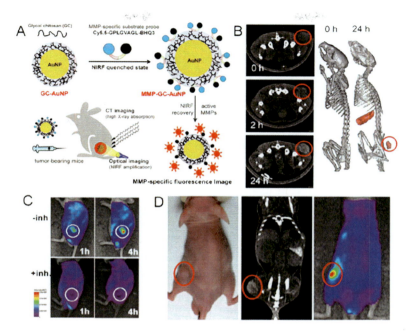

Figure 1.9 Gold nanoparticles for optical and CT imaging. (A) Schematic diagram of MMP peptide probe conjugated to glycol chitosan–coated gold nanoparticles (MMP-GC-AuNPs). (B) Cross-sectional CT images of tumor before and after tail vein injection of the GC-AuNPs and subsequent 3D reconstructed images at 0 h and 24 h. (C) Near-infrared fluorescent (NIRF) images of HT-29 tumor-bearing mice after injection of the MMP-GC-AuNPs with and without an inhibitor of matrix metalloproteinase. (D) Representative CT/optical dual imaging of the HT-29 tumor-bearing mouse model 24 h postinjection of the MMP-GC-AuNPs. Reprinted with permission from from Ref. [93]. Copyright © 2011 John Wiley & Sons, Inc.

of the nanoparticles in the tumor resulted in dual imaging of the tumors through the X-ray absorption of the gold nanoparticles, providing CT contrast and the evolution of Cy5.5 fluorescence upon the MMP degradation of the peptide for optical imaging (Fig. 1.9B–D) [93].

1.1.3.3 Magnetic resonance imaging

MRI is primarily a diagnostic tool that allows noninvasive visualization of organs and other structures within the body [94]. In

1946 two scientists, Felix Bloch and Edward Mills Purcell, through independent experiments, observed that when substances such as water or paraffin were placed in a strong magnetic field and then barraged with magnetic oscillations at radio frequencies, they would absorb and release energy [94]. This was the beginning of nuclear magnetic resonance (NMR), which in turn resulted in the development of MRI for the imaging of bodily tissues. Both Bloch and Purcell received the Nobel Prize in Physics in 1952 for their NMR discovery. The NMR phenomenon, which is the foundation of magnetic resonance image generation, is based on the interaction between an external magnetic field and nuclei, such as ^{1}H, which has a nonzero magnetic moment [95]. When such nuclei are placed in a large external magnetic field, they will either align parallel or antiparallel to the applied magnetic field and will precess at the Larmor frequency as they align [95, 96]. The Larmor or precession frequency is the rate at which these nuclei wobble when placed in a magnetic field, and it is directly proportional to the applied magnetic field that generates the nuclear spin alignment [96]. Although nuclear spins can align both parallel and antiparallel to the applied magnetic field, parallel alignment with the magnetic field is energetically favorable and hence a slightly larger fraction of spins align with the field [96]. The application of a radio frequency (rf) pulse perpendicular to the applied magnetic field will result in further precessional motion; this time the nuclei will precess about the axis of the rf pulse. Resonance between the frequency of the rf pulse and the Larmor frequency can be achieved if these frequencies are equal. This resonance results in a spiral motion of the nuclear spins into the plane, which is perpendicular to the applied field [97]. For example, if the applied field is orientated in the z direction, then a 90° rf pulse will force the nuclear spins into the xy plane. This pulse will force all of the spins to be in phase with one another and also for the system to now be in an excited state due to the addition of energy from the rf pulse [97].

The key to MRI is how this additional energy is released as the spins relax and return to align with the initial applied magnetic field [95, 96]. There are two mechanisms for which this spin relaxation can occur, T_1 relaxation, a result of spin–lattice interactions (longitudinal), and T_2 or T_2* relaxations resulting from spin–spin (transverse) relaxation [96, 98]. These relaxation times vary greatly depending on the immediate chemical environment surrounding the nuclei, which is the reason that differences in tissue provide slightly different contrast [98]. However, often differences in T_1 or T_2 of the tissue alone are not great enough to discern certain anatomical differences, tissue differences, or changes in pathology. To improve the visibility of abnormal pathology in MRI, contrast agents are applied to shorten relaxation times and in turn improve contrast between tissues [99].

1.1.3.4 Magnetic resonance contrast agents

The use of contrast-enhancing agents has become an integral part of MRI and its application in a clinical setting [99]. Under most conditions, differences in longitudinal and transverse relaxation times are usually high enough to provide sufficient contrast in magnetic resonance images. However, some pathological conditions do not display sufficient differences in tissue to clearly discriminate from surrounding healthy tissue. All MRI contrast agents work by shortening the T_1 or the T_2 relaxation times of the target tissue, and as a result they are often classified as T_1 agents or T_2 agents, depending on the signal that is predominantly influenced [99]. The ability for these agents to reduce T_1 and T_2 are described by the r_1 and r_2 relaxivity values of the agent, respectively. A higher relaxivity value means a greater effect of the contrast agent on nearby nuclear spins and, thus, a faster relaxation time observed [96, 99]. MRI contrast agents can be based broadly into two main categories, those based on paramagnetic materials, which mainly induce a shortening of the T_1 relaxation signal, and those based on superparamagnetic materials, which produce a more pronounced effect on the T_2 relaxation times.

Metal ions with one or more unpaired electrons are considered to be paramagnetic and as a result have a permanent magnetic moment [99]. The metal ion Gd^{3+} contains seven unpaired electrons and due to this is the most popular choice as a T_1 contrast agent, with significant research also being conducted on Mn^{2+} [96]. Although these ions are able to produce high r_1 relaxivities, their use must be carefully considered due to the high toxicity these elements produce in their ionic form. Hence they must be chelated or chemically bound in a nanoformulation for safe use as contrast agents [99]. Despite this, there is a range of contrast agents based on gadolinium currently on the market, including Magnevist®, Dotarem®, and Gadovist®, which are approved for clinical use.

Agents that shorten the T_2 relaxation times usually consist of iron oxide nanoparticles with magnetite (Fe_3O_4) and maghemite (γ-Fe_2O_3), both seen as the most popular candidates for this application. Nanoparticles of iron oxide can consist of several thousand magnetic ions and as a result of this are said to have superparamagnetic properties if these magnetic ions within the particle are aligned [99, 100]. If the magnetic moments of the iron ions within the nanoparticle are mutually aligned this will result in a permanent net magnetic moment for the nanoparticle, which when exposed to a magnetic field is very large [99]. Iron oxides are considered to be advantageous due to their relatively low toxicity, with the majority of these particles being endocytosed by Kupffer cells (specialized macrophages of the liver) where they are degraded within lysosomes within approximately seven days [99]. Sinorem®, Feridex®, Resovist®, and Endorem® are all examples of commercially available magnetic resonance contrast agents based on iron oxide nanoparticles.

Recent studies have endeavored to combine both T_1 and T_2 contrast agents in a single construct to produce nanoparticles suitable for the enhancement of both imaging signals. A study in 2010 by Bae et al. synthesized gadolinium-labeled magnetite nanoparticles (GMNPs) through a bioinspired method to be used as dual T_1- and T_2-weighted contrast agents in MRI [101]. The success of these dual contrast agents was demonstrated in vivo in mice when their contrast was compared to commercially available contrast agents for T_1- and T_2-weighted MRI, respectively (Fig. 1.10) [101].

1.1.3.5 Fluorescent probes for biological imaging

Fluorescence microscopy still stands as one of the most common and powerful techniques for both in vitro and in vivo imaging due to the ability to image intracellular events and differing tissues

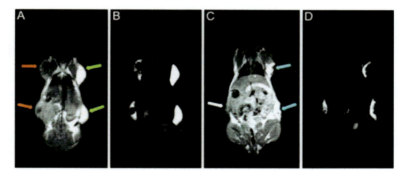

Figure 1.10 (A) T_1-weighted and (B) T_2-weighted magnetic resonance images of a mouse injected with Feridex® and Magnevist® (left: orange arrows indicate the injection sites of Feridex®; right: green arrows indicate the injection sites of Magnevist®). (C) T_1-weighted and (D) T_2-weighted magnetic resonance images of a mouse injected with GMNPs and the hydrogel solution as a control (left: white arrow indicates the injection site of the hydrogel solution; right: blue arrows indicate the injection sites of GMNPs). Reprinted with permission from Ref. [101], Copyright 2010 American Chemical Society.

with high specificity. The synthesis of traditional organic dyes and fluorescent quantum dot nanoparticles has seen these two imaging probes being developed to have emission spectra that cover the entire visible spectrum as well as going into the near-infrared region [102]. Organic fluorophores, the most commonly used imaging probes in biology, suffer from fast photobleaching and broad, sometimes overlapping emission and excitation spectra [103]. This limits the application of these probes for long-term imaging and/or when used as one of multiple probes due to the spectral overlap. Colloidal semiconductor nanoparticles, more commonly known as quantum dots, are robust, bright fluorescence emitters with size-dependent emission wavelengths. The extreme brightness of these nanoparticles and resistance to photobleaching make them ideal candidates for long-term imaging requirements such as the acquisition of z stacks or 3D reconstruction imaging [103]. The size-dependent, narrow, and tunable emission wavelength is also advantageous in the application of these imaging probes for multispectral imaging as they can often be tuned to avoid overlap unlike that of the traditional organic dyes [103]. However, despite the considerable upside to the use of quantum dots for biological imaging concerns have been raised with regard to their toxicity, with the majority of quantum dot cores usually containing highly toxic elements such as cadmium and selenium [103]. Care must be taken to ensure proper capping of these cores is achieved with biocompatible coatings such as ZnS (a common capping agent) to ensure these toxic elements do not leach [103].

Another interesting fluorescence imaging tool is that of fluorescent proteins. Naturally fluorescent proteins have become an incredibly useful tool for biologists and biochemists alike, especially in the fields of cancer research, neuroscience, and drug delivery. These proteins have allowed researchers to visualize important aspects of cancer in living animals, including tumor cell mobility, metastasis, and angiogenesis, all in real time [104]. Fluorescent proteins of many different colors have now been characterized, which in turn can be used to label cells of specific genotypes or phenotypes [104]. This allows for single-cell resolution and the ability to easily differentiate between a range of different biological processes. One area where this has promising applications is that of neuroscience, for the specific mapping of synaptic connections. Researchers through accurate mapping of neural circuits can learn how these account for mental activities and behaviors and more importantly how alterations to this circuitry can ultimately result in neurological or psychiatric disorders [105]. Recently, Livet et al. developed a technique that could allow neurologists to draw a detailed wiring plan of the mammalian brain through the insertion of genes coding for a range of fluorescent proteins in mice [106]. This technique, nicknamed "brainbow," can reveal individual neurons within the nervous system in high resolution and up to 160 distinctly different colors (Fig. 1.11) [105, 106]. This differential expression allowed researchers to map glial territories and follow glial cells and neurons independently over time in vivo [106].

1.1.4 Assessing Nanoparticle Toxicity

The assessment of nanoparticle toxicity is of paramount importance for all nano-engineered materials, not just for those prepared for

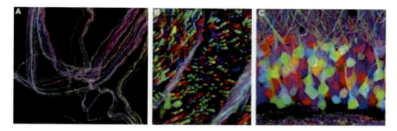

Figure 1.11 (A) A motor nerve innervating the ear muscle. (B) An axon tract in the brainstem. (C) The hippocampal dentate gyrus. In the brainbow mice from which these images were taken, up to ~160 colors were observed as a result of the co-integration of several tandem copies of the transgene into the mouse genome and the independent recombination of each by *Cre* recombinase. Reprinted by permission from Macmillan Publishers Ltd: Nature Reviews Neuroscience (Ref. [105]), copyright (2008).

intended biomedical applications. Due to the infancy of this science, the effects of nanoparticles on human health in general, as well as on the environment and ecosystems that these nanoparticles can potentially inadvertently reach, are integral to the future of the technology. The evolution of nanoparticle synthesis and technology has historically developed faster than testing and protocol development for the assessment of nanoparticle toxicity. However, this is changing with the ever-increasing interest in the field of nanotoxicology, which deals with the assessment of nanoparticles for their toxicity and environmental effects. An evaluation of this rapid growth is provided in Fig. 1.12, where it is clear that the rate of peer-reviewed publications mentioning the term "nanotoxicology" has shown strong growth within the past decade.

A recent report published by the US National Science Foundation in conjunction with the US Environmental Protection Agency identified five critical areas of risk associated with manufactured nanoparticles [107]. These five critical areas include:

- Exposure measurement and assessment of manufactured nanoparticles
- Toxicology of manufactured nanoparticles
- Ability to extrapolate manufactured nanoparticle toxicity using existing particle and fiber toxicological databases

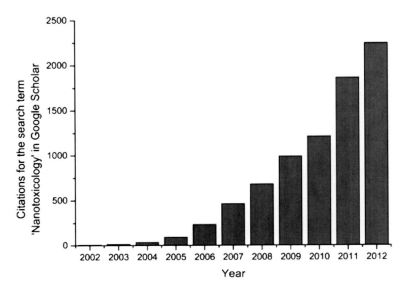

Figure 1.12 Number of citations recorded per year (2002–2012) for the search term "nanotoxicology," as assessed in Google Scholar.

- Environmental and biological fate, transport, persistence, and transformation of manufactured nanoparticles
- Recyclability and overall sustainability of manufactured nanomaterials

One of the main reasons that our understanding of nanotoxicology has lagged behind the production of nanoparticles is the difficulty of accurately predicting toxicity of specific nanomaterials. Toxicity is highly dependent on the dose, exposure, and pathway of cellular entry of the nanoparticles, not to mention the array of permutations possible for nanoparticles with regard to composition, size, shape, structure, and morphology, all adding to the potential for variation [108].

The most common approach to assess the toxicity of nanoparticles and nanomaterials alike is through in vitro toxicity tests for cell viability or by indirectly measuring cell numbers through the use of cell metabolism assays such as tetrazolium-based assays [108]. However, these in vitro assays only provide preliminary data, and to better understand the toxicology, including distribution, fate, and clearance of nanoparticles from a biological system, in vivo comparisons are required.

Two recent studies investigating comparative toxicological assessments of single-walled carbon nanotubes (SWCNTs) in rodent models found that the severity of the induced pulmonary granulomas followed a dose-dependent response [109, 110]. Current material safety data sheets classify SWCNTs as "a new form of graphite." However, results from these studies would suggest that simply extrapolating exposure limits from those set out for graphite would not be sufficient for protection against SWCNT exposure [107]. With the above in mind, it is clearly evident that before practical applications of nanoparticles for diagnosis or therapeutic purposes in humans, comprehensive assessments for potential toxicity of the nanoparticles must be carefully considered [15].

1.2 Multifunctional Poly(Glycidyl Methacrylate) Nanoparticles and Their Application in Cardiac Ischemia-Reperfusion Injuries

This section provides a research highlight of a multifunctional nanoparticle system we recently developed and how this nanoparticle was successfully used as a delivery vehicle for a therapeutic peptide. The nanoparticle was tested for efficacy by delivering to an ex vivo cardiac ischemia-reperfusion injury model, an important precursor to the majority of heart attack injuries worldwide.

1.2.1 *Rationale and Design of PGMA Nanoparticles for Therapeutic Delivery*

From the previous section, it is evident that a plethora of nanoparticle constructs have been developed for the biomedical industry to address areas such as drug delivery, therapy, diagnosis, and biological imaging. Advantages and disadvantages of a particular construct depend on the choice of material used to formulate the nanoparticle and the intended final use. Questions remain with regard to bionanotechnology and the safety of engineered nanomaterials and also their incorporation into clinical settings. Furthermore, nanoparticles developed for drug delivery applications must incorporate some form of a probe suitable for imaging in a clinical setting for tracking the nanoparticles in vivo. The application of targeting moieties to ensure site-specific targeting of nanoparticles is also an interesting concept that requires further exploration. Questions remain with regard to the importance of the attachment of targeting ligands for site-specific nanoparticle targeting in comparison to making use of known biological phenomena such as the EPR effect, which can aid in passive nanoparticle uptake. Furthermore, previous studies have successfully shown that nanoparticles with positively charged surfaces can enable rapid cellular attachment without targeting moeities. Finally, a nanoparticle construct developed for drug delivery must have the potential for encapsulation, protection, and delivery of a range of therapeutics, while achieving high levels of therapeutic loading. It is with these criteria in mind that we designed the poly(glycidal methacrylate) (PGMA) nanoparticles (presented in the following section) in order to combat some of these limiting characteristics seen with previously designed nanoparticle systems.

Multifunctional polymeric nanoparticles for drug delivery are an exciting area of research. The use of polymers to form nanoparticles provides structural rigidity and integrity to the nanoparticles, allowing for therapeutic protection and integrity when compared to other nanoparticle delivery methods. Further to this, the ability to easily modify the nanoparticle chemistry for the attachment of ligands and imaging probes makes polymeric particles an ideal core structure to build from. The choice of a polymer core is important to allow for fast and easy surface modification to occur. PGMA is an ideal choice, the epoxide functionality of this polymer being well suited for epoxide ring-opening reactions, thus making the addition of functionalized ligands and imaging probes straightforward.

PEI is a polyplex that has been shown to be able to enhance cellular uptake of a range of therapeutics both in vitro and in vivo. However, issues remain surrounding free PEI and its toxicity. Covalently binding this polymer to a polymeric surface of a nanoparticle has allowed for excellent transfection capabilities to remain without the inherent toxicity associated with free PEI. Furthermore, polymeric nanoparticles provide an ideal platform for the incorporation of multiple imaging probes, a limiting factor of other nanoparticle technologies where functionality is an issue.

The emulsion technique used to synthesize polymeric nanoparticles is well suited to the incorporation of hydrophobic drugs and therapeutics within the nanoparticle core. Furthermore, post-modification of the surfaces of these nanoparticles with PEI can enhance the electrostatic attachment of a range of biologically relevant payloads, including plasmid DNA, peptides, and proteins, to the nanoparticle surface. These methods and modifications, respectively, produce a nanosystem that has the potential for dual-drug delivery. The following section provides details of the characterization of these PGMA nanoparticles, their loading with a therapeutic peptide, and application in an ex vivo model of cardiac ischemia-reperfusion injury. The results from this study provide exciting prospects for future treatment of cardiac ischemia-reperfusion injury.

1.2.2 Current Treatment of Cardiac Ischemia-Reperfusion Injuries

Heart disease is the leading cause of death worldwide. Myocardial ischemia-reperfusion injury is the primary contributor to morbidity and mortality associated with heart disease [111]. Previous studies have shown that ischemia-reperfusion injury can lead to increases in both reactive oxygen species (ROS) and intracellular calcium within the heart, both of which directly contribute to the development of cardiac hypertrophy and potentially cardiac failure [112–115]. Intracellular Ca^{2+} is an integral component of normal cell function; however, significant increases in intracellular Ca^{2+} that occur during ischemia-reperfusion injury can be harmful, resulting in elevated ROS production and, subsequently, activation of apoptotic and necrotic cellular pathways [114, 116]. Therapeutic intervention with antioxidants aimed to counteract elevated ROS production that occurs during reperfusion has yielded mixed results, with some studies demonstrating a reduction in infarct size with antioxidant treatment [117–119] and others showing no significant difference [120–122]. Similarly the use of calcium-blocking agents to attenuate the sharp increase in calcium levels that occurs following ischemia-reperfusion injury have also had varied success [123, 124].

This study makes use of a novel peptide designed to bind to and regulate function of the cardiac L-type Ca^{2+} channel. The L-type Ca^{2+} channel is the main route of calcium influx into cardiac myocytes. Cardiac L-type Ca^{2+} channels are heterotetrameric polypeptide complexes comprising α_{1C}, $\alpha_2\delta$, and β_2 subunits. The α_{1C} subunit forms the pore of the channel, which regulates ion conductance and voltage sensing. The β_2 subunit plays an important role in regulating the probability of the channel being open and activation and inactivation kinetics [125–127]. The β_2 subunit is tightly bound to the α_{1C} subunit via the α-interacting domain (AID) [128, 129]. The peptide used in this study is designed to bind irreversibly to the AID region of the L-type Ca^{2+} channel (AID peptide). The AID of the L-type Ca^{2+} channel plays a role in modulating channel activation and inactivation kinetics. Binding of the AID peptide to the AID region of the channel can regulate channel activation and inactivation kinetics [130] (Fig. 1.13). Since activation of the L-type Ca^{2+} channel following oxidative stress can lead to further oxidative stress and induction of myocyte hypertrophy [112, 113], it is hypothesized that effective delivery of the therapeutic AID peptide to regulate channel function following reperfusion may hold the key to protection against myocardial damage.

The rationale for this approach is to manipulate L-type Ca^{2+} channel function at a concentration of the therapeutic AID peptide that does not alter calcium influx, thereby preventing negative inotropic effects, while still providing cardioprotection following ischemia-reperfusion. The AID peptide is designed against the 18-amino-acid sequence of AID of the cardiac L-type Ca^{2+} channel, a feature that is preserved across rodents and humans [129]. It has no homology to neuronal or skeletal muscle L-type Ca^{2+} channel AID, making this intervention highly specific to cardiac tissue and translatable to a human clinical setting.

The AID peptide, like most therapeutic proteins and peptides, does not readily cross the formidable barrier of the cell membrane without the assistance of a suitable delivery vehicle or transfection vector. This study aimed to compare the efficacy of the delivery of the therapeutic AID peptide bound to our multifunctional PGMA

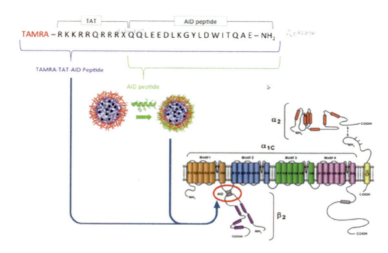

Figure 1.13 Schematic representation of nanoparticles loaded with AID peptide (AID-NPs) and TAT-bound AID peptide (AID-TAT) for delivery to the alpha-interacting domain (AID) of the L-type Ca^{2+} channel. Carboxytetramethyl rhodamine (TAMRA) was also covalently bound to the AID-TAT to facilitate peptide tracking of the TAT-conjugated peptide. Reprinted with permission from Ref. [131], Copyright 2013 American Chemical Society.

nanoparticles with that of the therapeutic peptide conjugated to the *trans*-activator of a transcription (TAT, described previously in Section 1.1.2.2 strategies to enhance cellular internalization) CPP (AID-TAT, see Fig. 1.13) [131]. TAT is an 11-residue-long peptide taken from the HIV-1 TAT protein that activates transcription of the viral genome and is a responsible factor for the virus's transfection [63]. The TAT peptide has been used for the delivery of a range of cargoes from peptides through nanoparticles. However, the potential therapeutic use of TAT is still uncertain, with questions remaining about its toxicity as well as poor public perception due to the origins of the peptide being from HIV-1 [63, 132–134].

1.2.3 PGMA Nanoparticle Characterization and Surface Peptide Loading

The PGMA nanoparticles used in this work were synthesized by the polymer emulsion method The nanoparticle core consists of the epoxide-functionalized polymer PGMA premodified with the fluorescent dye rhodamine B (RhB) to provide fluorescent imaging capabilities [131]. During the emulsion process, magnetite was encapsulated within the nanoparticle core. The presence of magnetite served two important purposes. The first function was for its suitability as an MRI contrast agent for in vivo tracking of the nanoparticles throughout the target tissue. Secondly, and most importantly, the presence of magnetite provided a means to separate, wash, and concentrate the nanoparticles using a magnetic fractionation column in preparation for peptide conjugation.

The final step in nanoparticle production is covalent surface decoration with the cationic polymer PEI to give the nanoparticle an overall net positive surface charge. This attachment also serves two integral purposes. The first is the cationic polymer chains allow for strong electrostatic binding between the negative residues in the therapeutic AID peptide and the amino groups of the PEI chains. Furthermore the attachment of the PEI allows for strong cellular association and cellular uptake, as previously reported [54].

That the nanoparticles used in this study consisted of magnetite encapsulated within the PGMA core of the particle is evident from transmission electron microscopy (Fig. 1.14A) [131]. The

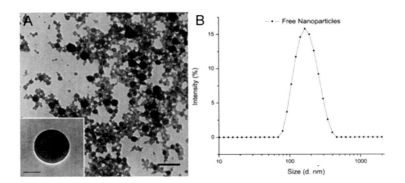

Figure 1.14 (A) Low-magnification transmission electron microscopy of PGMA nanoparticles (scale 500 nm) with high-magnification inset (scale 50 nm). (B) Size distribution of PGMA nanoparticles with PEI functionalization assessed by dynamic light scattering. Reprinted with permission from Ref. [131], Copyright 2013 American Chemical Society.

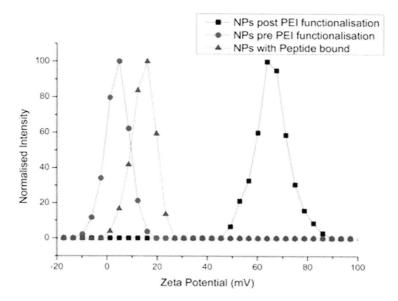

Figure 1.15 Zeta potential of the nanoparticles before PEI functionalization (circles), with PEI functionalization (squares), and with AID peptide conjugated to the PEI-functionalized nanoparticle surface (triangles). Reprinted with permission from Ref. [131], Copyright 2013 American Chemical Society.

nanoparticles with PEI functionalization had an average size of 160 nm (95% confidence interval 85–342 nm) when assessed by dynamic light scattering (Fig. 1.14B). The nanoparticles were surface-decorated with linear PEI chains to produce a nanoparticle with a net overall positive charge of 65 mV (Fig. 1.15). Successful PEI binding was determined by comparing the shift in the nanoparticle zeta potential post-PEI modification to the zeta potential of the nanoparticles prior to this functionalization (Fig. 1.15).

The AID peptide was conjugated to the nanoparticles through the favorable electrostatic interactions between the negative residues on the peptide and the cationic PEI grafted to the nanoparticle surface. Nanoparticles were assessed again for zeta potential with the peptide loaded onto the PEI-functionalized nanoparticles, and a significant reduction in the surface charge was observed, as was expected with the incorporation of the peptide (Fig. 1.15).

Peptide loading on the nanoparticles with the PEI surface coating was determined to be 0.072 nM AID peptide/µg nanoparticles (0.16% w/w), which was approximately a threefold increase when compared to nanoparticles without the PEI surface modification (AID peptide loading on nanoparticles minus PEI functionalization was 0.024 nM AID peptide/µg nanoparticles [0.05% w/w]). Due to the superior loading, and previous work that had demonstrated rapid cellular internalization of the PEI-functionalized nanoparticles [54], the PEI-functionalized nanoparticles were used throughout all aspects of this study [54]. The nanoparticle–AID peptide complexes containing magnetite and RhB (RhB-AID-NPs) were compared to AID-TAT at the same concentration of therapeutic peptide in subsequent in vitro studies and in the ex vivo ischemia-reperfusion injury model.

1.2.4 A Comparison of Cellular Uptake and Biodistribution

Both delivery systems were initially investigated for their rate of association with cardiac myocytes [131]. The AID-TAT was labeled with carboxytetramethyl rhodamine (TAMRA) (TAMRA-AID-TAT). Fluorescent labeling of the AID-TAT allowed for tracking of the TAT-mediated delivery in vitro and ex vivo and therefore allowed for comparisons to be made with the nanoparticle-mediated delivery of the peptide. Initial studies made use of primary isolates of guinea pig cardiac myocytes, which were incubated with either 1 µM TAMRA-AID-TAT or 1 µM RhB-AID-NPs. Uptake was assessed by fluorescence as an increase in the intensity of the fluorescence signal associated with cells, with respect to time, when compared to background levels prior to the addition of the peptide samples. Maximal association of TAMRA-AID-TAT with myocytes occurred at 35 minutes in contrast to the AID peptide conjugated to nanoparticles (RhB-AID-NPs), which associated with cells more rapidly, with the maximal fluorescent signal occurring at 15 minutes (Fig. 1.16A).

Furthermore, unloaded nanoparticles (RhB-NP) were also able to achieve rapid cellular association similar to that seen with the AID peptide–loaded nanoparticles (Fig. 1.16A). Nanoparticles loaded with the AID peptide still maintained a net positive surface exterior

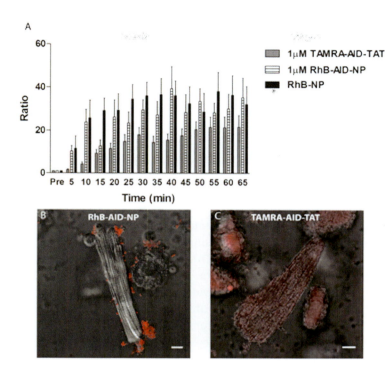

Figure 1.16 (A) Uptake of AID-TAT or AID nanoparticles (AID-NPs) was assessed as changes in fluorescence following addition of TAMRA-AID-TAT, RhB-AID-NPs, or nanoparticles not containing AID (RhB-NPs), compared to a fluorescence reading taken prior to application of peptides, in isolated cardiac myocytes. Representative confocal microscopy of rhodamine fluorescence with differential interference contrast (DIC) overlay for myocytes incubated with (B) AID-tethered nanoparticles, and (C) TAMRA-AID-TAT (scale = 10 μm). Reprinted with permission from Ref. [131], Copyright 2013 American Chemical Society.

(18 mV, Fig. 1.15), and it is anticipated that the preservation of this positive surface despite peptide loading was the major contributing factor associated with the rapid cellular association observed.

Confocal imaging of peptide conjugated to nanoparticles (labeled with RhB) and TAMRA-labeled TAT peptide demonstrated similar cellular association for both modes of delivery after 5 and 4.5 hours of incubation with cardiac myocytes, respectively (Fig. 1.16B,C) [131]. Additionally, confocal analysis revealed that the two modes of delivery operated differently in an in vitro setting. The TAT-based delivery showed cellular internalization of the peptide following incubation with myocytes. However, despite rapid cellular association, the nanoparticles were only evident on the cell surface. They did not appear to be internalized within the cells over the time frames investigated (Fig. 1.16B). The AID region of the cardiac L-type calcium channel is found proximal to but within the cellular membrane [123, 129]. Therefore we anticipated that both modes of delivery would be suitable for effective AID peptide delivery to its intended delivery target.

Distribution of the peptide in the myocardium ex vivo using the two delivery modes was also investigated. Healthy hearts were perfused with either buffer containing no treatment or buffer containing the AID peptide conjugated with nanoparticles (1 µM RhB-AID-NPs) or TAT (1 µM TAMRA-AID-TAT) directly into the coronary arteries via the aorta. Perfusion of 1 µM RhB-AID-NPs resulted in a dense and wide distribution of nanoparticles throughout the tissue, as indicated by fluorescence microscopy and supported by MRI, when compared to hearts perfused with buffer only (Fig. 1.17A,B). A very different pattern was observed with perfusion of 1 µM TAMRA-AID-TAT, which resulted in punctate

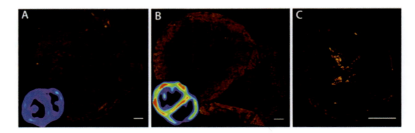

Figure 1.17 The biodistribution of both delivery methods was assessed in hearts perfused with either AID-tethered nanoparticles or AID-TAT-TAMRA. (A) Fluorescent microscopy of healthy guinea pig heart with buffer reperfusion (no therapeutic delivery), R_2-weighted MRI inset, (B) fluorescent microscopy of healthy guinea pig heart with reperfusion of 1 µM AID-tethered nanoparticles (RhB-AID-NPs), R_2-weighted MRI inset, and (C) fluorescent microscopy of healthy mouse heart perfused with 1 µM TAMRA-AID-TAT (scale = 1 mm). Reprinted with permission from Ref. [131], Copyright 2013 American Chemical Society.

(spotted) and sparse distribution, with very little uptake evident in the sectioned muscle tissue (Fig. 1.17C). These studies demonstrate that PEI-coated nanoparticles were able to penetrate further, and throughout the entire cross section, in comparison to TAT-mediated delivery.

A major limitation of the TAT-mediated delivery in this study was the inability for the peptide conjugates to produce MRI contrast, further highlighting a key advantage of the multifunctional polymeric nanoparticles with respect to multimodal imaging capabilities. From comparison of the R_2 maps (Fig. 1.17A,B) it is evident that the MRI analysis for the buffer-only and nanoparticle-treated hearts agree with the fluorescence signal from the nanoparticles with regard to localization within the tissue. These data suggest that the multifunctional PGMA nanoparticles were able to produce strong MRI contrast, a result of the superparamagnetic properties of the magnetite nanoparticles incorporated within the PGMA polymer core of the nanoparticles.

This study was one of the first to demonstrate multimodal imaging capabilities of PGMA nanoparticles, and it demonstrated agreement of fluorescent and MRI signals in a tissue sample [131]. The results from this study demonstrate the strengths of nanoparticle-mediated multimodal imaging capabilities when compared to TAT-mediated delivery. Multifunctional PGMA nanoparticles were able to produce strong MRI contrast. MRI is a widely used, noninvasive imaging technique that does not cause significant damage or side effects to samples or patients. The ability to image nanoparticle-mediated delivery of AID in this manner may therefore prove advantageous in the clinical setting.

1.2.5 Nanoparticle and TAT-Mediated Delivery of the AID Peptide Reduces Damage Following Ischemia-Reperfusion Injury

After assessing delivery potential through both cellular attachment and cardiac biodistribution, we investigated efficacy of the nanoparticle and TAT-mediated delivery of the AID peptide in alleviating damage following cardiac ischemia-reperfusion injury [131]. For damage assessments an ex vivo ischemia-reperfusion injury model

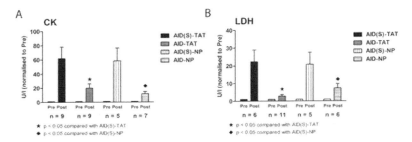

Figure 1.18 Comparison of effects of AID-TAT and AID-NPs on damage assessment ex vivo in an ischemia-reperfusion injury. (A) Creatine kinase (CK), and (B) lactate dehydrogenase (LDH) levels were assessed in perfusate taken before (pre-) and after (post-) ischemia-reperfusion in the presence of AID(S)-TAT, AID-TAT, AID(S)-NPs, or AID-NPs, as indicated. Results are reported as mean ± SE. Statistical comparisons were made using a student's t-test (*$p \leq 0.05$). Reprinted with permission from Ref. [131], Copyright 2013 American Chemical Society.

was used. Hearts were isolated from adult guinea pigs and perfused retrogradely on a Langendorff apparatus with Ca^{2+}-containing KHB solution for 30 minutes. Following this perfusion phase no flow ischemia was induced for 30 minutes, followed by reperfusion for 30 minutes in the presence of either 1 µM AID-TAT peptide (AID-TAT), 1 µM scrambled AID-TAT peptide (AID(S)-TAT), AID-tethered nanoparticles (AID-NPs), or scrambled AID peptide tethered to nanoparticles (AID(S)-NPs). Damage was assessed by comparing the release of creatine kinase (CK) and lactate dehydrogenase (LDH) in the perfusate collected during reperfusion to CK and LDH release during the initial perfusion phase (pre-reperfusion). Release of CK and LDH provides indications of cardiac tissue damage following ischemia-reperfusion injury. Both 1 µM AID-NPs and 1 µM AID-TAT were effective at reducing the levels of CK following ischemia-reperfusion compared to respective controls (AID(S)-TAT and AID(S)-NPs) (Fig. 1.18A). Similarly, both delivery methods of the therapeutic AID peptide resulted in significant reductions in the level of LDH released, following ischemia-reperfusion, when compared to control treatments (Fig. 1.18B).

1.2.6 Conclusions and Future Work

Nanotechnology and nanoparticle drug delivery vehicles provide an exciting prospect for the delivery of therapeutics in the treatment of disease and injury. This includes the treatment of heart disease. Heart disease is the leading cause of death worldwide. However, the application of nanotechnology to improve outcomes postinjury has been limited in comparison to other diseases such as cancer. This study compared the efficacy of TAT-mediated delivery of the therapeutic AID peptide to delivery of the AID peptide via conjugation to multifunctional PGMA nanoparticles [131]. Effectiveness of these two delivery systems was assessed using both in vitro and ex vivo models.

The AID peptide conjugated to PGMA nanoparticle was more rapidly taken up into cardiac myocytes and more widely distributed in the myocardium than the AID peptide delivered using the HIV-derived TAT sequence. Although in vitro studies suggested association of the nanoparticles occurred only with the cell membrane of cardiac myocytes, ex vivo studies suggested this was sufficient for the AID peptide to produce a therapeutic benefit and reduce cardiac damage following ischemia-reperfusion injury. This study also demonstrates the effectiveness of multimodal imaging capabilities of multifunctional PGMA nanoparticles compared to the TAT delivery method, as evidenced by biodistribution and localization studies.

Overall we find that AID-TAT and AID-tethered nanoparticles provide effective modes of delivery of the AID peptide in the heart. Both modes of delivery were efficacious in reducing damage associated with ischemia-reperfusion injury. However, nanoparticle delivery of the peptide appeared to be more effective with regard to multimodal imaging capabilities. An additional advantage of the nanoparticle-based system compared to the TAT-mediated delivery system may be the potential to carry multiple payloads combined within a single-nanoparticle delivery platform. This study provides justification for further development of both delivery systems for tolerance as a therapy in the clinical setting.

Acknowledgments

We would like to thank the Centre for Microscopy, Characterization and Analysis at the University of Western Australia and the MRI unit at Sir Charles Gardner Hospital, Perth Western Australia, for their support with imaging and analysis. We would also like to thank the financial support that made this research possible, including funding from the Australian Research Council, the National Health and Medical Research Council (APP1073180), the University of Western Australia, and the Australian Nanotechnology Network.

References

1. Cooper, D. R., and Nadeau, J. L. Nanotechnology for *in vitro* neuroscience, *Nanoscale*, **1**, 2009, 183–200.
2. Eustis, S., and El-Sayed, M. Why gold nanoparticles are more precious than pretty gold: noble metal surface plasmon resonance and its enhancement of the radiative and non radiative proerties of nanocrystals of different shapes, *Chem. Soc. Rev.*, **35**, 2006, 209–217.
3. Silva, G. A. Neuroscience nanotechnology: progress, opportunities and challenges, *Nat. Rev. Neurosci.*, **7**, 2006, 65–74.
4. Shi, J. J., Votruba, A. R., Farokhzad, O. C., and Langer, R. Nanotechnology in drug delivery and tissue engineering: from discovery to applications, *Nano Lett.*, **10**, 2010, 3223–3230.
5. Zrazhevskiy, P., and Gao, X. H. Multifunctional quantum dots for personalized medicine, *Nano Today*, **4**, 2009, 414–428.
6. Niu, J. L., Azfer, A., Rogers, L. M., Wang, X. H., and Kolattukudy, P. E. Cardioprotective effects of cerium oxide nanoparticles in a transgenic murine model of cardiomyopathy, *Cardiovasc. Res.*, **73**, 2007, 549–559.
7. Scott, R. C., Crabbe, D., Krynska, B., Ansari, R., and Kiani, M. F. Aiming for the heart: targeted delivery of drugs to diseased cardiac tissue, *Expert Opin. Drug Delivery*, **5**, 2008, 459–470.
8. Kamaly, N., Xiao, Z. Y., Valencia, P. M., Radovic-Moreno, A. F., and Farokhzad, O. C. Targeted polymeric therapeutic nanoparticles: design, development and clinical translation, *Chem. Soc. Rev.*, **41**, 2012, 2971–3010.

9. Cheng, Z. L., Al Zaki, A., Hui, J. Z., Muzykantov, V. R., and Tsourkas, A. Multifunctional nanoparticles: cost versus benefit of adding targeting and imaging capabilities, *Science*, **338**, 2012, 903–910.
10. Yan, Y., Such, G. K., Johnston, A. P. R., Best, J. P., and Caruso, F. Engineering particles for therapeutic delivery: prospects and challenges, *ACS Nano*, **6**, 2012, 3663–3669.
11. Sanna, V., Siddiqui, I. A., Sechi, M., and Mukhtar, H. Nanoformulation of natural products for prevention and therapy of prostate cancer, *Cancer Lett.*, **334**, 2013, 142–151.
12. Orive, G., Anitua, E., Pedraz, J. L., and Emerich, D. F. Biomaterials for promoting brain protection, repair and regeneration, *Nat. Rev. Neurosci.*, **10**, 2009, 682–692.
13. Cho, K. J., Wang, X., Nie, S. M., Chen, Z., and Shin, D. M. Therapeutic nanoparticles for drug delivery in cancer, *Clin. Cancer Res.*, **14**, 2008, 1310–1316.
14. Gilmore, J. L., Yi, X., Quan, L., and Kabanov, A. V. Novel nanomaterials for clinical neuroscience, *J. Neuroimmune Pharmacol.*, **3**, 2008, 83–94.
15. Lee, D. E., Koo, H., Sun, I. C., Ryu, J. H., Kim, K., and Kwon, I. C. Multifunctional nanoparticles for multimodal imaging and theragnosis, *Chem. Soc. Rev.*, **41**, 2012, 2656–2672.
16. Koo, H., et al. In vivo tumor diagnosis and photodynamic therapy via tumoral pH-responsive polymeric micelles, *Chem. Commun.*, **46**, 2010, 5668–5670.
17. Tannock, I. F., and Rotin, D. Acid pH in tumors and its potential for therapeutic exploitation, *Cancer Res.*, **49**, 1989, 4373–4384.
18. Markman, M. PEGylated liposomal doxorubicin in the treatment of cancers of the breast and ovary, *Expert Opin. Pharmacother.*, **7**, 2006, 1469–1474.
19. Rivera, E. Liposomal anthracyclines in metastatic breast cancer: clinical update, *Oncologist*, **8**, 2003, 3–9.
20. Rosenthal, E., Poizot-Martin, I., Saint-Marc, T., Spano, J. P., Cacoub, P., and Grp, D. S. Phase IV study of liposomal daunorubicin (DaunoXome) in AIDS-related Kaposi sarcoma, *Cancer Clin. Trials*, **25**, 2002, 57–59.
21. Hajos, F., Stark, B., Hensler, S., Prassl, R., and Mosgoeller, W. Inhalable liposomal formulation for vasoactive intestinal peptide, *Int. J. Pharm.*, **357**, 2008, 286–294.
22. Svenson, S., and Tomalia, D. A. Commentary: dendrimers in biomedical applications; reflections on the field, *Adv. Drug Delivery Rev.*, **57**, 2005, 2106–2129.

23. Malik, N., Evagorou, E. G., and Duncan, R. Dendrimer-platinate: a novel approach to cancer chemotherapy, *Anti-Cancer Drugs*, **10**, 1999, 767–776.
24. Wijagkanalan, W., Kawakami, S., and Hashida, M. Designing dendrimers for drug delivery and imaging: pharmacokinetic considerations, *Pharm. Res.*, **28**, 2011, 1500–1519.
25. Lockman, P. R., Mumper, R. J., Khan, M. A., and Allen, D. D. Nanoparticle technology for drug delivery across the blood-brain barrier, *Drug Dev. Ind. Pharm.*, **28**, 2002, 1–13.
26. Soppimath, K. S., Aminabhavi, T. M., Kulkarni, A. R., and Rudzinski, W. E. Biodegradable polymeric nanoparticles as drug delivery devices, *J. Controlled Release*, **70**, 2001, 1–20.
27. Grabnar, P. A., and Kristl, J. The manufacturing techniques of drug-loaded polymeric nanoparticles from preformed polymers, *J. Microencapsul.*, **28**, 2011, 323–335.
28. Malam, Y., Loizidou, M., and Seifalian, A. M. Liposomes and nanoparticles: nanosized vehicles for drug delivery in cancer, *Trends Pharmacol. Sci.*, **30**, 2009, 592–599.
29. Menei, P., Pean, J. M., Nerriere-Daguin, V., Jollivet, C., Brachet, P., and Benoit, J. P. Intracerebral implantation of NGF-releasing biodegradable microspheres protects striatum against excitotoxic damage, *Exp. Neurol.*, **161**, 2000, 259–272.
30. Jackanicz, T., Nash, H., Wise, D., and Gregory, J. Polylactic acid as a biodegradable carrier for contraceptive steroids, *Contraception*, **8**, 1973, 227–234.
31. Anderson, L., Wise, D., and Howes, J. An injectable sustained release fertility control system, *Contraception*, **13**, 1976, 375–384.
32. Gradishar, W. J., Tjulandin, S., Davidson, N., Shaw, H., Desai, N., Bhar, P., Hawkins, M., and O'Shaughnessy, J. Phase III trial of nanoparticle albumin-bound paclitaxel compared with polyethylated castor oil-based paclitaxel in women with breast cancer, *J. Clin. Oncol.*, **23**, 2005, 7794–7803.
33. Green, M. R., Manikhas, G. M., Orlov, S., Afanasyev, B., Makhson, A. M., Bhar, P., and Hawkins, M. J. Abraxane((R)), a novel Cremophor((R))-free, albumin-bound particle form of paclitaxel for the treatment of advanced non-small-cell lung cancer, *Ann. Oncol.*, **17**, 2006, 1263–1268.
34. Nyman, D. W., Campbell, K. J., Hersh, E., Long, K., Richardson, K., Trieu, V., Desai, N., Hawkins, M. J., and Von Hoff, D. D. Phase I and

pharmacokinetics trial of ABI-007, a novel nanoparticle formulation of paclitaxel in patients with advanced nonhematologic malignancies, *J. Clin. Oncol.*, **23**, 2005, 7785–7793.

35. Black, C. D. V., and Gregoriadis, G. Intracellular fate and effect of liposome-entrapped actinomycin-D injected into rats, *Biochem. Soc. Trans.*, **2**, 1974, 869–871.
36. Couvreur, P., Tulkens, P., Roland, M., Trouet, A., and Speiser, P. Nanocapsules: new type of lysosomotropic carrier, *FEBS Lett.*, **84**, 1977, 323–326.
37. Torchilin, V. P. Cell penetrating peptide-modified pharmaceutical nanocarriers for intracellular drug and gene delivery, *Biopolymers*, **90**, 2008, 604–610.
38. Conner, S., and Schmid, S. Regulated portals of entry into the cell, *Nature*, **422**, 2003, 37–44.
39. Zhao, F., Zhao, Y., Liu, Y., Chang, X. L., Chen, C. Y., and Zhao, Y. L. Cellular uptake, intracellular trafficking, and cytotoxicity of nanomaterials, *Small*, **7**, 2011, 1322–1337.
40. Hillaireau, H., and Couvreur, P. Nanocarriers' entry into the cell: relevance to drug discovery, *Cell. Mol. Life Sci.*, **66**, 2009, 2873–2896.
41. Aderem, A., and Underhill, D. M. Mechanisms of phagocytosis in macrophages, *Annu. Rev. Immunol.*, **17**, 1999, 593–623.
42. Mellman, I. Endocytosis and molecular sorting, *Annu. Rev. Cell Dev. Biol.*, **12**, 1996, 575–625.
43. Mayor, S., and Pagano, R. Pathways of clathrin-independant endocytosis, *Nat. Rev. Mol. Cell Biol.*, **8**, 2007, 603–612.
44. Claus, V., Jahraus, A., Tjelle, T., Berg, T., Kirschke, H., Faulstich, H., and Griffiths, G. Lysosomal enzyme trafficking between phagosomes, endosomes, and lysosomes in J774 macrophages: enrichment of cathepsin H in early endosomes, *J. Biol. Chem.*, **273**, 1998, 9842–9851.
45. Rejman, J., Oberle, V., Zuhorn, I. S., and Hoekstra, D. Size-dependent internalization of particles via the pathways of clathrin-and caveolae-mediated endocytosis, *Biochem. J.*, **377**, 2004, 159–169.
46. Panyam, J., Zhou, W. Z., Prabha, S., Sahoo, S. K., and Labhasetwar, V. Rapid endo-lysosomal escape of poly(DL-lactide-co-glycolide) nanoparticles: implications for drug and gene delivery, *FASEB J.*, **16**, 2002, 1217–1226.
47. Hatakeyama, H., Ito, E., Akita, H., Oishi, M., Nagasaki, Y., Futaki, S., and Harashima, H. A pH-sensitive fusogenic peptide facilitates endosomal escape and greatly enhances the gene silencing of siRNA-containing

nanoparticles in vitro and in vivo, *J. Controlled Release*, **139**, 2009, 127–132.
48. Gratton, S. E. A., Ropp, P. A., Pohlhaus, P. D., Luft, J. C., Madden, V. J., Napier, M. E., and DeSimone, J. M. The effect of particle design on cellular internalization pathways, *Proc. Natl. Acad. Sci. U. S. A.*, **105**, 2008, 11613–11618.
49. Banquy, X., Suarez, F., Argaw, A., Rabanel, J. M., Grutter, P., Bouchard, J. F., Hildgen, P., and Giasson, S. Effect of mechanical properties of hydrogel nanoparticles on macrophage cell uptake, *Soft Matter*, **5**, 2009, 3984–3991.
50. Harush-Frenkel, O., Rozentur, E., Benita, S., and Altschuler, Y. Surface charge of nanoparticles determines their endocytic and transcytotic pathway in polarized MDCK cells, *Biomacromolecules*, **9**, 2008, 435–443.
51. Harush-Frenkel, O., Debotton, N., Benita, S., and Altschuler, Y. Targeting of nanoparticles to the clathrin-mediated endocytic pathway, *Biochem. Biophys. Res. Commun.*, **353**, 2007, 26–32.
52. Alexis, F., Lo, S. L., and Wang, S. Covalent attachment of low molecular weight poly(ethylene imine) improves tat peptide mediated gene delivery, *Adv. Mater.*, **18**, 2006, 2174–2178.
53. Boussif, O., Lezoualch, F., Zanta, M. A., Mergny, M. D., Scherman, D., Demeneix, B., and Behr, J. P. A versatile vector for gene and oligonucleotide transfer into cells in culture and *in vivo*: polyethylenimine, *Proc. Natl. Acad. Sci. U. S. A.*, **92**, 1995, 7297–7301.
54. Evans, C. W., et al. Multimodal analysis of PEI-mediated endocytosis of nanoparticles in neural cells, *ACS Nano*, **5**, 2011, 8640–8648.
55. Fuller, J. E., Zugates, G. T., Ferreira, L. S., Ow, H. S., Nguyen, N. N., Wiesner, U. B., and Langer, R. S. Intracellular delivery of core-shell fluorescent silica nanoparticles, *Biomaterials*, **29**, 2008, 1526–1532.
56. Whitehead, K. A., Langer, R., and Anderson, D. G. Knocking down barriers: advances in siRNA delivery, *Nat. Rev. Drug Discovery*, **8**, 2009, 129–138.
57. Gary, D. J., Puri, N., and Won, Y. Y. Polymer-based siRNA delivery: perspectives on the fundamental and phenomenological distinctions from polymer-based DNA delivery, *J. Controlled Release*, **121**, 2007, 64–73.
58. Bonner, D. K., Zhao, X. Y., Buss, H., Langer, R., and Hammond, P. T. Crosslinked linear polyethylenimine enhances delivery of DNA to the cytoplasm, *J. Controlled Release*, **167**, 2013, 101–107.

59. Ko, Y. T., Kale, A., Hartner, W. C., Papahadjopoulos-Sternberg, B., and Torchilin, V. P. Self-assembling micelle-like nanoparticles based on phospholipid-polyethyleneimine conjugates for systemic gene delivery, *J. Controlled Release*, **133**, 2009, 132–138.
60. Akinc, A., Thomas, M., Klibanov, A. M., and Langer, R. Exploring polyethylenimine-mediated DNA transfection and the proton sponge hypothesis, *J. Gene Med.*, **7**, 2005, 657–663.
61. Sonawane, N. D., Szoka, F. C., and Verkman, A. S. Chloride accumulation and swelling in endosomes enhances DNA transfer by polyamine-DNA polyplexes, *J. Biol. Chem.*, **278**, 2003, 44826–44831.
62. Jones, S. W., Christison, R., Bundell, K., Voyce, C. J., Brockbank, S. M., Newham, P., and Lindsay, M. A. Characterisation of cell-penetrating peptide-mediated peptide delivery, *Br. J. Pharmacol.*, **145**, 2005, 1093–1102.
63. Rapoport, M., and Lorberboum-Galski, H. TAT-based drug delivery system: new directions in protein delivery for new hopes?, *Expert Opin. Drug Delivery*, **6**, 2009, 453–463.
64. Brooks, H., Lebleu, B., and Vives, E. Tat peptide-mediated cellular delivery: back to basics, *Adv. Drug Delivery Rev.*, **57**, 2005, 559–577.
65. Herce, H., and Garcia, A. Molecular dynamics simulations suggest a mechanism for translocation of the HIV-1 TAT peptide across lipid membranes, *Proc. Natl. Acad. Sci. U. S. A.*, **104**, 2007, 20805–20810.
66. Lundin, P., Johansson, H., Guterstam, P., Holm, T., Hansen, M., Langel, U., and Andaloussi, S. Distinct uptake routes of cell-penetrating peptide conjugates, *Bioconjug. Chem.*, **19**, 2008, 2535–2542.
67. Farokhzad, O. C., Cheng, J. J., Teply, B. A., Sherifi, I., Jon, S., Kantoff, P. W., Richie, J. P., and Langer, R. Targeted nanoparticle-aptamer bioconjugates for cancer chemotherapy in vivo, *Proc. Natl. Acad. Sci. U. S. A.*, **103**, 2006, 6315–6320.
68. Sanvicens, N., and Marco, M. P. Multifunctional nanoparticles: properties and prospects for their use in human medicine, *Trends Biotechnol.*, **26**, 2008, 425–433.
69. Zhou, J., Patel, T. R., Fu, M., Bertram, J. P., and Saltzman, W. M. Octa-functional PLGA nanoparticles for targeted and efficient siRNA delivery to tumors, *Biomaterials*, **33**, 2012, 583–591.
70. Moghimi, S. M., Hunter, A. C., and Murray, J. C. Long-circulating and target-specific nanoparticles: theory to practice, *Pharmacol. Rev.*, **53**, 2001, 283–318.
71. Torchilin, V. P. Drug targeting, *Eur. J. Pharm. Sci.*, **11**, 2000, S81–S91.

72. Maeda, H., Wu, J., Sawa, T., Matsumura, Y., and Hori, K. Tumor vascular permeability and the EPR effect in macromolecular therapeutics: a review, *J. Controlled Release*, **65**, 2000, 271–284.
73. Peer, D., Karp, J. M., Hong, S., FaroKHzad, O. C., Margalit, R., and Langer, R. Nanocarriers as an emerging platform for cancer therapy, *Nat. Nanotechnol.*, **2**, 2007, 751–760.
74. Huang, M., Wu, W., Qian, J., Wan, D. J., Wei, X. L., and Zhu, J. H. Body distribution and *in situ* evading of phagocytic uptake by macrophages of long-circulating poly (ethylene glycol) cyanoacrylate-co-n-hexadecyl cyanoacrylate nanoparticles, *Acta Pharmacol. Sin.*, **26**, 2005, 1512–1518.
75. Li, S. D., and Huang, L. Stealth nanoparticles: high density but sheddable PEG is a key for tumor targeting, *J. Controlled Release*, **145**, 2010, 178–181.
76. Socha, M., Bartecki, P., Passirani, C., Sapin, A., Damge, C., Lecompte, T., Barre, J., El Ghazouani, F., and Maincent, P. Stealth nanoparticles coated with heparin as peptide or protein carriers, *J. Drug Targeting*, **17**, 2009, 575–585.
77. Zambaux, M. F., Faivre-Fiorina, B., Bonneaux, F., Marchal, S., Merlin, J. L., Dellacherie, E., Labrude, P., and Vigneron, C. Involvement of neutrophilic granulocytes in the uptake of biodegradable non-stealth and stealth nanoparticles in guinea pig, *Biomaterials*, **21**, 2000, 975–980.
78. Adiseshaiah, P. P., Hall, J. B., and McNeil, S. E. Nanomaterial standards for efficacy and toxicity assessment, *Wiley Interdiscip. Rev. Nanomed. Nanobiotechnol.*, **2**, 2010, 99–112.
79. Tan, Y. F., Chandrasekharan, P., Maity, D., Yong, C. X., Chuang, K. H., Zhao, Y., Wang, S., Ding, J., and Feng, S. S. Multimodal tumor imaging by iron oxides and quantum dots formulated in poly (lactic acid)-D-alpha-tocopheryl polyethylene glycol 1000 succinate nanoparticles, *Biomaterials*, **32**, 2011, 2969–2978.
80. Akiyama, Y., Mori, T., Katayama, Y., and Niidome, T. The effects of PEG grafting level and injection dose on gold nanorod biodistribution in the tumor-bearing mice, *J. Controlled Release*, **139**, 2009, 81–84.
81. Niidome, T., Yamagata, M., Okamoto, Y., Akiyama, Y., Takahashi, H., Kawano, T., Katayama, Y., and Niidome, Y. PEG-modified gold nanorods with a stealth character for in vivo applications, *J. Controlled Release*, **114**, 2006, 343–347.
82. Lankveld, D. P. K., Rayavarapu, R. G., Krystek, P., Oomen, A. G., Verharen, H. W., van Leeuwen, T. G., De Jong, W. H., and Manohar, S. Blood

clearance and tissue distribution of PEGylated and non-PEGylated gold nanorods after intravenous administration in rats, *Nanomedicine*, **6**, 2011, 339–349.
83. Danhier, F., Feron, O., and Preat, V. To exploit the tumor microenvironment: passive and active tumor targeting of nanocarriers for anticancer drug delivery, *J. Controlled Release*, **148**, 2010, 135–146.
84. Jain, R. K., and Stylianopoulos, T. Delivering nanomedicine to solid tumors, *Nat. Rev. Clin. Oncol.*, **7**, 2010, 653–664.
85. Blanco, E., Hsiao, A., Mann, A. P., Landry, M. G., Meric-Bernstam, F., and Ferrari, M. Nanomedicine in cancer therapy: innovative trends and prospects, *Cancer Sci.*, **102**, 2011, 1247–1252.
86. Poon, Z., Lee, J. A., Huang, S. W., Prevost, R. J., and Hammond, P. T. Highly stable, ligand-clustered "patchy" micelle nanocarriers for systemic tumor targeting, *Nanomedicine*, **7**, 2011, 201–209.
87. Low, P. S., Henne, W. A., and Doorneweerd, D. D. Discovery and development of folic-acid-based receptor targeting for Imaging and therapy of cancer and inflammatory diseases, *Acc. Chem. Res.*, **41**, 2008, 120–129.
88. McNeeley, K. M., Annapragada, A., and Bellamkonda, R. V. Decreased circulation time offsets increased efficacy of PEGylated nanocarriers targeting folate receptors of glioma, *Nanotechnology*, **18**, 2007, 385101–385112.
89. Louie, A. Y. Multimodality imaging probes: design and challenges, *Chem. Rev.*, **110**, 2010, 3146–3195.
90. de Rosales, R. T. M., Tavare, R., Paul, R. L., Jauregui-Osoro, M., Protti, A., Glaria, A., Varma, G., Szanda, I., and Blower, P. J. Synthesis of Cu-64(II)-bis(dithiocarbamatebisphosphonate) and its conjugation with superparamagnetic iron oxide nanoparticles: in vivo evaluation as dual-modality PET-MRI agent, *Angew. Chem., Int. Ed.*, **50**, 2011, 5509–5513.
91. Willmann, J. K., van Bruggen, N., Dinkelborg, L. M., and Gambhir, S. S. Molecular imaging in drug development, *Nat. Rev. Drug Discovery*, **7**, 2008, 591–607.
92. Ritman, E. L. Micro-computed tomography-current status and developments, *Annu. Rev. Biomed. Eng.*, **6**, 2004, 185–208.
93. Sun, I. C., et al. Tumor-targeting gold particles for dual computed tomography/optical cancer imaging, *Angew. Chem., Int. Ed.*, **50**, 2011, 9348–9351.

94. Carr, M., and Grey, M. Magnetic resonance imaging, *Am. J. Nurs.*, **102**, 2002, 26–33.
95. Kuperman, V. *Magnetic Resonance Imaging: Physical Principles and Applications*, Academic Press, San Diego, 2000.
96. Weishaupt, D., Kochli, V., and Marincek, B. *How Does MRI Work? An Introduction to the Physics and Function of Magnetic Resonance Imaging*, 2nd Ed., Springer, Berlin, 2008.
97. Hashemi, R., Bradley, J., William, G., and Lisanti, C. *MRI: The Basics*, 2nd Ed., Lippincott Williams and Wilkins, Philadelphia, 2004.
98. Bruns, O. T., et al. Real-time magnetic resonance imaging and quantification of lipoprotein metabolism in vivo using nanocrystals, *Nat. Nanotechnol.*, **4**, 2009, 193–201.
99. Merbach, A., and Toth, E. (eds.) *The Chemistry of Contrast Agents in Medical Magnetic Resonance Imaging*, John Wiley and Sons, West Sussex, 2001.
100. Sun, S., Zeng, H., Robinson, D., Raoux, S., Rice, P., Wang, S., and Li, G. Monodisperse MFe_2O_4 (M = Fe, Co, Mn) nanoparticles, *J. Am. Chem. Soc.*, **126**, 2004, 273–279.
101. Bae, K. H., Kim, Y. B., Lee, Y., Hwang, J., Park, H., and Park, T. G. Bioinspired synthesis and characterization of gadolinium-labeled magnetite nanoparticles for dual contrast T-1- and T-2-weighted magnetic resonance imaging, *Bioconjug. Chem.*, **21**, 2010, 505–512.
102. Hahn, M., Singh, A., Sharma, P., Brown, S., and Moudgil, B. Nanoparticles as contrast agents for *in vivo* bioimaging: current status and future perspectives, *Anal. Bioanal. Chem.*, **399**, 2011, 3–27.
103. Alivisatos, P., Gu, W., and Larabell, C. Quantum dots as cellular probes, *Annu. Rev. Biomed. Eng.*, **7**, 2005, 55–76.
104. Hoffman, R. The multiple uses of fluorescent proteins to visualize cancer *in vivo*, *Nat. Rev. Cancer*, **5**, 2005, 796–806.
105. Lichtman, J. W., Livet, J., and Sanes, J. R. Progress: a technicolour approach to the connectome, *Nat. Rev. Neurosci.*, **9**, 2008, 417–422.
106. Livet, J., Weissman, T. A., Kang, H. N., Draft, R. W., Lu, J., Bennis, R. A., Sanes, J. R., and Lichtman, J. W. Transgenic strategies for combinatorial expression of fluorescent proteins in the nervous system, *Nature*, **450**, 2007, 56–62.
107. Dreher, K. L. Health and environmental impact of nanotechnology: toxicological assessment of manufactured nanoparticles, *Toxicol. Sci.*, **77**, 2004, 3–5.

108. Suh, W. H., Suslick, K. S., Stucky, G. D., and Suh, Y. H. Nanotechnology, nanotoxicology, and neuroscience, *Prog. Neurobiol.*, **87**, 2009, 133–170.
109. Lam, C. W., James, J. T., McCluskey, R., and Hunter, R. L. Pulmonary toxicity of single-wall carbon nanotubes in mice 7 and 90 days after intratracheal instillation, *Toxicol. Sci.*, **77**, 2004, 126–134.
110. Warheit, D. B., Laurence, B. R., Reed, K. L., Roach, D. H., Reynolds, G. A. M., and Webb, T. R. Comparative pulmonary toxicity assessment of single-wall carbon nanotubes in rats, *Toxicol. Sci.*, **77**, 2004, 117–125.
111. Rosamond, W., et al. Heart disease and stroke statistics: 2008 update; a report from the American Heart Association Statistics Committee and Stroke Statistics Subcommittee, *Circulation*, **117**, 2008, E25–E146.
112. Viola, H. M., Arthur, P. G., and Hool, L. C. Transient exposure to hydrogen peroxide causes an increase in mitochondria-derived superoxide as a result of sustained alteration in L-type Ca_2^+ channel function in the absence of apoptosis in ventricular myocytes, *Circ. Res.*, **100**, 2007, 1036–1044.
113. Seenarain, V., Viola, H. M., Ravenscroft, G., Casey, T. M., Lipscombe, R. J., Ingley, E., Laing, N. G., Bringans, S. D., and Hool, L. C. Evidence of altered guinea pig ventricular cardiomyocyte protein expression and growth in response to a 5 min *in vitro* exposure to H_2O_2, *J. Proteome Res.*, **9**, 2010, 1985–1994.
114. Brookes, P. S., Yoon, Y. S., Robotham, J. L., Anders, M. W., and Sheu, S. S. Calcium, ATP, and ROS: a mitochondrial love-hate triangle, *Am. J. Physiol. Cell Physiol.*, **287**, 2004, 817–833.
115. Frey, N., and Olson, E. N. Cardiac hypertrophy: the good, the bad and the ugly, *Annu. Rev. Physiol.*, **65**, 2003, 45–79.
116. Chernyak, B. V. Redox regulation of the mitochondrial permeability transition pore, *Biosci. Rep.*, **17**, 1997, 293–302.
117. Bandyopadhyay, D., Chattopadhyay, A., Ghosh, G., and Datta, A. Oxidative stress-induced ischemic heart disease: protection by antioxidants, *Curr. Med. Chem.*, **11**, 2004, 369–387.
118. Dhalla, N. S., Elmoselhi, A. B., Hata, T., and Makino, N. Status of myocardial antioxidants in ischemia-reperfusion injury, *Cardiovasc. Res.*, **47**, 2000, 446–456.
119. Kilgore, K. S., Friedrichs, G. S., Johnson, C. R., Schasteen, C. S., Riley, D. P., Weiss, R. H., Ryan, U., and Lucchesi, B. R. Protective effects of the Sod-mimetic Sc-52608 against ischemia-reperfusion damage in the rabbit isolated heart, *J. Mol. Cell. Cardiol.*, **26**, 1994, 995–1006.

120. Downey, J. M., Omar, B., Ooiwa, H., and Mccord, J. Superoxide-dismutase therapy for myocardial-ischemia, *Free Radical Res. Commun.*, 12(3), **1991**, 703–720.
121. Ooiwa, H., Stanley, A., Felaneousbylund, A. C., Wilborn, W., and Downey, J. M. Superoxide-dismutase conjugated to polyethylene-glycol fails to limit myocardial infarct size after 30 min ischemia followed by 72 h of reperfusion in the rabbit, *J. Mol. Cell. Cardiol.*, **23**, 1991, 119–125.
122. Vanhaecke, J., Vandewerf, F., Ronaszeki, A., Flameng, W., Lesaffre, E., and Degeest, H. Effect of superoxide-dismutase on infarct size and postischemic recovery of myocardial-contractility and metabolism in dogs, *J. Am. Coll. Cardiol.*, **18**, 1991, 224–230.
123. Striessnig, J. Pharmacology, structure and function of cardiac L-type Ca_2^+ channels, *Cell. Physiol. Biochem.*, **9**, 1999, 242–269.
124. Fitzpatrick, D. B., and Karmazyn, M. Comparative effects of calcium-channel blocking-agents and varying extracellular calcium-concentration on hypoxia reoxygenation and ischemia reperfusion-induced cardiac injury, *J. Pharmacol. Exp. Ther.*, **228**, 1984, 761–768.
125. Cingolani, E., Ramirez Correa, G., Kizana, E., Murata, M., Cheol Cho, H., and Marban, E. Gene therapy to inhibit the calcium channel β subunit. Physiological consequences and pathophysiological effects in models of cardiac hypertrophy, *Circ. Res.*, **101**, 2007, 166–175.
126. Dolphin, A. β subunits of voltage-gated calcium channels, *J. Bioenerg. Biomembr.*, **35**, 2003, 599–620.
127. Kobrinsky, E., Tiwari, S., Maltsev, V., Harry, J., Lakatta, E., Abernethy, D., and Soldatov, N. Differential role of the α1C subunit tails in regulation of the Cav1.2 channel by membrane potential, β subunits, and Ca_2^+ ions, *J. Biol. Chem.*, **280**, 2005, 12474–12485.
128. Bodi, I., Mikala, G., Koch, S. E., Akhter, S. A., and Schwartz, A. The L-type calcium channel in the heart: the beat goes on, *J. Clin. Invest.*, **115**, 2005, 3306–3317.
129. Pragnell, M., Dewaard, M., Mori, Y., Tanabe, T., Snutch, T. P., and Campbell, K. P. Calcium-channel beta-subunit binds to a conserved motif in the I-II cytoplasmic linker of the alpha(1)-subunit, *Nature*, **368**, 1994, 67–70.
130. Viola, H. M., Arthur, P. G., and Hool, L. C. Evidence for regulation of mitochondrial function by the L-type Ca_2^+ channel in ventricular myocytes, *J. Mol. Cell. Cardiol.*, **46**, 2009, 1016–1026.
131. Clemons, T., Viola, H., House, M., Swaminathan, I., and Hool, L. Examining efficacy of "TAT-less" delivery of a peptide against the L-

type calcium channel in cardiac ischemia-reperfusion injury, *ACS Nano*, **7**, 2013, 2212–2220.
132. Fawell, S., Seery, J., Daikh, Y., Moore, C., Chen, L. L., Pepinsky, B., and Barsoum, J. Tat-mediated delivery of heterologous proteins into cells, *Proc. Natl. Acad. Sci. U. S. A.*, **91**, 1994, 664–668.
133. Krpetic, Z., Saleemi, S., Prior, I. A., See, V., Qureshi, R., and Brust, M. Negotiation of intracellular membrane barriers by TAT-modified gold nanoparticles, *ACS Nano*, **5**, 2011, 5195–5201.
134. de la Fuente, J., and Berry, C. Tat peptide as an efficient molecule to translocate gold nanoparticles into the cell nucleus, *Bioconjug. Chem.*, **16**, 2005, 1176–1180.

Biography

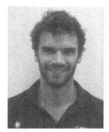

Tristan Clemons was born in Bunbury, Western Australia, and did his BSc (Hons.) in nanotechnology at Curtin University of Technology, graduating in 2008. He obtained his graduate diploma of education following this, before beginning his PhD studies within the BioNano research group in the School of Chemistry and Biochemistry at the University of Western Australia. He completed his thesis entitled "Applications of Multifunctional Poly(Glycidyl Methacrylate) (PGMA) Nanoparticles in Enzyme Stabilization and Drug Delivery" in 2013. He has continued his research on nanoparticles for drug delivery, currently working as a postdoctoral researcher at the University of Western Australia.

Chapter 2

Yolk–Shell-Structured Nanoparticles: Synthesis, Surface Functionalization, and Their Applications in Nanomedicine

Tianyu Yang,[a] Jian Liu,[a,b] and Michael J. Monteiro[a]

[a]*Australian Institute for Bioengineering and Nanotechnology, University of Queensland, QLD 4072, Australia*
[b]*Department of Chemical Engineering, Curtin University, Perth, WA 6845, Australia*
tianyu.yang@deakin.edu.au

Nanosized particles are promising candidates as delivery vehicles in nanomedicine applications. They can be designed to be colloidally stable under diverse environmental conditions found in the body, they have an excellent drug-loading capacity, and their biodistribution can be controlled through size and shape [1]. One unique nanoparticle (NP) with a yolk–shell structure represents a new generation of smart NPs. The yolk–shell nanoparticles (YSNs) or "nanorattles" have a distinctive core–void–shell structure, generally indicated as A–B. The multilevel structure consists of a shell, a void, and a core and could be used for therapy and diagnosis, as first demonstrated by Xu et al. in 2007 [2]. Controlling the physical and chemical properties of the yolk and shell makes YSNs attractive in

---

Nanomaterials: Science and Applications
Edited by Deborah Kane, Adam Micolich, and Peter Roger
Copyright © 2016 Pan Stanford Publishing Pte. Ltd.
ISBN 978-981-4669-72-6 (Hardcover), 978-981-4669-73-3 (eBook)
www.panstanford.com

the delivery of therapeutics, targeting agents, imaging agents, and hyperthermia agents.

Since the first synthetic procedure by Xia and coworkers in 2003 [2], who made YSNs via the conventional hard-template method, various synthetic routes, such as selective-etching hard templating and soft templating, have been developed. In addition, great efforts have been made by researchers to fabricate YSNs with various core/shell compositions, such as inorganic/organic hybrid materials.

This book chapter will highlight recent literature as well as our own developments in YSNs' synthetic approaches and their applications in the nanomedicine area. We will first discuss the synthesis of various YSNs, including the methods developed to control the growth of both the yolk and the shell, surface chemical functionality, and properties of the shell. Their biomedical applications for both therapy and diagnosis will then be discussed. These applications are categorized on the basis of the number of different active medical agents delivered by YSNs, including chemotherapeutic drug and gene delivery, molecular imaging by incorporating different magnetic and fluorescent contrast agents, and photothermal therapy by encapsulating various photoheat-converting agents. We will comment on their safety and toxicity in both in vitro and in vivo, which is important for potential clinical application. Finally, some perspectives on the future developments and directions in the synthesis, characterization, and commercial applications will be briefly discussed. It is the intention of this contribution to provide a brief account of these research activities and some of our recent work in this area.

2.1 Controllable Synthesis of Yolk–Shell-Structured Nanoparticles

Since the first report of yolk–shell nanoparticles (YSNs) via the hard template method, the approaches to synthesize YSNs have been widely developed. In this section, the typical synthetic approaches to make YSNs will be presented in detail and their advantages and

Table 2.1 An overview of yolk–shell-structured nanoparticles synthesized from template methods

Method	Template	Chemicals	Shell structure	Particle size (nm)	Ref.
Hard template	Resorcinol formaldehyde polymer	Resorcinol formaldehyde, TEOS, NH_3, H_2O, alcohol, water	Mesoporous	>100	[4]
Hard template	Silica	TEOS, TMSPAM, PNIPAM	Nonporous	>100	[14]
Hard template	Silica	C_{18}TMS, TEOS	Mesoporous	>100	[7]
Soft template	Vesicles	SDBS, LSB, APTES, TEOS	Nonporous	>100	[15]
Soft template	Vesicles	SDBS, LSB, APTES, TMAPS, TEOS	Mesoporous	>100	[11]
Soft template	Vesicles	FC4, F127, TEOS	Mesoporous	>100	[12]
Soft template	Vesicles	FC4, CTAB, BTME	Ordered mesoporous	>100	[13]
Soft template	Microemulsions	Triton X-100, hexane, cyclohexane, water	Mesoporous	40	[16]
Soft template	Double emulsions	P(AA-DSA), THF/CH_3Cl, water	Nonporous	>100	[17]

drawbacks will be discussed (Table 2.1). In addition, the method to control the shell composition will also be introduced.

In general, synthetic approaches could be classified into six major categories: (1) the selective-etching hard-templating method, (2) the soft-templating method, (3) the ship-in-a-bottle method, and (4–6) methods based on Ostwald ripening, galvanic replacement, and the Kirkendall effect. The principles and approaches of the different methods have been introduced in our recent review [3]. Here, we will update the recent progress based on the selective-etching hard-templating and soft-templating methods.

2.1.1 The Hard-Template Method

The selective-etching hard-templating method is based on the compositional difference between the sacrificial hard template and the remaining shell(s) and core(s) (Fig. 2.1). For example, we recently developed a method to prepare Ag, AgBr–meso-silica YSNs, and Ag–carbon–meso-silica YSNs using resorcinol formaldehyde (RF) crosslinked polymers as a sacrificial template [4]. As illustrated

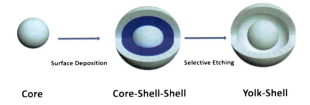

Figure 2.1 Illustration of the hard-template method.

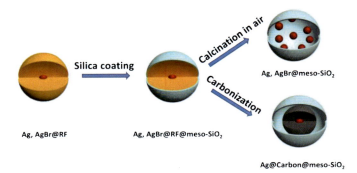

Figure 2.2 Scheme illustration of the preparation of Ag, AgBr-meso-SiO$_2$ and Ag-carbon-meso-SiO$_2$.

in Fig. 2.2, first, a general RF-coating method was developed to make a Ag, AgBr–RF core–shell-structured nanoparticle (NP). Thereafter, another mesoporous silica layer was uniformly coated on the surface of the RF polymer to fabricate a Ag, AgBr–RF–meso-silica core–shell–shell "sandwich" structure using the surfactant cetyltrimethylammonium bromide (CTAB) as a phase transfer agent and a mesopore-directing agent. Both the rattle-type (Ag, AgBr–meso-SiO$_2$) and the yolk–shell (Ag–carbon–meso-SiO$_2$) structures were made from the corresponding Ag, AgBr–RF–meso-SiO$_2$ by calcination in air and carbonization under nitrogen, respectively. Removal of the RF polymer template in Ag, AgBr–RF–meso-SiO$_2$ and further calcination results in a greater number of Ag particles trapped within the mesoporous silica shell. On the other hand, conversion of the RF template to carbon results in maintenance of the number and size of the Ag particles. The void and shell thickness of YSNs can be further controlled by adjusting the thickness of the first RF shell and/or the thickness of the second silica shell through a judicious choice of precursor concentration.

Conventionally, selective etching of silica/organosilica is a widely accepted approach to fabricate YSNs. The reason stems from the ease of silica to encapsulate metals, metal oxides, and quantum dot NPs with various cores. This is done through a modified Stöber method established by Liz-Marzan's group [5]. Hydrofluoric acid (HF) is commonly employed as the etching agent that degrades the Si–O–Si framework. Lu et al. [6] demonstrated the synthesis of hybrid microrattles to encapsulate gold (Au) NPs within a crosslinked thermal-responsive polymer, poly(N-isopropylacrylamide) (PNIPAM), shell. First, they encapsulated the metal NPs with a thick silica shell with an acrylate functional group on the surface. Second, the monomer N-isopropylacrylamide (NIPAM) and a crosslinker N, N'-methylene-bisacrylamide (BIS) were crosslinked and formed a thermal-responsive shell via free-radical polymerization. Finally, the silica shell was selectively etched by HF to form a yolk–shell-structured Au–PNIPAM NP.

The so-called *structural difference–based selective-etching method* was reported for the synthesis of yolk–shell-structured mesoporous silica shell NPs [7]. Initially, the mesoporous silica shell was coated on the surface of a metal–solid silica core in the presence of a pore-directing agent, octadecyltrimethoxysilane ($C_{18}TMS$). Because of the differences in the electrostatic/covalent interactions during the hydrolysis/condensation of the silica precursor under the absence/presence of the pore-directing agent, its mesoporous silica shell showed a high degree of condensation compared to that of the silica core. As a result, the inner solid silica layer could be selectively etched with a mild Na_2CO_3 solution, while the mesoporous silica shell still remained. On the basis of this strategy, YSNs with various core compositions like Au, Fe_2O_3, and Fe_3O_4 NPs have been successfully prepared.

Similarly, Yin's group developed a facile *surface-protected etching method* to prepare YSNs with enhanced surface stability [8]. The typical surface-protected etching process involved precoating of solid oxide shells with a protecting agent, poly(vinylpyrrolidone) (PVP); this protective polymer layer allowed the silica shell to retain its original morphology, whereas the interior silica could be selectively etched to produce the porous structure. The carbonyl group of PVP could form strong hydrogen bonds with the hydroxyl groups of the surface of the silica NP. In this case, the multiactive groups on the PVP polymer chains bind with the hydroxyl groups on the silica surface to strongly increase the stability against etching agents like NaOH. This surface-protected etching method is general and has been applied to other oxide shell such as TiO_2.

The advantages of the sacrificial template method in fabricating YSNs lies in their facial procedure, scalable yield, and controllability of porosity, morphology, and core(s)/shell(s) structures by simply adjusting the calcination environments or etching agents.

Because both calcination and etching methods require a multistep process to remove the sacrificial templates, which induce particle aggregation or broken shells, researchers overcome these drawbacks through a template-free strategy or self-template method. For example, a swelling-evaporation process was adopted to transform a core–shell structure to a yolk–shell structure [9]. The NP consists of a gold core and a conductive polymer, poly(o-methoxyaniline) (POMA), shell. The idea of this method relies on the fact that the chosen solvent should swell but not dissolve the polymer. A good solvent can dissolve the polymer shell, leading to a deformed core–shell nanostructure, whereas a poor solvent cannot penetrate into polymer shell and thus will not form a void during the evaporation process. Typically the Au–POMA core–shell structure could be in a swollen state in an ethanol solvent and then turn into a yolk–shell structure induced by ethanol evaporation under ambient conditions. This morphology transformation is also core independent, as confirmed by replacing Ag cores by Au cores. The void space could also be tailored by changing the ratio between water and ethanol.

In the absence of any surface-protecting agent, silica NPs with a yolk–shell structure could also be realized due to the inhomogeneous structural property of the modified Stöber coating method [10]. It is identified that a solid silica shell could transform to a porous yolk–shell structure after being treated in water at 90°C. A solid silica shell with a multilayered structure could be rationally designed from this standard etching test. It is believed that the mechanism for the formation of these yolk–shell particles is through the harder outer silica shell being more resistant to etching compared to the softer inner silica. This is a result of the inhomogeneous crosslinking, and thus structural property, radiating from the center of the particle. It is intriguing to re-examine the structural difference between the inner space and outer surface in a solid silica shell using the Stöber method. Researchers could take advantage of this to obtain YSNs in a silica shell in a very simple way.

Even a self-template method to fabricate YSNs has many advantages, like simplicity, saving of time, an environment-friendly chemical system, and low-cost chemical reagents. Currently the major limitation of this method is that it is still difficult to obtain a mesoporous shell that allows fast mass transfer from the shell to the active core and further allows high cargo loading in the capsule void.

2.1.2 The Soft-Template Assembly Method

Various soft templates have also been employed for the synthesis of hollow nanostructures. These include microemulsions formed in a two-phase solution, micelles, vesicles, and gas bubbles in liquid. Soft templates are assembled by surfactants or supermacromolecules. The synthesis of YSNs by a soft template needs to form a complex between the presynthesized core and vesicle for simultaneously building a shell and an interior void (Fig. 2.3).

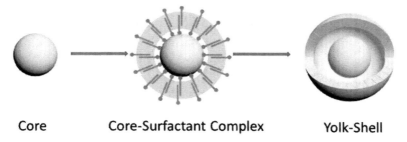

Figure 2.3 Illustration of the soft-template method.

In 2008, Xu and coworkers were the first to report a novel method to fabricate YSNs by using mixed surfactant vesicles to encapsulate silica, gold, and Fe_2O_3 NPs as movable cores in hollow silica capsules [11]. The combination of zwitterionic co-surfactant lauryl sulfonate betaine (LSB) and anionic surfactant sodium dodecyl benzene sulfonate (SDBS) formed vesicles with movable cores under the assistance of co-structure-directing agents (CSDAs), namely 3-aminopropyl-triethoxysilane (APTES). The APTES was then attached to the surface of the vesicles through electrostatic interactions. Finally, the sol–gel process was performed between APTES and tetraethyl orthasilicate (TEOS) to form a silica shell. Adjusting the molar ratio between NPs and the surfactant mixture resulted in each core being encapsulated by a silica shell. The porosity could also be tailored by replacing CSDAs from only APTES to a mixture of *N*-trimethoxysilypropyl-*N*, *N*, *N*-trimethylammonium chloride (TMAPS) and APTES. In addition, the multishell-structured YSNs could be synthesized by using soft-template-extracted single-layer YSNs as the cores to repeat this whole process.

We have also explored a general soft-template method [12] by using a fluorocarbon surfactant, FC4, as the template to synthesize YSNs with different particle sizes (200–700 nm), various types of cores (e.g., silica spheres, mesoporous silica spheres or rods, gold NPs, magnetic Fe_3O_4 particles), and tunable shell thickness (10–50 nm). The hierarchical mesoporous yolk/shell structures were obtained for the first time by encapsulating mesoporous silica with different pore sizes into the mesoporous silica shell. A three-step drug release profile was observed when these unique mesoporous rattle-type structures were used as drug carriers. Following this method, we prepared YSNs with a periodic mesoporous organosilica (PMO) shell [13]. We have conducted extensive investigations on the preparation of magnetic YSN–PMO by embedding the monodisperse magnetic nanocrystals into the cavities of highly ordered PMO hollow spheres, where the particle size, thickness of the hollow shell, and magnetization value are controllable. The YSN–PMO material possesses advantageous characteristics such as small particle size, low density, high surface area, large pore volume, and most importantly a high saturation magnetization value.

2.2 Approaches to Composition Control

2.2.1 Yolk–Shell-Structured Nanoparticles with an Inorganic Material Shell

2.2.1.1 Silica-shell-based yolk–shell-structured nanoparticles

Silica-shell-based YSNs have attracted considerable attention in recent years due to their following structural properties: high surface area and pore volume, tunable shell thickness, thermal stability, and ease for specific functionalization of both the inner core and the outer shell. These highly attractive features make silica-shell-based YSNs a promising and widely applicable platform for diverse biomedical applications, including controlled drug/gene delivery, bioimaging for diagnostics, and photothermal/chemothermal therapy. Tang and coworkers fabricated an organic–inorganic hybrid solid silica sphere (HSSS) with a three-layer sandwich structure [18]. The core and outer shell layer of the particles were pure silica frameworks hydrolyzed from TEOS, and the organic–inorganic hybrid silica middle layer was formed from the co-condensation of TEOS and N-[3-(trimethoxysilyl) propyl]ethylenediamine (TSD). Because the middle layer had a less compact structure than the core and shell of the pure silica framework, HF as an etchant had a tendency to selectively etch the middle layer of HSSSs, forming silica YSNs. The particle size, core diameter, and shell thickness can be tuned from over a broad range, from sub-100 nm to micrometer length, by simply controlling the precursor amount. The other major advantage is that one can synthesize up to 10 g of monodispersed silica nanorattles in one batch. It provides a sufficient sample for the study of long-term toxicity and the application in drug delivery. On the basis of this method, the resultant YSNs have been used as anticancer drugs, proteins, and near-infrared (NIR) imaging probe molecules.

2.2.1.2 Yolk–shell-structured nanoparticles with an organosilica shell

PMO-shell-based YSNs have also been developed in our group [13]. The PMO shell endows some features like preferential delivery of a hydrophobic drug and sustainable release due to the organic/inorganic components (silsesquioxane, $O_{1.5}$Si–R–Si$O_{1.5}$, R = organic group) within the framework. PMO-shell-based YSNs have been rationally developed through the hard-template method [19]. Metal–silica core–shell-structured NPs were prepared via extension of the Stöber coating method. Then another PMO shell was coated on the surface of silica to form metal–silica–POM core–shell–shell-structured NPs. After that, the silica shell could be selectively etched with the assistance of adding an organosilane precursor, 1,2-bis(trimethoxysilyl)ethane (BTME). Moreover, multi-layer structured PMO-shell-based YSNs have also been developed via this organosilane-assisted etching approach [20]. Interestingly, functional groups such as amines and sulfate groups could be selectively functionalized in the yolk and shell, respectively, by the organosilane co-condensation method.

PMO-based YSNs have also been realized via the soft-template method. We have developed silica–PMO YSNs by using FC4 and CTAB as co-surfactants as the soft template [13]. First, a monodispersed solid silica core is assembled with co-structure-directing agents FC4 and CTAB to form a core–vesicle complex. Then the organosilica precursor BTME was introduced to form a PMO shell. A PMO shell YSN was obtained after removal of both the FC4 and CTAB templates via solvent extraction. In addition, hybrid PMO–silica complexes as yolk- and shell-based YSNs have been developed using the soft-template method [21]. By using CTAB as the structure-directing agent, the PMO–silica hybrid YSNs were formed via co-condensation of the PMO precursor BTSE and the silica precursor TEOS. The hemocompatibility of the resulting YSNs has been evaluated. The lower acidity and silanol density exposed on the PMO–silica YSN surface showed significantly lower hemolysis performance compared to mesoporous silica and solid silica NPs.

2.2.1.3 Other inorganic-material-shell-based yolk–shell-structured nanoparticles

Along with silica-shell-based YSNs, other inorganic-material-shell-based YSNs, such as TiO_2-, carbon-, gold-, and SnO_2-based YSNs, have been developed (Table 2.2).

Table 2.2 Summary of inorganic-material-shell-based yolk–shell-structured nanoparticles, excluding those that are silica based

Yolk–shell composition	Method	Shell structure	Chemicals	Particle size	Ref.
TiO_2–TiO_2	Oswald ripening	Mesoporous	Titanium(IV) isopropoxide (TIP)	2.5 μm	[22]
Fe_3O_4–TiO_2	Hard template	Mesoporous	Tetrabutyl-titanate (TBOT)	250 nm	[23]
Metal–carbon	Hard template	Mesoporous	Phenol	200–250 nm	[24]
Au–carbon	Hard template	Mesoporous	Divinylbenzene	200 nm	[25]
Au–carbon	Hard template	Nanoporous	Dopamine	300 nm	[26]
Metal–carbon	Hard template	Mesoporous	Fufuryl alcohol, divylbenzene, pitch	100 nm	[27]
SiO_2–gold	Hard template	Mesoporous	Chloroauric acid	150 nm	[28]
Co–Au	Galvanic replacement	Mesoporous	Chloroauric acid	150 nm	[29]
SnO_2–SnO_2	Spray pyrolysis	Nonporous	SnO_2 powder	1.1 μm	[30]

2.2.2 Yolk–Shell-Structured Nanoparticles with a Polymer Shell

Polymer-shell-based YSNs have also attracted wide interest. For example, magnetic-core thermal-responsive-polymer PNIPAM-shell YSNs have been developed via a selective-etching approach. At first, an Fe_3O_4–SiO_2 microsphere was prepared via the well-known Stöber process [10]. Then the microspheres were coated with PNIPAM by polymerization. Finally, the silica was selectively etched to form the target YSNs. In a later work, a soft-template method has also been developed to fabricate Fe_3O_4–PNIPAM YSNs [31]. Butyl acetate (BA) oil beads containing Fe_3O_4 NPs and the oil-soluble initiator 2,2-azobisisobutyronitrile (AIBN) were first made. The oil beads acted like a soft template to be coated by a crosslinked PNIPAM shell using the layer-by-layer polymerization method in aqueous solution. The soft template could be easily removed by volatilization in order to obtain the yolk–shell-structured Fe_3O_4–PNIPAM NPs.

Moreover, YSNs with a polymer both in the core and in the shell have also been developed in a one-pot synthesis. For instance, Pan et al. have pioneered a method for the synthesis of polymeric yolk–shell microspheres by one-pot reversible addition-fragmentation chain transfer (RAFT) polymerization via polymerization-induced self-assembly and recognition [32]. This system consisted of a polystyrene and poly(4-vinylpyridine-co-styrene) (P4VP-PS) copolymer. During the formation process of P4VP-PS vesicles via fusion and reorganization of the spherical micelles, the polystyrene (PS) NPs existing in the system could be encapsulated in the vesicles, forming PS-yolk/P4VP-shell NPs. In addition, organic yolk-/shell-composition NPs could also be formed, as demonstrated from the emulsion polymerization reported in Zhang's group [33]. The typical polymeric yolk–shell microspheres of PS–PS-co-PAM, which contain a spherical core of PS and a hollow shell of poly(styrene-co-acrylamide) (PS-co-PAM), are initially synthesized by seed emulsion polymerization employing the polystyrene-co-poly(methylacrylic acid) (PS-co-PMAA) core–shell microspheres as seeds.

2.3 Control of Surface Properties in Silica-Based YSNs

Control of the surface properties on the NP will allow specific functionalities necessary for biomedical applications. These include controlled drug release, targeted therapy, and early disease diagnosis and detection. "Living" radical polymerization techniques and silane chemistry provide various methods to control the surface properties of NPs with controlled chemical functionality, hydrophilicity, and biocompatibility.

2.3.1 Modification of Silica-Based Nanoparticle Surface by Living Radical Polymerization Techniques

The versatility of a polymer shell as a coating for a silica NP could provide many functional properties for a biomedical nanovehicle, such as intelligent control of therapeutic release via pH, temperature, and light stimulation; biocompatibility in a cellular environment; and stability in biomedical media. To design a smart polymer shell on the surface of a silica NP for various biomedical applications, a high degree of control over the size and uniformity of the polymer chain is critical. Living radical polymerization (LRP) such as RAFT, atom transfer radical polymerization (ATRP), and nitroxide-mediated radical polymerization (NMP) offers control over the polymer, including molecular weight and molecular weight distribution (quantified by its polydispersity index, PDI), the functional groups on the chain ends or on the side chains, and molecular architecture [34].

2.3.1.1 Living radical polymerization techniques

RAFT polymerization is mediated by a RAFT chain transfer agent (CTA) in a conventional free-radical polymerization system. The CTA consists of a thiocarbonylthio backbone with a stabilizing Z-group and a re-initiating R-group (Fig. 2.4). The Z-group should be designed to increase the reactivity of the growing polymeric radical toward the RAFT agent. The R-group should be far less stable and have fast re-initiation toward the monomer. The continuous reversible deactivation of the R-group allows the polymerization to be controlled as a rapid exchange of propagating radicals between the (macro)CTA and the growing chain.

ATRP is controlled by equilibrium of the reversible activation-deactivation reaction between a propagating polymer chain and a metal/ligand complex. The ATRP initiator (typically alkyl halides/dormant species) (Fig. 2.4) is activated in the presence of a complex of a metal catalyst, such as Cu(I) salts and N-containing ligands, to reversibly form propagating radicals and the radical deactivator Cu(II) species. The equilibrium between Cu(I) and Cu(II) allows control over the molecular weight distribution of the resultant polymer. The revolutionary single-electron transfer–living radical polymerization (SET-LRP) developed by Percec and coworkers [35] provides an ultrafast method to make polymers with a controlled chain length and close to 100% end-group functionality. It is believed that the mechanism relies on the rapid disproportionation of Cu(I) to form Cu(II) and Cu(0), resulting in a self-regulated process.

NMP is based on the concept of activation-deactivation equilibrium between dormant species and a small fraction of propagating macroradicals. The polymerization is carried out at high temperatures where initiation is rapid and all the polymer chains grow at

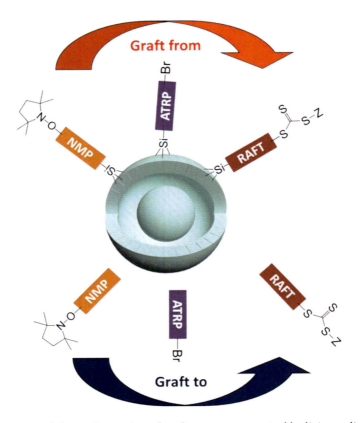

Figure 2.4 Scheme illustration of surface property control by living radical polymerization.

the same rate. The initiated polymer chains are reversibly capped by a stable free radical to give a dormant polymer chain.

Generally, there are two approaches to achieving polymer binding on the surface of silica by LRP, the graft-from and the graft-to methods. The graft-from approach immobilizes the initiators (or RAFT agent) on the surface of silica such that the monomers grow directly on the silica surface in situ. The graft-to method relies on the attachment of the preformed polymer to the silica surface through surface coupling chemistry. The progress of each method will be discussed in detail next.

2.3.1.2 Graft-from methods

2.3.1.2.1 RAFT

Among the LRP techniques, RAFT, ATRP, and NMP have been widely used to graft various polymers from silica NPs. Compared to NMP and ATRP, RAFT polymerization displays the advantage of compatibility for a wide range of monomers and is free from metal catalyst contamination. Pan and coworkers have successfully grafted PS on the surface of solid silica NPs [36] and mesoporous silica nanoparticles (MSNs) [37], respectively, by using the graft-from method of the RAFT technique. The RAFT agent was anchored to the exterior surface of the silica NP through esterification between the RAFT acid and the alkyl hydroxyl functional group obtained from the reduction of epoxysilane attached on the surface of silica [37]. In this method, the RAFT agent's packing density was 0.6 RAFT agent/nm^2. The thickness of the PS shell was increased from 19 to 29 nm with an increase in the molecular weight of each chain from 12,300 to 23,700. They also grafted a pH-responsive polymer poly(acrylic acid) (PAA) shell on the surface of MSNs as a nanovalve [38]. This nanovalve could transfer from the open state and the close state as the pH decreased from 8 to 4. Additionally, the thermoresponsive polymer PNIPAM could also be introduced using this methodology [39]. The grafted PNIPAM shell could be intelligently controlled to close or open by simply turning the temperature above or below its lower critical solubility temperature (LCST) at 32°C. Similarly, the Lin group also used the graft-from method to coat thermoresponsive PNIPAM on the MSNs' surface [40]. The RAFT agent was coupled between the amine functional group on the silica surface and the carboxylic acid group in the RAFT agent through the amidation reaction. The resulting PNIPAM-functionalized MSNs showed a shuttling ability in the biphasic toluene/water solution by changing the temperature above or below PNIPAM's LCST. The thermal sensitivity of PNIPAM provided unique properties in controlled therapeutic release and the ability to recycle. Perrier and coworkers successfully developed a silane RAFT agent by adding a trimethoxysilane functional group on the R-group of the trithiocarbonate RAFT agent [41]. This new RAFT agent could be facilely attached to the silica surface through an azeotropic distillation reaction, achieving a high grafting density of 0.8 RAFT agent/nm^2. This resulted in a polymer (poly(butyl acrylate) [PBA], PNIPAM, poly(methyl methacrylate) [PMMA]) grafting density of around 0.27–0.38 chains/nm^2. Recently, this RAFT agent methodology was used to make a block copolymer poly(VBC-co-PyAc) by using 4-vinylbenzyl chloride (VBC) and pyren-1-ylmethyl acrylate (PyAc) as monomers [42]. The pyrenic moieties in the polyPyAc block have a fluorescence capability for biosensor application, while the chloride end group in polyVBC can be quaternized to provide a positive charge for better cellular uptake performance. Therefore, the resulting fluorescent, quaternized particles are capable of being taken up into the endosomes of human colon cancer cells and the excited fluorescence used to image the cells in vitro.

2.3.1.2.2 ATRP
ATRP is another efficient strategy to graft a polymer shell on the silica surface. Ohno and coworkers have developed a saline ATRP initiator that can be facilely attached to the surface of silica NPs, in the size range from 100 nm to 1.5 µm, without any particle aggregation [43]. The resulting initiator-functionalized silica NPs have been coated with well-defined PMMA with a molecular weight of up to 480,000 with a graft density as high as 0.65 chains/nm^2. This methodology could also be applicable in small silica NP less than 100 nm [44]. Two typical particle sizes of around 55 and 15 nm were selected to coat on a PMMA polymer shell through the surface-initiated ATRP technique. The PMMA packing density on the 55 nm silica core was 0.8 chains/nm^2. That on the 15 nm silica core decreased to 0.4 to 0.5 chains/nm^2. Interestingly, they also extended this strategy to graft hydrophilic polymer poly(poly[ethylene glycol] methyl ether methacrylate) (PPEGMA) brushes with different packing densities on silica cores with various particle sizes ranging from 15 nm to 1.5 µm [45]. Their research reported the circulation lifetime of polymer-functionalized particles was highly reliant on their structural features. The smaller silica core size with a long polymer chain length (upper limit of 500,000 for PPEGMA) exhibited more favorable biodistribution. However, hybrid particles with a relatively short circulation lifetime were easily trapped by immune-responsive organs like the liver and spleen.

Their results showed, by contrasting two types of hybrid NPs with the same hydrodynamic particle size of 480 nm, that 70% of hybrid particles with a silica core of 130 nm and a 289,000 PPEGMA brush shell remained in the blood 1 h after injection. Only 20% of hybrid particles with a 290 nm silica core and a 113,000 PPEGMA brush shell remained in the blood under the same conditions. Moreover, the hybrid particles with 15 nm silica cores and a 68,000 PPEGMA polymer brush shell exhibited an extremely long circulation period with a 20-hour half-life in the blood. Such long-circulation-lifetime hybrid particles labeled with fluorescence molecules like Cy5.5 were found to preferentially accumulate in tumor tissue through passive targeting, as investigated by near-infrared fluorescence (NIRF) optical bioimaging. These in vivo results further indicate the significance of precise control of the chain length and surface functionalization of silica NPs by controlled radical polymerization techniques. The surface-initiated ATRP technique could also be used to fabricate cationic polymer shells to endow gene delivery capability. The Schmalz group report a graft density of 0.04 poly(2-[dimethylaminoethylmethacrylate]) (PDMAEMA) polymer chains/nm^2 of 2-(dimethylaminoethylmethacrylate) (DMAEMA) monomer units on each particle could be synthesized [46]. The hybrid NPs as a plasmid DNA delivery carrier have been tested under standard conditions in CHO-K1 and L929 cells, revealing transfection efficiencies higher than 50% and low cytotoxicity at NP-to-plasmid ratios of 10 and 15.

2.3.1.2.3 NMP

Recently, NMP has also been used to graft a polymer from a silica surface. The Charleux group [47] did a very interesting study on functionalizing PMMA on the surface of mesoporous silica in various nanoporous structures such as MSU-Brij56, hexagonal ordered SBA-15, core–shell NPs with a solid silica core–mesoporous silica shell-MCM41 in different mesoporous shell thicknesses and Stöber solid silica NPs.

First, the initiator derived from BlocBuilder alkoxyamine was covalently grafted via a dimethylethoxysilane functional group coupled with a hydroxyl group on the silica surface. The polymerizations were conducted in the presence of a free alkoxyamine with a chemical structure similar to that of the grafted one. It was found that the difference in surfactants' structure-directing agents, the pores size of MSN cores could be well controlled. For example, the pore sizes of the MCM41 silica NP porous shell directed by CTAB, SBA-15 silica NPs directed by P123, and Michigan State University (MSU) silica NPs directed by Brij56 were well tuned in 2, 5, and 10 nm, respectively. According to their results, polymers grafted onto Stöber solid silica NPs have the best symmetric gel permission chromatography (GPC) trace. The trace has a narrow peak and no tailing. However, among the mesoporous structure silica substrates, MSU with 5 nm pores and a highly connected mesoporous network have the most preferable pore size and porous structure. Their results showed pores of 2 nm diameter in MCM-41-based mesopores are too small to ensure good diffusion of the reactants. However, SBA-15 with pores of 10 nm, that is, large compared to MSU, showed less pore connectivity (highly ordered hexagonal mesostructure) and were limited to rapid diffusion of the reactive species.

2.3.1.2.4 Combined CRP technique

The molecular architecture and chain length of a polymer on the silica surface are very critical for rational design of therapeutic delivery vehicles. Thus, the precise regulation of surface properties by bi- or multifunctionalization is necessary and interesting.

The Voit group reported a method to functionalize MSNs by combining the ATRP and RAFT techniques to allow anchoring two heteropolymers on the surface of MSNs via attaching a Y-shaped initiator with a RAFT agent and an ATRP initiator double head [48]. The two independently grown polymers could provide more choice to regulate the MSNs' surface properties. The pH-sensitive polymer poly(2-diethylaminoethylmethacrylate) (PDEAEMA) was used as a gatekeeper to control the drug by pH variation. The drug is capped or released by simply changing the pH value. The other hydrophilic polymer poly(2-hydroxypropypl methacrylamide) (PHPMA) could provide enhanced hydrophilicity and biocompatibility to MSNs. The anticancer drug doxorubicin (Dox) was used as a model drug loaded in these dipolymer-functionalized MSNs, and the pharmacokinetics profile showed the drug releasing rate was increased significantly with a pH value dropdown from a physiological condition of 7.4 to an acid condition of 5. Additionally, the toxicity studies also indicated good biocompatibility of the MSN and polymer. Concentrations ranging up to 20 μg/mL in MCF7 and 293T cells were well tolerated.

2.3.1.3 Graft-to method

The graft-to method is more likely to graft well-defined polymer chains onto the surface of particles because the polymer chains can be produced with control over the molecular weight distribution. Subsequently, the click reaction techniques such as copper-catalyzed azide-alkyne cycloaddition (CuAAC) or thiol-ene reaction have been researched for attaching the polymer onto silica NPs.

Ranjan and Brittain firstly prepared azide-functionalized silica via direct conversion from bromide-functionalized silica [49]. Thereafter, PS or polyacrylamide with an alkyne end group was clicked with azide silica to obtain PS-coated silica NPs. Calculated from their elemental analysis data, the grafting density of PS is 0.31 chains/nm^2 and polyacrylamide is 0.37 chains/nm^2. This methodology was also successfully extended to alkyne-end-group ATRP-initiator-polymerized PS and PMA to achieve silica–PS and silica–PMA hybrid NPs, respectively.

It should be noted that the polymer grafting density from the graft-to method cannot be as high as that from the graft-from method. This is because the graft-to method depends on the diffusion of large polymeric chains to the silica surface, and as a result, the functional end group in the macromolecule will not be as easily accessible as the monomer to the active site on the surface of silica NPs.

2.3.1.4 Combined graft-to/graft-from method

Interestingly, rationally combining the graft-to and graft-from methods has been used to prepare asymmetric Janus particles. Synytska and coworkers [50] reported PtBA or PNIPAM grafted on one side of silica particles using the surface-initiated ATRP graft-from method, while the second polymer, carboxy-terminated rhodamine-labeled poly(2-vinylpyridine) (P2VP), was immobilized using the amidation reaction between the amine-functionalized silica and the carboxylic end group P2VP. The resulting janus particles could be pH responsive and, therefore, controlled for aggregation and disaggregation.

2.3.2 Silica Surface Modification via Silane Chemistry

Organosilanes used as silica NP surface-modifying agents for varying chemical and physical properties have been widely developed (Table 2.3). Generally, two approaches are available for organosilane incorporation with a silica matrix, (i) subsequent modification of naked silica NP surface (the postgrafting method) and (ii) simultaneous condensation of corresponding siliane and organosilane precursors (one step co-condensation method). The postgrafting method is carried out primarily by reaction of organosilanes of the type $(R'O)_3SiR$, with free silanol groups on the silica NP surface. However, the co-condensation of tetraalkoxysilane and one or more organoalkoxysilanes with Si–C bonds is an alternative method of producing inorganic-organic hybrid networks by sol–gel chemistry. The postgrafting method is preferable for maintaining the size distribution and morphology of silica NPs during the synthesis, while the co-condensation method provides uniform distribution of functional groups. Recently, reactive functional groups such as amine [40, 51–55], thiol [56, 57], vinyl [58, 59], azide [60], alkyne [61], maleimide [62], alkyl halide [63], mannose [64], and azobenzene [65] have been introduced onto the surface of silica NPs. Surface-modified silica NPs via silane chemistry can provide various surface functional groups in biomedical applications. The direct condensation of silane-functionalized molecules, such as organic dyes or polymers coupling to a silanol group, on the surface of silica NPs has been reported. Amino-functionalized silica NPs can be conjugated with metal NPs, small organic molecules, proteins, peptides, nucleic acids, and fluorescent dyes by coupling with functional moieties such as carboxylic acids, alkyl halides, and N-hydroxysuccinimide (NHS) esters. Wisely using reductive addition, disulfide coupling, or maleimide reaction chemistry, thiol-functionalized silica NPs could further conjugate with gold NPs, proteins, antibodies, peptides, fluorophores, and polymers. For example, a thiol-functionalized molecule could couple with

Table 2.3 Summary of silane chemistry approaches for surface functionalization

Functional group	Functionalization method	Silane species	Conjugation molecule	Coupling chemistry	Ref.
Amine	Postgrafting	3-aminopropyl trimethoxysilane	FITC	Amide bonding	[54]
Amine	Postgrafting	3-aminopropyl trimethoxysilane	Metal nanoparticle	Nucleophilic substitution	[51]
Amine	Postgrafting	3-aminopropyl trimethoxysilane	Organic molecule	NHS ester	[55]
Amine	Postgrafting	3-aminopropyl trimethoxysilane	DNA	Electrostatic interaction	[52]
Amine	Postgrafting	3-aminopropyl trimethoxysilane	Polypeptide	N-carboxyanhydride	[53]
Amine	Postgrafting	3-aminopropyl trimethoxysilane	Polymer	Amide bonding	[40]
Thiol	Co-condensation	3-mercaptopropyl trimethoxysilane	DNA	Electrostatic interaction	[57]
Thiol	Postgrafting	3-mercaptopropyl trimethoxysilane	Polymer	Disulfide bond	[56]
Vinyl	Postgrafting	3-(methacryloxy)propyl trimethoxysilane	Dextran maleic acid	Ether bond	[59]
Vinyl	Postgrafting	3-(methacryloxy)propyl trimethoxysilane	Polymer	Thiol-ene	[58]
Azide	Postgrafting	3-(Azidopropyl) triethoxysilane	DNA	CuAAc	[60]
Alkyne	Postgrafting	Propiolic acid (3-propyltriethoxysilane) amide	Azobenze molecule	CuAAc	[61]
Maleimide	Postgrafting	Maleimel silane	Melittin	Acetal bond	[62]
Iodine	Postgrafting	(3-iodopropyl) trimethoxysilane	Sulfasalazine	Substitution	[63]
Mannose	Postgrafting	Mannose-silane	Concanayaline A	Affinity	[64]
Azobenzene	Postgrafting	Azobeneze silane	Cyclodextrin	Inclusion	[65]

thiol groups on silica to form redox-responsive disulfide bonds, which are good candidates for redox-responsive controlled drug delivery. Similarly, maleimide-functionalized molecules react with thiol groups on the surface of silica NPs to form stable thioether bonds. Moreover, introduction of azide groups and the subsequent click reaction with alkyne-substituted molecules could also be an efficient method to conjugate with fluorescent probes or polymers via a Cu-catalyzed Huisgen cycloaddition reaction.

2.4 YSNs for Biomedicine Applications

Multifunctional YSNs have attracted substantial attention in recent years due to their advantageous structural properties, such as high internal surface area and pore volume, tunable void size, hierarchical pore size, selective functionalization sites on core and shell, and colloidal stability. These highly attractive features make YSNs a promising platform with excellent performance in diverse biomedicine applications, including chemotherapeutic delivery, gene and protein delivery, photothermal therapy, and bioimaging (Fig. 2.5). Compared to other biomedicine materials, a unique rattle-type structure enables YSNs to have synergistic effects by efficiently combining diverse therapies together in one NP via rational designs.

2.4.1 *YSNs for Chemotherepy*

In 2007, an FePt–CoS$_2$ yolk–shell-structured nanocrystal was first reported as a potent drug delivery agent to be applicable to HeLa cancer cells [66]. Although the ultrahigh cytotoxicity of the uncoated FePt core and the FePt–CoS$_2$ nanocrystals was evaluated by the MTT assay, this work still inspired researchers to develop a multifunctional therapeutic agent in a rationally designed yolk–shell structure. Later, a magnetic core–mesoporous silica shell YSN was synthesized via a hydrothermal method [67]. The resultant YSNs showed high magnetization strength (>20 emu/g) and drug-loading capacity (ibuprofen 302 mg/g) because of their large void between the core and the shell. Their drug-releasing profile shows an initial burst in the first 20 h with a sustainable release thereafter.

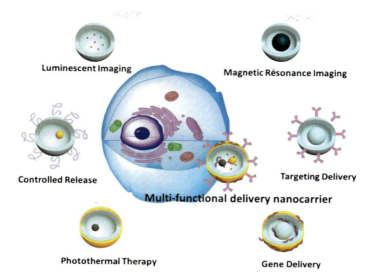

Figure 2.5 Illustration of yolk–shell-structured nanoparticles for biomedicine applications.

It also shows a faster release rate and higher release capacity in a neutral environment (pH = 7.1) than in an acidic condition (pH = 2.4). SiO_2–SiO_2 YSNs were also investigated as a drug delivery carrier with a hydrophobic antitumor drug (docetaxel, DOC) for in vitro and in vivo liver cancer therapy (Fig. 2.6). Efficient cellular internalization was achieved as fluorescein isothiocyanate (FITC)-labeled YSNs monitored by fluorescence microscopy. The resulting YSNs could successfully penetrate the plasma membrane of Hep-G2 cells and translocate into the cytoplasm with high efficiency. Moreover, the DOC-loaded YSNs showed greater antitumor activity with about a 15% enhanced tumor inhibition rate compared to taxotere on the marine hepatocarcinoma 22 subcutaneous model [68].

Interestingly, rationally designed YSNs with various surface modifications have achieved improved therapeutic efficacy via a controlled release system. A superparamagnetic Fe_3O_4 core with amino group–functionalized mesoporous-silica-shell rattle-type structure NPs were prepared via the water-in-oil microemulsion method. The amino group on the surface could bind with an

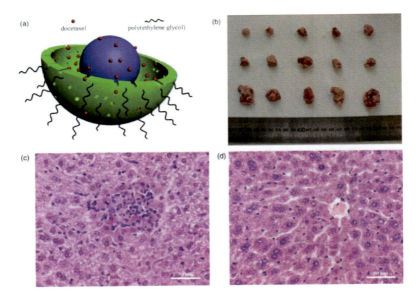

Figure 2.6 Silica nanorattles as a drug delivery system of docetaxel for liver cancer therapy with low toxicity and high efficacy. (a) Schematic diagram of the drug delivery system based on silica nanorattles for docetaxel. (b) In vivo antitumor activities of SN-PEG-Dtxl and Taxotere (clinical formulation of docetaxel) on H22 liver cancer subcutaneous model. Photographs of tumors after therapy from (a) SN-PEG-Dtxl group, (b) Taxotere group, and (c) control group. Systematic toxicity of Taxotere and SN-PEG-Dtxl on healthy ICR mice. Histological section stained with H&E of liver samples of (c) SN-PEG-Dtxl and (d) Taxotere group. H&E: hematoxylin and eosin. Reproduced with permission from Ref. [68]. Copyright 2010, American Chemical Society.

anticancer drug Dox molecule with assistance by a dicarboxylic anhydride linker. The resulting pH-sensitive amide bond–conjugated Dox molecule could have pH-triggered controlled release. The release kinetics profile is clearly matched with pH-triggered hydrolysis kinetics of the amide bonds. A high drug loading of 1.53 mg/g was achieved and an efficient release capacity could be obtained in a pH-triggered manner. About 73.2% of the Dox content was effectively released at pH 5, whereas only 21.8% was released at pH 7.4 in 10 h [69].

In addition, light-triggered controlled release from YSNs has also been reported [70]. The YSNs were fabricated by coating an upconversion nanocrystal NaYF$_4$:Tm^{3+},Yb^{3+}–NaLuF$_4$ with mesoporous silica via the soft-template method. Then a phototrigger-conjugated prodrug (combined anticancer drug chlorambucil and phototrigger agent amino-coumarin) was loaded into the cavities. This hydrophobic prodrug is designed to be embedded inside the YSNs without any premature release until an NIR laser triggers the upconversion cleavage of the amino coumarin phototrigger-conjugated prodrug. This releases the anticancer drug chlorambucil from the cavity of YSNs to cancer cells. This innovative photostimuli-responsive YSN possesses the advantages of a high drug-loading capacity, zero premature release in nontargeted tissue, and sensitivity to NIR light with a wavelength that has a large penetration depth in tissue [70].

Scientists are also developing multiresponsive NP systems to better control drug release. A temperature and pH dual-response YSN drug delivery system [71] was successfully fabricated by combining a pH-responsive polymer poly(methacrylic acid-co-ethyleneglycol dimethacrylate) (P(MAA-co-EGDMA)) microgel core and a temperature-responsive polymer (PNIPAM) shell together via the selective-etching silica sacrificial template method. The resulting Dox-loaded YSNs exhibited temperature and pH dual-controlled release in HEpG2 tumor cells. Their particle size could be easily controlled by changing the degree of crosslinking of the thermoresponsive polymer shell.

It has been accepted that targeted delivery is very necessary for anticancer drug delivery systems, as most of the commonly used anticancer drugs have serious side effects due to nonspecific action on healthy cells. Moreover, targeted delivery enhances the therapeutic efficacy. One strategy to achieve it is to prepare magnetic hollow mesoporous silica spheres as delivery vehicles for delivering the anticancer drug to the cancerous organs or tissues by using a magnetic field [72]. Magnetic targeting could enable drug delivery systems to reach the targeted organs or tissues quickly, but it did not effectively enhance nanocarriers' cell uptake in cancer cells. Another strategy is to utilize antibodies or specific ligands to selectively bind to the cell surface to trigger receptor-mediated endocytosis. Kaskel et al. conjugated folic acid (FA) on the surface of Fe$_3$O$_4$–SiO$_2$ YSNs via the amidation reaction [73]. An in vitro cell uptake experiment indicated a nearly four times' increase for FA YSNs as compared to FA-free YSNs acting in HeLa cells. Additionally, the Dox-loaded Fe_3O_4–SiO_2-FA NPs exhibited higher cytotoxicity than free Dox and Dox-loaded Fe_3O_4–SiO_2 NPs due to the increase of cell uptake of anticancer drug delivery vehicles mediated by the FA receptor. In a later report, Tang et al. developed a tumor-targeted drug delivery system to efficiently anchor mesenchymal stem cells (MSCs) by specific antibody–antigen recognitions at the cytomembrane interface without any cell preconditioning [74]. In vivo experiments proved that the burdened MSCs can track down the U251 glioma tumor cells more efficiently and deliver Dox with a wider distribution and longer retention lifetime in the tumor tissues as compared to free Dox and silica nanorattle-encapsulated Dox. The increased and prolonged Dox intratumoral distribution further contributed to a significantly enhanced tumor cell apoptosis (Fig. 2.7).

2.4.2 YSNs for Gene/Protein Delivery

Use of YSNs for therapeutic biomolecule delivery has attracted significant research attention in the field of human disease treatment. For example, Co–Au YSNs have been prepared via a one-step galvanic replacement method [29]. The resulting Co–Au YSNs have good biocompatibility in an MTT cytotoxicity assay and could be monodispersed in endosomes and in the cytosol. Plasmid-enhanced green fluorescence protein (pEGFP) plasmid DNA has been successfully delivered into the cells with these Co–Au YSNs in a transfection experiment and the expressed green fluorescent protein was observed. Their strong two-photon fluorescence and superparamagnetic property lead to potential applications in cellular optical imaging and in vivo magnetic resonance tracking. In a later work, magnetic poly(ethyleneimine) (PEI)-functionalized Fe_3O_4–mesoporous silica YSNs have been employed for small interfering RNA (siRNA) delivery [75]. The cationic PEI polymer can provide a positive charge to bind with negatively charged siRNA in order to prevent rapid degradation and to enable siRNA to penetrate the negatively charged cell membrane. These results indicate PEI–Fe_3O_4–$mSiO_2$ YSNs, used as a siRNA delivery nanocarrier, can

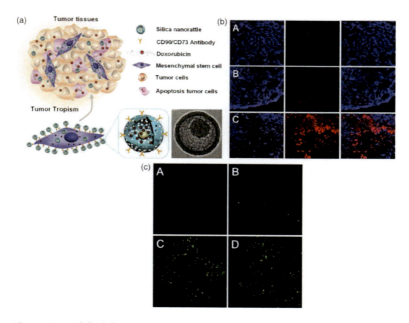

Figure 2.7 (a) Schematic illustration of silica nanorattle-doxorubicin-anchored mesenchymal stem cells (MSC-SN-Ab(CD90)-Dox) for tumor-tropic therapy. (b) Fluorescent microscopy images of tissue sections 7 days after intratumoral injection of (A) Dox, (B) SN-Dox, and (C) MSC-SN-Ab(CD90)-Dox. Blue fluorescence shows nuclear staining with DAPI and red fluorescence shows the location of doxorubicin. (c) TUNEL staining assay showing cell apoptosis by (A) control, (B) Dox, (C) SN-Dox, and (D) MSC-SN-Ab(CD90)-Dox at 7 days after intratumoral injection. Reproduced with permission from Ref. [74]. Copyright 2011, American Chemical Society.

efficiently deliver siRNA into the cytoplasm. The delivered siRNA is released for effective silencing of the targeted mRNA. Consequently, the targeted protein expression was effectively suppressed to 77% in HeLa cells by using Fe_3O_4–$mSiO_2$ YSNs under an external magnetic field. Furthermore, YSNs may be a good candidate for protein delivery. For instance, mesoporous SiO_2–SiO_2 YSNs have been shown to efficiently load the model protein ovalbumin (OVA), relying on their porous structure and surface charge [76]. The adjuvant effect of the resulting YSNs on the immune response was evaluated by using OVA as an antigen model. The results suggest they can not only induce the production of antigen-specific antibody responses, including antigen-specific Th2 allergic immune responses, but also improve the antibody level of OVA after a single dose vaccination. This was confirmed by the enzyme-linked immunosorbent assay (ELISA) of the antibody of OVA.

2.4.3 YSNs for Photothermal Therapy

Photothermal cancer therapy using NIR light has attracted wide attention. This technique provides many advantages such as easy operation, fast recovery, fewer complications, and shorter hospital stays. Two biological transparency windows are located in 650–950 nm (first NIR window) and 1000–1350 nm (second NIR window) in the NIR region. The second window is recognized to offer deeper tissue penetration than the first window by experiencing less absorption and scattering in tissue. YSNs with a tailored void size and a controllable yolk–shell composition experience enhanced thermal conductivity and diffraction of the laser light in a confined nanostructure. Thus, they are considered a good candidate for photothermal therapy. Yeh et al. reported that Au–AgAu rod-shaped YSNs less than 100 nm in size could be fabricated via galvanic replacement [77]. The void size can be tailored from 2 to 6.5 nm by simply changing the $HAuCl_4$ amount. $HAuCl_4$ triggers Ag nanoshell etching through galvanic corrosion. With additional $HAuCl_4$, the gap distances decrease and an increased Au-to-Ag ratio is achieved. The resulting Au–AgAu YSNs were used to perform hyperthermia therapy in both the first and second NIR windows. The in vitro experiment indicated high efficacy in the NIR photothermal destruction of cancer cells. Large cells experienced damage beyond the directly laser irradiated area. Moreover, the yolk–shell-structured Au–AgAu nanorod has highly efficient therapeutic effect by laser ablation of solid tumors, as confirmed in the in vivo mouse model [77].

2.4.4 YSNs for Bioimaging

The introduction of imaging to the biomedical field has significantly improved the accuracy of medical diagnosis. Magnetic resonance imaging (MRI) is one of the most representative imaging techniques to provide high-resolution and superior-contrast images for differentiating different tissues. Typically, MRI relies on the relaxation time of protons triggered by an external magnetic field pulse or pulse sequence. There are several advantages for yolk-shell nanostructures for bioimaging applications such as MRI: The confinement of magnetic metal species within the hollow cage prevents toxic leakage of the toxic metal ions in vivo; the surface porosity of the shell allows easy penetration of small molecules rather than biomacromolecules. For example, a Gd–SiO_2 YSN was reported by Mou's group [78]. Firstly, the Gd–SiO_2 core–shell-structured NP was formed through coating silica on the citrate–Gd(III) complex. Thereafter, yolk–shell-structured Gd–SiO_2 was fabricated via a selective-etching method. The resulting Gd–SiO_2 YSNs have an extremely high payload of the Gd(III) species (10.5%, wt%) and could allow a very high amplified signal. Thus, a better signal-to-noise ratio in the imaging would be obtained. However, as discussed above, the selective-etching template method often suffers from difficulty in controlling the silica shell morphology and a decrease of magnetic property due to template removal.

The ship-in-a-bottle method has been applied to fabricate magnetic rattle-type silica (MRS) NPs for cancer imaging [79]. The essence of this method is based on choosing a suitable iron precursor with good solubility in water and insolubility in ethanol. The embedded iron precursor can reside inside the nanocavity due to this combination of solubilities. Finally, magnetite NPs were formed in the interior of silica shells via co-precipitation of Fe^{2+} and Fe^{3+} ions under alkaline conditions. In this method, the amount of magnetic material can be enriched in the rattle-type silica as there is a 76.7% increase in its magnetic saturation value. The intravenously injected MRS can be effectively accumulated in the tumor tissue via the enhanced passive targeting effect and can show strong enhancement in contrast to MRI. One hour after injection of magnetic YSNs, significant tissue darkening, corresponding to a T_2 signal intensity drop of 39.5% at the tumor site, was observed.

2.4.5 YSNs with Dual Functions for Bioimaging and Chemotherapy

YSNs for simultaneous anticancer drug delivery and cell MRI have been developed. One such is composed of functional inorganic nanocrystals as cores, a thin porous shell, and a large cavity in between. In 2008, Xu and coworkers firstly reported YSNs with both MRI contrast and anticancer agent capability [80]. The FePt–Fe_2O_3 YSNs were fabricated through the Kirkendall effect with FePt NPs serving as the seeds. The FePt yolk could form Pt ions under certain redox reactions, and the porous Fe_2O_3 shell could ensure the Pt ions could diffuse out of the shell. Their ultralow IC_{50} value (238 ng of Pt/mL) also indicated the slow oxidation and release from FePt yolks increasing the cytotoxicity. Magnetic resonance relaxation enhancement effects of the Fe_2O_3 nanoshell could provide a direct means for measuring the cancerous tissue in real time during cancer treatment. Shi's group conducted a series of projects by using magnetic YSNs as delivery vehicles to perform MRI and anticancer drug delivery simultaneously. Fe_3O_4–SiO_2 YSNs with an ellipsoidal shape were prepared via the silica-etching method [81]. The increased surface area and pore volume of the resulting YSNs provided high drug-loading capacity (20%) and encapsulation efficiency (100%) for the anticancer drug Dox. The cytotoxicity of Dox-loaded Fe_3O_4–SiO_2 against human breast cancer MCF-7 cells was higher than free Dox at a relatively low drug concentration because of the intracellular release of the drug. Application of the Fe_3O_4–SiO_2 YSNs as the contrast agent for MRI indicates the cells exposed to the magnetic YSNs for 6 h could be easily detected in vitro. In vivo experiment showed a darkened area at the injection site and confirmed the imaging capability. The darkened area extended through the tumor with time and increased concentration. In a later work, magnetic spherical YSNs functionalized with a hydrophilic polymer poly(ethylene glycol) (PEG) and targeting molecular FA on a mesoporous silica shell surface were prepared. The MRI study revealed the FA grafting on the particle surface enhanced the cellular uptake capability of the resulting YSNs by folate receptor HeLa cells in a dose-dependent manner. In contrast, there was very low uptake in folate-receptor-deficient MCF-7 cells. In addition, the magnetic YSNs could be in vivo transported to the designated organ under an external magnetic field, suggesting the resulting magnetic YSNs could be an ideal platform for simultaneous imaging and therapeutic applications.

Optical imaging techniques have also been widely used to monitor therapeutic release and distribution in real time. For example, a fluorescent dye like FITC has been combined with YSNs via various methods such as absorption [82], covalent amidation conjugation [54], and in situ co-condensation [75]. Covalent bonding between YSNs and FITC is considered the best method to accurately track YSNs' intercellular trace [54]. FITC-labeled YSNs have been tracked through the whole process of endocytosis: from cellular membrane penetration, to endosomes, then escape to the cytosol, and finally expulsion by lysosomes. The drug release pharmacokinetics could also be traced by this methodology in order to inform better design for the release of an anticancer drug in the cytoplasm rather than premature leakage. As a result, improved biocompatibility and low-side-effect delivery can be obtained by taking advantage of the optical imaging. Interestingly, the new-generation clinically approved NIRF molecule indocyanine green (ICG), has been successfully attached to silica nanorattles in Tang's group [83]. Because NIRF imaging has advantages such as high tissue penetration and low autofluorescence, it is applicable to noninvasive in vivo tracking for tumor-specific delivery and biodistribution in living animals. In this case, the targeting peptide, luteinizing hormone–releasing hormone–*Pseudomonas aeruginosa* exotoxin 40 (LHRH-PE40), was also bioconjugated with a multifunctional nanocomposite. From the NIRF-guided imaging, the targeting ability and drug delivery ability of the targeting peptide and NIRF molecule–functionalized silica nanorattles were evaluated in vivo. The resulting silica nanocomposites could be specifically directed to an A549 xenograft tumor and accumulated there 24 h postinjection. The antitumor drugs were efficiently and specifically delivered into the tumor cells.

2.4.6 YSNs with Dual Function: Photothermal Therapy and Chemotherapy

Due to superior performance of gold material in photothermal therapy and the wide interest in MSNs for drug delivery, a novel material for gold–nanoshell-on-drug-loaded-silica nanorattles has been reported. This hybrid YSN could combine hyperthermia therapy with chemotherapy to optimize cancer treatment. The effect of the combined treatment is greater than either of the individual treatments [28]. Firstly, the silica nanorattles were synthesized via the selective-etching method, and then a gold shell was coated on these silica nanorattles via gold seeds catalyzed by further reduction with chloroauric acid. The gold nanoshell could induce a temperature of tumor increase from 25°C to 50°C using 2W/cm^2 NIR laser irradiation for 3 minutes. High amount of hydrophobic anticancer drug DOC (52%) could be loaded, and it is released in a sustainable behavior to reduce side effects. In vitro experiments indicate that the combined hyperthermia and chemotherapy give a significantly enhanced cell-killing effect toward HepG2 cells. About an 82.1% inhibition rate was obtained as compared with 51.8% in pure chemotherapy treatment and 40.5% in photothermal treatment only. In addition, the tumor weight loss from in vivo experiment data indicated that the inhibition rate in combined photothermal and chemotherapy treatment was 85.4%, significantly higher than the 57.4% for chemotherapy treatment only. In a later work, a targeting ligand, transferrin (tf), was attached to a gold-shell–silica nanorattle in order to preferentially bind to receptor-rich breast cancer cells, rather than normal cells, to increase the efficiency of thermochemotherapy ablation with NIR laser irradiation [84]. The content of tf-targeted nanorattles in MCF-7 cells could be nearly 15 times higher than for nontargeted nanorattles. More importantly, the half-maximum inhibiting concentration (IC_{50} value) of combined hyperthermia and chemotherapy based on tf-targeted gold-shell–silica nanorattle is extremely low. It is only 36.2% of the IC_{50} value with nontargeted gold-shell–silica nanorattles, 21% of that for chemotherapy alone, and 7.9% of that for phototherapy only. Last but not least, after one irradiation treatment with an NIR laser light (808 nm, 2 Wcm^{-2}, 3 minutes), the in vivo breast tumors in mice show complete regression due to the combination of selective targeting, photothermal therapy, and chemotherapy with the NPs. In contrast tumors treated with NIR laser irradiation only, or drug therapy only, regrow after the an initial period of inhibited growth [84].

All these results demonstrate the importance of the synergetic effect of combined photothermal therapy and chemotherapy.

2.4.7 Multifunction YSNs: Multimodal Imaging, Photothermal Therapy, and Delivery to Therapeutic Site

YSNs have promising prospects for application in multifunctional nanomedicine due to their unique hierarchical structure with movable cores and mesoporous shells; their high thermal, chemical, and mechanical stability; and their large surface-to-volume ratio, controllable mesoporous pores, and good biocompatibility.

Polymer-functionalized magnetic YSNs are being researched, which combine controlled drug delivery, imaging, targeting, and even gene therapy using one NP carrier. For instance, PEI-functionalized magnetic YSNs were developed via electrostatic interaction. Then the targeting molecule lactobionic acid (LA) was linked with PEI via the amidation reaction, and the anticancer drug Dox was encapsulated inside the void [72]. The resulting YSNs, with concurrent use of the LA groups and the magnetic field, were observed to migrate into the HepGII cells and to achieve a pharmacokinetic effect as measured by MTT assays, compared to no LA group and without a magnetic field group. Moreover, this general synthesis method could be extended to encapsulated gold cores or upconversion nanoparticle (UCNP) cores, which construct a potential platform for the simultaneous targeted delivery of drug and gene therapeutics monitored by bimodal imaging. In another case, the thermally sensitive polymer, PNIPAM derivative hydrogel, could also be functionalized into the inner cavity of Gd_2O_3:Eu–mesoSiO$_2$ YSNs. This allows the advantages of thermal-responsive drug delivery and optical and magnetic bimodal imaging to be integrated [85]. Similarly, yolk–shell-structured nanoellipsoids were fabricated by Shi's group by assembling CdTe quantum dots on the surface of magnetic YSNs via a novel layer-by-layer self-assembly technique [86]. The resulting nanoellipsoids showed a relatively high $r2$ value (143/mM·s) as contrast agents for MRI and excellent contrast from confocal fluorescent microscopic images as fluorescent imaging magnets. Taking advantage of magnetic resonance and fluorescent bimodal imaging, the mechanism of resulting nanoellipsoids as an anticancer drug delivery carrier causing cell apoptosis is fully investigated. In a later work, a rattle-structured theranostic nanocarrier consisting of a Gd-doped UCNP core and a nanoporous silica shell has been developed [87]. The rare-earth UCNPs have been considered to be promising fluorescent probes, while a Gd-doped UCNPs also can be applied to MRI. Therefore, the Gd-doped UCNP core can serve as a magnetic and luminescent imaging probe. More importantly, the anticancer drug cisplatin can be delivered by this nanorattle due to its yolk-shell structure. Thus, the resulting nanorattles have been found to be an ideal platform for synergetic chemo-/radiotherapy and simultaneous magnetic/luminescenst dual-mode imaging.

Plasmonic nanorattles are also being considered for multimodal imaging and chemotherapeutics. For example, Au–porous Ag, Au–shell rattle-like NPs with two precisely placed surface-enhanced Raman scattering (SERS) probes (1,4-benzenethiol [BDT] and naphthalenethiol [NT]) have been reported [88]. Irradiation with an NIR laser triggered release of the encapsulated drug accompanied by a dramatic switch in the SERS signal between two reporters (BDT and NT) via outer shell fragmentation. Therefore, these novel nanorattles can enable targeted delivery of the payload combined with simultaneous monitoring of payload release and the therapy process using SERS. The localization of therapy and cell killing has been confirmed by SKBR3 cells via simple laser irradiation and Raman signal monitoring

YSNs can be further researched and used as the chemo- and photothermal therapeutics carriers for in vivo combined therapeutics and diagnosis (theranostic) purposes. For example, Shi's group reported assembled Au nanorods on the surface of magnetic mesoporous NPs to obtain a multifunctional platform with magnetic resonance/thermal dual-modality bioimaging and simultaneous NIR-induced hyperthermia and chemotherapy [89]. The T2 MRI was evaluated in vivo. It showed the tumor carried in a mouse host exhibits an apparently darkened area at the injection site compared to the control. In addition, NIR thermal imaging indicates a photothermal effect could induce cell death by heating and cause irreversible tumor damage using a 808 nm wavelength laser beam at

2 Wcm^{-2} for a 1-minute exposure. The combined photothermal and chemotherapy anticancer therapeutic effect was also investigated in an MCF-7 cell line. The hybrid YSNs showed a synergistic effect (54% inhibition rate) under combined anticancer drug therapy and photothermal therapy compared to the single therapies (40% inhibition rate), at low anticancer drug dosage and moderate NIR laser intensity.

2.5 Conclusion

In this review, strategies to fabricate YSNs, especially the selective-etching hard-templating method and the soft-template method, have been selected and proposed. YSNs with various particle sizes, pore sizes, void sizes, shell thicknesses, porous geometry, and structural compositions have been synthesized by using these methods. Furthermore, the importance of silica surface chemistry in biomedicine applications has been widely recognized. Therefore, techniques for surface functionalization of silica-based NPs such as LRP and rich silane condensation have also been illustrated in this chapter. More importantly, their properties in biomedical applications have been classified and introduced in terms of their multifunctions in both therapy and diagnosis.

Although extensive research has greatly promoted the development of YSNs in nanomedicine, methods to synthesize YSNs with active therapeutic and diagnosing core agents with a rational combination in a facial and scalable way are still a challenging topic. In addition, surface modification strategies for NPs in mild condition in order to keep therapeutic and diagnosing core agents in high activity and large loading amounts are also worth of updating. More importantly, although YSNs could be an ideal platform in multifunctional nanomedicine with magnetic resonance/thermal dual-modality bioimaging, simultaneous NIR-induced hyperthermia, and chemotherapy, better combinations for these multifunctions to obtain synergistic theranostic effects are highly desired and worth investigating. Furthermore, biosafety parameters such as biodegradation behavior, excretion routes, and long-term toxicity assessments still lack enough evidence for further clinical evaluation. Therefore, much more efforts should be devoted to exploring YSNs with high biologically active synthesis routes, specific surface functionalities in high density, and long-term biocompatibility and theranostic efficiency in the near future.

Acknowledgments

We are grateful to the editors for their kind invitation to contribute to this book. We are pleased to acknowledge the work that has been done by our colleagues, who have worked with us in this area and whose names can be found in the references. TY would like to thank the University of Queensland's international scholarship and is sincerely grateful to Prof. Michael Monteiro and Dr. Jian Liu's great supervision and advice. Dr. Tianyu Yang sincerely appreciates Prof. Deb Kane's thoughtful suggestions and careful revision for this chapter.

References

1. Peer, D., Karp, J. M., Hong, S., Farokhzad, O. C., Margalit, R., and Langer, R. Nanocarriers as an emerging platform for cancer therapy, *Nat. Nanotechnol.*, **2**, 2007, 751–760.
2. Kamata, K., Lu, Y., and Xia, Y. Synthesis and characterization of monodispersed core–shell spherical colloids with movable cores, *J. Am. Chem. Soc.*, **125**, 2003, 2384–2385.
3. Liu, J., Qiao, S. Z., Chen, J. S., Lou, X. W., Xing, X., and Lu, G. Q. Yolk/shell nanoparticles: new platforms for nanoreactors, drug delivery and lithium-ion batteries, *Chem. Commun. (Camb.)*, **47**, 2011, 12578–12591.
4. Yang, T., Liu, J., Zheng, Y., Monteiro, M. J., and Qiao, S. Z. Facile fabrication of core–shell-structured Ag@carbon and mesoporous yolk–shell-structured Ag@carbon@silica by an extended Stöber method, *Chem.: Eur. J.*, **19**, 2013, 6942–6945.
5. Guerrero-Martínez, A., Pérez-Juste, J., and Liz-Marzán, L. M. Recent progress on silica coating of nanoparticles and related nanomaterials, *Adv. Mater. (Weinheim, Ger.)*, **22**, 2010, 1182–1195.

6. Wu, S., Dzubiella, J., Kaiser, J., Drechsler, M., Guo, X., Ballauff, M., and Lu, Y. Thermosensitive Au-PNIPA yolk–shell nanoparticles with tunable selectivity for catalysis, *Angew. Chem., Int. Ed.*, **51**, 2012, 2229–2233.
7. Chen, Y., Chen, H., Guo, L., He, Q., Chen, F., Zhou, J., Feng, J., and Shi, J. Hollow/rattle-type mesoporous nanostructures by a structural difference-based selective etching strategy, *ACS Nano*, **4**, 2009, 529–539.
8. Zhang, Q., Zhang, T., Ge, J., and Yin, Y. Permeable silica shell through surface-protected etching, *Nano Lett.*, **8**, 2008, 2867–2871.
9. Han, J., Chen, R., Wang, M., Lu, S., and Guo, R. Core-shell to yolk-shell nanostructure transformation by a novel sacrificial template-free strategy, *Chem. Commun. (Camb.)*, **49**, 2013, 11566–11568.
10. Wong, Y. J., Zhu, L., Teo, W. S., Tan, Y. W., Yang, Y., Wang, C., and Chen, H. Revisiting the Stöber method: inhomogeneity in silica shells, *J. Am. Chem. Soc.*, **133**, 2011, 11422–11425.
11. Wu, X.-J., and Xu, D. Soft template synthesis of yolk/silica shell particles, *Adv. Mater. (Weinheim, Ger.)*, **22**, 2010, 1516–1520.
12. Liu, J., Qiao, S. Z., Budi Hartono, S., and Lu, G. Q. Monodisperse Yolk–shell nanoparticles with a hierarchical porous structure for delivery vehicles and nanoreactors, *Angew. Chem., Int. Ed.*, **49**, 2010, 4981–4985.
13. Liu, J., Yang, H. Q., Kleitz, F., Chen, Z. G., Yang, T., Strounina, E., Lu, G. Q., and Qiao, S. Z. Yolk–shell hybrid materials with a periodic mesoporous organosilica shell: ideal nanoreactors for selective alcohol oxidation, *Adv. Funct. Mater.*, **22**, 2012, 591–599.
14. Li, G. L., Xu, L. Q., Neoh, K., and Kang, E. Hairy hybrid microrattles of metal nanocore with functional polymer shell and brushes, *Macromolecules*, **44**, 2011, 2365–2370.
15. Wu, X.-J., and Xu, D. Formation of Yolk/SiO_2 shell structures using surfactant mixtures as template, *J. Am. Chem. Soc.*, **131**, 2009, 2774–2775.
16. Lin, Y.-S., Wu, S.-H., Tseng, C.-T., Hung, Y., Chang, C., and Mou, C.-Y. Synthesis of hollow silica nanospheres with a microemulsion as the template, *Chem. Commun. (Camb.)*, 3542–3544.
17. Chiu, H.-C., Lin, Y.-W., Huang, Y.-F., Chuang, C.-K., and Chern, C.-S. Polymer vesicles containing small vesicles within interior aqueous compartments and pH-responsive transmembrane channels, *Angew. Chem., Int. Ed.*, **47**, 2008, 1875–1878.
18. Chen, D., Li, L., Tang, F., and Qi, S. Facile and scalable synthesis of tailored silica "nanorattle" structures, *Adv. Mater. (Weinheim, Ger.)*, **21**, 2009, 3804–3807.

19. Yang, Y., Liu, J., Li, X., Liu, X., and Yang, Q. Organosilane-assisted transformation from core–shell to yolk–shell nanocomposites, *Chem. Mater.*, **23**, 2011, 3676–3684.
20. Yang, Y., Liu, X., Li, X., Zhao, J., Bai, S., Liu, J., and Yang, Q. A Yolk–shell nanoreactor with a basic core and an acidic shell for cascade reactions, *Angew. Chem., Int. Ed.*, **51**, 2012, 9164–9168.
21. Teng, Z., Wang, S., Su, X., Chen, G., Liu, Y., Luo, Z., Luo, W., Tang, Y., Ju, H., Zhao, D., and Lu, G. Facile synthesis of yolk–shell structured inorganic–organic hybrid spheres with ordered radial mesochannels, *Adv. Mater. (Weinheim, Ger.)*, **26**, 2014, 3741–3747.
22. Cao, L., Chen, D., and Caruso, R. A. Surface-metastable phase-initiated seeding and ostwald ripening: a facile fluorine-free process towards spherical fluffy core/shell, yolk/shell, and hollow anatase nanostructures, *Angew. Chem., Int. Ed.*, **52**, 2013, 10986–10991.
23. Li, W., Deng, Y., Wu, Z., Qian, X., Yang, J., Wang, Y., Gu, D., Zhang, F., Tu, B., and Zhao, D. Hydrothermal etching assisted crystallization: a facile route to functional yolk-shell titanate microspheres with ultrathin nanosheets-assembled double shells, *J. Am. Chem. Soc.*, **133**, 2011, 15830–15833.
24. Kim, M., Sohn, K., Na, H. B., and Hyeon, T. Synthesis of nanorattles composed of gold nanoparticles encapsulated in mesoporous carbon and polymer shells, *Nano Lett.*, **2**, 2002, 1383–1387.
25. Kim, J. Y., Yoon, S. B., and Yu, J.-S. Fabrication of nanocapsules with Au particles trapped inside carbon and silica nanoporous shells, *Chem. Commun. (Camb.)*, 2003, 790–791.
26. Liu, R., Mahurin, S. M., Li, C., Unocic, R. R., Idrobo, J. C., Gao, H., Pennycook, S. J., and Dai, S. Dopamine as a carbon source: the controlled synthesis of hollow carbon spheres and yolk-structured carbon nanocomposites, *Angew. Chem., Int. Ed.*, **50**, 2011, 6799–6802.
27. Galeano, C., Baldizzone, C., Bongard, H., Spliethoff, B., Weidenthaler, C., and Meier, J. C., Mayrhofer, K. J. J., Schüth, F. Carbon-based yolk–shell materials for fuel cell applications, *Adv. Funct. Mater.*, **24**, 2013, 220–232.
28. Liu, H., Chen, D., Li, L., Liu, T., Tan, L., Wu, X., and Tang, F. Multifunctional gold nanoshells on silica nanorattles: a platform for the combination of photothermal therapy and chemotherapy with low systemic toxicity, *Angew. Chem., Int. Ed.*, **50**, 2011, 891–895.
29. Lu, Y., Zhao, Y., Yu, L., Dong, L., Shi, C., Hu, M.-J., Xu, Y.-J., Wen, L.-P., and Yu, S.-H. Hydrophilic Co@Au yolk/shell nanospheres: synthesis, assembly,

and application to gene delivery, *Adv. Mater. (Weinheim, Ger.)*, **22**, 2010, 1407–1411.
30. Hong, Y. J., Son, M. Y., and Kang, Y. C. One-Pot facile synthesis of double-shelled SnO_2 yolk-shell-structured powders by continuous process as anode materials for Li-ion batteries, *Adv. Mater. (Weinheim, Ger.)*, **25**, 2013, 2279–2283.
31. Chen, L.-B., Zhang, F., and Wang, C.-C. Rational synthesis of magnetic thermosensitive microcontainers as targeting drug carriers, *Small*, **5**, 2009, 621–628.
32. Wan, W.-M., and Pan, C.-Y. Formation of polymeric yolk/shell nanomaterial by polymerization-induced self-assembly and reorganization, *Macromolecules*, **43**, 2010, 2672–2675.
33. Zhang, M., Lan, Y., Wang, D., Yan, R., Wang, S., Yang, L., and Zhang, W. Synthesis of polymeric yolk–shell microspheres by seed emulsion polymerization, *Macromolecules*, **44**, 2011, 842–847.
34. Monteiro, M. J., and Cunningham, M. F. Polymer nanoparticles via living radical polymerization in aqueous dispersions: design and applications, *Macromolecules*, **45**, 2012, 4939–4957.
35. Percec, V., Guliashvili, T., Ladislaw, J. S., Wistrand, A., Stjerndahl, A., Sienkowska, M. J., Monteiro, M. J., and Sahoo, S. Ultrafast synthesis of ultrahigh molar mass polymers by metal-catalyzed living radical polymerization of acrylates, methacrylates, and vinyl chloride mediated by SET at 25°C, *J. Am. Chem. Soc.*, **128**, 2006, 14156–14165.
36. Liu, C.-H., and Pan, C.-Y. Grafting polystyrene onto silica nanoparticles via RAFT polymerization, *Polymer*, **48**, 2007, 3679–3685.
37. Hong, C.-Y., Li, X., and Pan, C.-Y. Grafting polymer nanoshell onto the exterior surface of mesoporous silica nanoparticles via surface reversible addition-fragmentation chain transfer polymerization, *Eur. Polym. J.*, **43**, 2007, 4114–4122.
38. Hong, C.-Y., Li, X., and Pan, C.-Y. Fabrication of smart nanocontainers with a mesoporous core and a pH-responsive shell for controlled uptake and release, *J. Mater. Chem.*, **19**, 2009, 5155–5160.
39. Hong, C.-Y., Li, X., and Pan, C.-Y. Smart core–shell nanostructure with a mesoporous core and a stimuli-responsive nanoshell synthesized via surface reversible addition–fragmentation chain transfer polymerization, *J. Phys. Chem.*, **112**, 2008, 15320–15324.
40. Chung, P.-W., Kumar, R., Pruski, M., and Lin, V. S. Y. Temperature responsive solution partition of organic–inorganic hybrid poly(N-isopropylacrylamide)-coated mesoporous silica nanospheres, *Adv. Funct. Mater.*, **18**, 2008, 1390–1398.

41. Ohno, K., Ma, Y., Huang, Y., Mori, C., Yahata, Y., Tsujii, Y., Maschmeyer, T., Moraes, J., and Perrier, S. Surface-initiated reversible addition–fragmentation chain transfer (RAFT) polymerization from fine particles functionalized with trithiocarbonates, *Macromolecules*, **44**, 2011, 8944–8953.
42. Moraes, J., Ohno, K., Maschmeyer, T., and Perrier, S. Monodisperse, charge-stabilized, core–shell particles via silica-supported reversible addition–fragmentation chain transfer polymerization for cell imaging, *Chem. Mater.*, **25**, 2013, 3522–3527.
43. Ohno, K., Morinaga, T., Koh, K., Tsujii, Y., and Fukuda, T. Synthesis of monodisperse silica particles coated with well-defined, high-density polymer brushes by surface-initiated atom transfer radical polymerization, *Macromolecules*, **38**, 2005, 2137–2142.
44. Ohno, K., Akashi, T., Huang, Y., and Tsujii, Y. Surface-initiated living radical polymerization from narrowly size-distributed silica nanoparticles of diameters less than 100 nm, *Macromolecules*, **43**, 2010, 8805–8812.
45. Ohno, K., Akashi, T., Tsujii, Y., Yamamoto, M., and Tabata, Y. Blood clearance and biodistribution of polymer brush-afforded silica particles prepared by surface-initiated living radical polymerization, *Biomacromolecules*, **13**, 2012, 927–936.
46. Majewski, A. P., Stahlschmidt, U., Jérôme, V., Freitag, R., Müller, A. H. E., and Schmalz, H. PDMAEMA-grafted core–shell–corona particles for non-viral gene delivery and magnetic cell separation, *Biomacromolecules*, **14**, 2013, 3081–3090.
47. Blas, H., Save, M., Boissiere, C., Sanchez, C., and Charleux, B. Surface-initiated nitroxide-mediated polymerization from ordered mesoporous silica, *Macromolecules*, **44**, 2011, 2577–2588.
48. Huang, X., Hauptmann, N., Appelhans, D., Formanek, P., Frank, S., Kaskel, S., Temme, A., and Voit, B. Synthesis of hetero-polymer functionalized nanocarriers by combining surface-initiated ATRP and RAFT polymerization, *Small*, **8**, 2012, 3579–3583.
49. Ranjan, R., and Brittain, W. J. Combination of living radical polymerization and click chemistry for surface modification, *Macromolecules*, **40**, 2007, 6217–6223.
50. Berger, S., Synytska, A., Ionov, L., Eichhorn, K.-J., and Stamm, M. Stimuli-responsive bicomponent polymer janus particles by "grafting from"/"grafting to" approaches, *Macromolecules*, **41**, 2008, 9669–9676.

51. Kim, J., Lee, J. E., Lee, J., Jang, Y., Kim, S.-W., An, K., Yu, J. H., and Hyeon, T. Generalized fabrication of multifunctional nanoparticle assemblies on silica spheres, *Angew. Chem.*, **118**, 2006, 4907–4911.
52. Climent, E., Martínez-Máñez, R., Sancenón, F., Marcos, M. D., and Soto, J., Maquieira, A., Amorós, P. Controlled delivery using oligonucleotide-capped mesoporous silica nanoparticles, *Angew. Chem., Int. Ed.*, **49**, 2010, 7281–7283.
53. Borase, T., Iacono, M., Ali, S. I., Thornton, P. D., and Heise, A. Polypeptide core-shell silica nanoparticles with high grafting density by N-carboxyanhydride (NCA) ring opening polymerization as responsive materials and for bioconjugation, *Polym. Chem.*, **3**, 2012, 1267–1275.
54. Song, G., Li, C., Hu, J., Zou, R., Xu, K., Han, L., Wang, Q., Yang, J., Chen, Z., Qin, Z., Ruan, K., and Hu, R. A simple transformation from silica core-shell-shell to yolk-shell nanostructures: a useful platform for effective cell imaging and drug delivery, *J. Mater. Chem.*, **22**, 2012, 17011–17018.
55. Tang, L., Yang, X., Dobrucki, L. W., Chaudhury, I., Yin, Q., Yao, C., Lezmi, S., Helferich, W. G., Fan, T. M., and Cheng, J. Aptamer-functionalized, ultra-small, monodisperse silica nanoconjugates for targeted dual-modal imaging of lymph nodes with metastatic tumors, *Angew. Chem., Int. Ed.*, **51**, 2012, 12721–12726.
56. You, Y.-Z., Kalebaila, K. K., Brock, S. L., and Oupický, D. Temperature-controlled uptake and release in PNIPAM-modified porous silica nanoparticles, *Chem. Mater.*, **20**, 2008, 3354–3359.
57. Gandra, N., Wang, D.-D., Zhu, Y., and Mao, C. Virus-mimetic cytoplasm-cleavable magnetic/silica nanoclusters for enhanced gene delivery to mesenchymal stem cells, *Angew. Chem., Int. Ed.*, **52**, 2013, 11278–11281.
58. Kotsuchibashi, Y., Ebara, M., Aoyagi, T., and Narain, R. Fabrication of doubly responsive polymer functionalized silica nanoparticles via a simple thiol-ene click chemistry, *Polym. Chem.*, **3**, 2012, 2545–2550.
59. Sun, L., Zhang, X., Wu, Z., Zheng, C., and Li, C. Oral glucose- and pH-sensitive nanocarriers for simulating insulin release in vivo, *Polym. Chem.*, **5**, 2014, 1999–2009.
60. Chen, C., Geng, J., Pu, F., Yang, X., Ren, J., and Qu, X. Polyvalent nucleic acid/mesoporous silica nanoparticle conjugates: dual stimuli-responsive vehicles for intracellular drug delivery, *Angew. Chem., Int. Ed.*, **50**, 2011, 882–886.
61. Yan, H., Teh, C., Sreejith, S., Zhu, L., Kwok, A., Fang, W., Ma, X., Nguyen, K. T., Korzh, V., and Zhao, Y. Functional mesoporous silica nanoparticles

for photothermal-controlled drug delivery in vivo, *Angew. Chem., Int. Ed.*, **51**, 2012, 8373–8377.
62. Schlossbauer, A., Dohmen, C., Schaffert, D., Wagner, E., and Bein, T. pH-responsive release of acetal-linked melittin from SBA-15 mesoporous silica, *Angew. Chem., Int. Ed.*, **50**, 2011, 6828–6830.
63. Popat, A., Ross, B. P., and Liu, J., Jambhrunkar, S., Kleitz, F., Qiao, S. Z. Enzyme-responsive controlled release of covalently bound prodrug from functional mesoporous silica nanospheres, *Angew. Chem., Int. Ed.*, **51**, 2012, 12486–12489.
64. Wu, S., Huang, X., and Du, X. Glucose- and pH-responsive controlled release of cargo from protein-gated carbohydrate-functionalized mesoporous silica nanocontainers, *Angew. Chem., Int. Ed.*, **52**, 2013, 5580–5584.
65. Li, Q.-L., Wang, L., Qiu, X.-L., Sun, Y.-L., Wang, P.-X., Liu, Y., Li, F., Qi, A.-D., Gao, H., and Yang, Y.-W. Stimuli-responsive biocompatible nanovalves based on β-cyclodextrin modified poly(glycidyl methacrylate), *Polym. Chem.*, **5**, 2014, 3389–3395.
66. Gao, J., Liang, G., Zhang, B., Kuang, Y., Zhang, X., and Xu, B. FePt@CoS$_2$ yolk–shell nanocrystals as a potent agent to kill HeLa cells, *J. Am. Chem. Soc.*, **129**, 2007, 1428–1433.
67. Zhao, W., Chen, H., Li, Y., Li, L., Lang, M., and Shi, J. Uniform rattle-type hollow magnetic mesoporous spheres as drug delivery carriers and their sustained-release property, *Adv. Funct. Mater.*, **18**, 2008, 2780–2788.
68. Li, L., Tang, F., Liu, H., Liu, T., Hao, N., Chen, D., Teng, X., and He, J. In vivo delivery of silica nanorattle encapsulated docetaxel for liver cancer therapy with low toxicity and high efficacy, *ACS Nano*, **4**, 2010, 6874–6882.
69. Zhang, X., Clime, L., Roberge, H., Normandin, F., Yahia, L. H., Sacher, E., and Veres, T. pH-triggered doxorubicin delivery based on hollow nanoporous silica nanoparticles with free-standing superparamagnetic Fe$_3$O$_4$ cores, *J. Phys. Chem.*, **115**, 2010, 1436–1443.
70. Zhao, L., Peng, J., Huang, Q., Li, C., Chen, M., Sun, Y., Lin, Q., Zhu, L., and Li, F. Near-infrared photoregulated drug release in living tumor tissue via yolk-shell upconversion nanocages, *Adv. Funct. Mater.*, **24**, 2014, 363–371.
71. Du, P., Yang, H., Zeng, J., and Liu, P. Folic acid-conjugated temperature and pH dual-responsive yolk/shell microspheres as a drug delivery system, *J. Mater. Chem. B*, **1**, 2013, 5298–5308.

72. Zhang, L., Wang, T., Yang, L., Liu, C., Wang, C., Liu, H., Wang, Y. A., and Su, Z. General Route to multifunctional uniform yolk/mesoporous silica shell nanocapsules: a platform for simultaneous cancer-targeted imaging and magnetically guided drug delivery, *Chem.: Eur. J.*, **18**, 2012, 12512–12521.
73. Zhu, Y., Fang, Y., and Kaskel, S. Folate-conjugated $Fe_3O_4@SiO_2$ hollow mesoporous spheres for targeted anticancer drug delivery, *J. Phys. Chem.*, **114**, 2010, 16382–16388.
74. Li, L., Guan, Y., Liu, H., Hao, N., Liu, T., Meng, X., Fu, C., Li, Y., Qu, Q., Zhang, Y., Ji, S., Chen, L., Chen, D., and Tang, F. Silica nanorattle–doxorubicin-anchored mesenchymal stem cells for tumor-tropic therapy, *ACS Nano*, **5**, 2011, 7462–7470.
75. Zhang, L., Wang, T., Li, L., Wang, C., Su, Z., and Li, J. Multifunctional fluorescent-magnetic polyethyleneimine functionalized Fe_3O_4-mesoporous silica yolk-shell nanocapsules for siRNA delivery, *Chem. Commun. (Camb.)*, **48**, 2012, 8706–8708.
76. Liu, T., Liu, H., Fu, C., Li, L., Chen, D., Zhang, Y., and Tang, F. Silica nanorattle with enhanced protein loading: a potential vaccine adjuvant, *J. Colloid Interface Sci.*, **400**, 2013, 168–174.
77. Tsai, M.-F., Chang, S.-H. G., Cheng, F.-Y., Shanmugam, V., Cheng, Y.-S., Su, C.-H., and Yeh, C.-S. Au nanorod design as light-absorber in the first and second biological near-infrared windows for in vivo photothermal therapy, *ACS Nano*, **7**, 2013, 5330–5342.
78. Lin, W.-I., Lin, C.-Y., Lin, Y.-S., Wu, S.-H., Huang, Y.-R., Hung, Y., Chang, C., and Mou, C.-Y. High payload Gd(iii) encapsulated in hollow silica nanospheres for high resolution magnetic resonance imaging, *J. Mater. Chem.B*, **1**, 2013, 639–645.
79. Qiang, L., Meng, X., Li, L., Chen, D., Ren, X., Liu, H., Ren, J., Fu, C., Liu, T., Gao, F., Zhang, Y., and Tang, F. Preparation of magnetic rattle-type silica through a general and facile pre-shell-post-core process for simultaneous cancer imaging and therapy, *Chem. Commun. (Camb.)*, **49**, 2013, 7902–7904.
80. Gao, J., Liang, G., Cheung, J. S., Pan, Y., Kuang, Y., Zhao, F., Zhang, B., Zhang, X., Wu, E. X., and Xu, B. Multifunctional yolk–shell nanoparticles: a potential mri contrast and anticancer agent, *J. Am. Chem. Soc.*, **130**, 2008, 11828–11833.
81. Chen, Y., Chen, H., Zeng, D., Tian, Y., Chen, F., Feng, J., and Shi, J. Core/Shell structured hollow mesoporous nanocapsules: a potential platform for simultaneous cell imaging and anticancer drug delivery, *ACS Nano*, **4**, 2010, 6001–6013.

82. Wang, T.-T., Chai, F., Wang, C.-G., Li, L., Liu, H.-Y., Zhang, L.-Y., Su, Z.-M., and Liao, Y. Fluorescent hollow/rattle-type mesoporous Au@SiO$_2$ nanocapsules for drug delivery and fluorescence imaging of cancer cells, *J. Colloid Interface Sci.*, **358**, 2011, 109–115.
83. Gao, F., Li, L., Fu, C., Nie, L., Chen, D., and Tang, F. LHRH-PE40 Fusion protein tethered silica nanorattles for imaging-guided tumor-specific drug delivery and bimodal therapy, *Adv. Mater. (Weinheim, Ger.)*, **25**, 2013, 5508–5513.
84. Liu, H., Liu, T., Wu, X., Li, L., Tan, L., Chen, D., and Tang, F. Targeting gold nanoshells on silica nanorattles: a drug cocktail to fight breast tumors via a single irradiation with near-infrared laser light, *Adv. Mater. (Weinheim, Ger.)*, **24**, 2012, 755–761.
85. Kang, X., Cheng, Z., Yang, D., Ma, P. a., Shang, M., Peng, C., Dai, Y., and Lin, J. Design and synthesis of multifunctional drug carriers based on luminescent rattle-type mesoporous silica microspheres with a thermosensitive hydrogel as a controlled switch, *Adv. Funct. Mater.*, **22**, 2012, 1470–1481.
86. Chen, Y., Chen, H., Zhang, S., Chen, F., Zhang, L., Zhang, J., Zhu, M., Wu, H., Guo, L., Feng, J., and Shi, J. Multifunctional mesoporous nanoellipsoids for biological bimodal imaging and magnetically targeted delivery of anticancer drugs, *Adv. Funct. Mater.*, **21**, 2011, 270–278.
87. Fan, W., Shen, B., Bu, W., Chen, F., Zhao, K., Zhang, S., Zhou, L., Peng, W., Xiao, Q., Xing, H., Liu, J., Ni, D., He, Q., and Shi, J. Rattle-structured multifunctional nanotheranostics for synergetic chemo-/radiotherapy and simultaneous magnetic/luminescent dual-mode imaging, *J. Am. Chem. Soc.*, **135**, 2013, 6494–6503.
88. Gandra, N., Portz, C., and Singamaneni, S. Multifunctional plasmonic nanorattles for spectrum-guided locoregional therapy, *Adv. Mater. (Weinheim, Ger.)*, **26**, 2014, 424–429.
89. Ma, M., Chen, H., Chen, Y., Wang, X., Chen, F., Cui, X., and Shi, J. Au capped magnetic core/mesoporous silica shell nanoparticles for combined photothermo-/chemo-therapy and multimodal imaging, *Biomaterials*, **33**, 2012, 989–998.

Biography

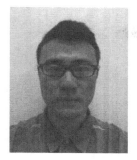

Tianyu Yang enrolled in a PhD at the University of Queensland in December 2010, supervised by Prof. Michael Monteiro, Dr. Jian Liu, and Prof. Shizhang Qiao from the University of Queensland (UQ), Curtin University, and the University of Adelaide (UoA), respectively. His research interests focus on the buildup of organic-inorganic hybrid nanoparticles as delivery vehicles and nanoreactors.

Chapter 3

Chemical and Biological Sensors Based on Microelectromechanical Systems

Gino Putrino,[a] Adrian Keating,[b] Mariusz Martyniuk,[a] Lorenzo Faraone,[a] and John Dell[a]

[a]*Microelectronics Research Group, University of Western Australia, 35 Stirling Highway, Crawley, WA 6009, Australia*
[b]*School of Mechanical and Chemical Engineering, University of Western Australia, 35 Stirling Highway, Crawley, WA 6009, Australia*
gino.putrino@uwa.edu.au

Microelectromechanical systems (MEMS) cantilevers can be used to detect trace gas elements. The surface of a cantilever is functionalized with a coating that preferentially bonds to the substance that is to be detected. When the coating adsorbs this substance, the cantilever will bend due to surface stresses, and the resonant frequency of the cantilever will change. The change is proportional to the additional mass of the adsorbed substance. To construct an effective cantilever sensor, a sensitive technique is required to read out the state of the cantilever. This chapter describes the operation of MEMS cantilever sensors and the readout techniques used to determine their state. The chapter also describes a novel optical readout technique suitable for determining the state of a cantilever sensor. A noise analysis is performed using theoretical and computational models, and it is found that the readout system

Nanomaterials: Science and Applications
Edited by Deborah Kane, Adam Micolich, and Peter Roger
Copyright © 2016 Pan Stanford Publishing Pte. Ltd.
ISBN 978-981-4669-72-6 (Hardcover), 978-981-4669-73-3 (eBook)
www.panstanford.com

is capable of a shot-noise-limited deflection noise density of 4.1 fm/$\sqrt{Hz}$. An implementation of the readout system has been experimentally demonstrated, which has a noise floor of 1 pm/$\sqrt{Hz}$.

3.1 Microelectromechanical Systems for Chemical/Biological Sensing and Atomic Force Microscopy

The rapid progress of the last few decades in electronics miniaturization has led to a new class of devices known as microelectromechanical systems (MEMS). These are characterized by having mechanical moving parts that are typically in the range of a tenth to a thousandth of a millimeter in size.

On the basis of current trends, the MEMS industry is expected to experience a compound annual growth rate (CAGR) of 13% over the next five years, becoming a US$22.5 billion market by 2018. Due to inherent similarities in the fabrication of MEMS and silicon microelectronics, it is possible to retrofit older microelectronics fabrication plants to produce MEMS. This has lowered the barrier to entry for MEMS foundries, leading to a number of such foundries establishing a foothold over the last 10 years.

There are many applications that need and benefit from the use of such tiny and robust devices, and so MEMS have been deployed into many devices and many environments, such as accelerometers in cars and portable electronics [1], lab-on-chip biological sensing [2], pressure sensors for applications in car tires and blood [3, 4], and actuating mirror parts for pico-projectors [5].

MEMS are typically fabricated using thin-film technology and often have a very large surface-to-volume ratio. This can have interesting physical effects. Forces that scale by volume, such as gravity and inertia, will be dominated by forces that scale by area, such as electrostatics or wetting.

3.1.1 MEMS Chemical and Biological Sensors

A particularly interesting MEMS subdiscipline that has arisen recently is that of chemical and biological sensing. Sensors based on MEMS have been shown to have the ability to measure mass with sensitivities in the zeptogram (10^{-21} g) regime [6]. This is well within the specification necessary to weigh single cells. These sensors are very robust and generally do not respond to environmental vibrations.

A basic chemical/biological MEMS sensor can be formed by taking a MEMS structure—such as a cantilever or doubly clamped beam—and coating it in a nanoparticle analyte that preferentially bonds to the substance that is to be detected. This coating process is termed "functionalization." The resulting change in the MEMS structure is observed as a detection event. These sensors are designed to operate in one of two main modes, either *static* or *dynamic*. This is described in further detail in the next two sections.

As individual MEMS sensors are tiny, multiple sensors can form a large array on a single silicon chip. This gives many benefits as listed below:

- Improved detection statistics. Increasing the number of sensors assists in avoiding false positives/negatives in gas sensing by improving the reliability of the measurement.
- The ability to perform thermal compensation. By not functionalizing some of the MEMS sensors on a chip, any measured change in their state can be attributed to thermal drift or other environmental effects. This provides the means to correct for these effects in the functionalized MEMS sensors.
- The potential for multianalyte testing. Different MEMS structures can be functionalized for different substances. This provides the ability to test for various gases using a single chip.

3.1.1.1 Static operation mode

Figure 3.1 shows an example of static mode operation of a cantilever-based MEMS sensor. Here the top surface of a cantilever has been uniformly coated with a nanoparticle functionalization layer, such as one made from antibody fragments, which will specifically bond to a protein it is desirable to detect. If this protein

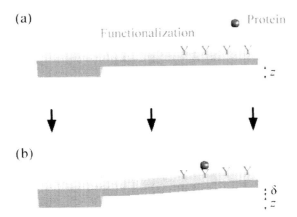

Figure 3.1 Example of the static mode operation of a MEMS cantilever protein sensor. (a) The MEMS cantilever has been functionalized, but no detection event has yet occurred. The cantilever beam is flat. In its normal state, the cantilever tip is a distance z above the substrate. (b) The protein has bonded to the antibody functionalization layer, and the resulting surface stress has led to the elastic stretching of the surface, causing the cantilever beam to deform. As a result, the tip of the cantilever beam is now a distance of $z + \delta$ above the substrate.

bonds to the top surface of the thin, flexible, MEMS cantilever beam, the surface stresses that occur will cause that cantilever beam to deform. Monitoring the change in the position of the cantilever tip in the z direction, due to this deformation, gives an indication of whether a sensing event has occurred. In aqueous environments, the bending of the cantilever due to surface stresses is approximately the same as bending in gaseous environments, so this technique is suitable for both these environments.

3.1.1.2 Dynamic operation mode

The alternative to static mode operation is dynamic mode operation. This is based on the knowledge that all mechanical structures have a characteristic frequency at which they will naturally vibrate in response to any perturbation. This is known as their natural resonance frequency. The resonance frequency of a structure is mainly influenced by the mass and physical dimensions of the structure. When a substance to be sensed bonds to a MEMS structure, the mass of that structure, and therefore its resonant frequency, will change. Dynamic-mode-operation MEMS sensors operate by measuring that frequency shift.

Two other response parameters are also available for a microcantilever operating in dynamic mode, the Q-factor and the amplitude of vibration [7]. The Q-factor, or quality factor, of a cantilever is defined in terms of the ratio of the energy stored in the cantilever to the energy supplied by the actuation technique in order to keep the amplitude of the motion of the cantilever constant. In most cases, both the Q-factor and the amplitude of vibration can be measured simultaneously via frequency measurement. These parameters can give additional information regarding the density and viscosity of the medium that the cantilever is vibrating in. This knowledge can be particularly useful in aqueous environments.

The dynamic mode technique is best used with thick, rigid MEMS beams with high resonance frequencies and high Q-factors, as these features allow determination of the resonance frequency of the MEMS beams with higher resolution. This technique is extremely effective in gaseous environments, due to the small amount of damping that occurs. In viscous mediums, larger damping of the cantilever movement occurs, lowering both the amplitude of the movement of the cantilever and the cantilever's Q-factor. This means that dynamic mode sensing in aqueous environments is not particularly effective unless an extremely sensitive position readout technique is used.

3.1.2 MEMS Sensor Implementations

Although not yet in common usage, a significant amount of work has been performed in the field of MEMS sensing. The first description of the use of a cantilever-based chemical sensor was by Norton in a US patent named "Gas Analyzer," which was submitted in 1939 and accepted in 1943 [8]. However, it was not until 1969 that Shaver used Norton's technique to demonstrate the detection of hydrogen gas at a sensitivity of 50 ppm by using large, 100 mm long, 125 µm thick cantilevers [9]. Although these cantilever beams were too large to be considered MEMS, this demonstration set the scene for what was to follow in later decades.

In 1983, Greenwood created a freestanding resonant pressure sensor [10] that was etched from silicon and could truly be considered the first MEMS environmental sensor. A few years later in 1986, Howe and Muller demonstrated the first MEMS gas sensor: a xylene vapor sensor created by depositing a polymer film (in this case a negative photoresist) on a polysilicon microbridge [11, 12]. The proven sensitivity of these devices triggered a large research effort into other sensing applications. Before long, several groups had demonstrated the sensing of simple chemicals and then moved toward applying this technique to more complex biological samples. The variety of chemicals these devices can sense is only limited by the ability of chemists to find specific functionalization layers [13, 14]. Laboratory demonstrations of MEMS sensing for explosives such as TNT and RDX [15], pesticides such as DDT [16], and melanoma skin cancer detection via nanomechanically detecting a specific mutation in the *BRAF* gene [17] are examples since 2003.

Gas sensing was not the only application considered. Many biological sensing applications require operation of the sensors in aqueous environments and so substantial work was also performed analyzing the behavior of microcantilever beams in viscous fluids [18]. Nieradka et al. [19] demonstrated microcantilever sensors operating immersed in a liquid cell. Burg [20] demonstrated the weighing of biomolecules, single cells, and single nanoparticles in fluid flowing through a microchannel embedded in a MEMS cantilever beam. Prior to Burg's demonstration, surface plasmon resonance (SPR) had been regarded as the most sensitive technique for biomolecular detection, as SPR had allowed a mass resolution of 1 picogram. Burg's technique enabled a resolution of 300 attograms, bettering SPR by almost 4 orders of magnitude. This ability has given rise to a strong, new field dubbed *nanomicrobiology* [21]. It has been used to measure the masses of individual live *Escherichia coli* and *Bacillus subtilis* bacteria with enough resolution to differentiate between them. This lays a path forward toward the development of label-free assays for the rapid detection of pathogens and toxins.

Due to the ease of mass fabrication of MEMS devices, arrays of cantilever beams on chips were soon implemented in order to realize the benefits described in Section 3.1.1: better detection statistics, the ability for simultaneous multianalyte sensing, and the provision of reference cantilevers that were not functionalized to provide a measure of thermal drift. At the turn of the millennium, several research groups demonstrated such arrays with up to eight cantilever sensors on a single device.

3.1.3 Example: Palladium-Coated Cantilever Hydrogen Sensor

To obtain an idea of the size of the movements that must be measured for MEMS sensors, it is instructive to consider the example of a palladium-coated cantilever.

An interesting property of palladium is that it expands when absorbing hydrogen. An expression for the change in radius of curvature, R, of a cantilever coated on one side with palladium when exposed to hydrogen was derived by Okuyama et al. [22]:

$$\frac{1}{R} = \frac{2\left(\Delta V/V_o\right)a_1 E_1}{K a_2^2 E_2}\sqrt{pH_2} \qquad (3.1)$$

where pH_2 is the partial pressure of hydrogen in Torr, V_o is the atomic volume of palladium, and ΔV is the characteristic volume change per hydrogen atom. The ratio $\Delta V/V_o$ is this situation is 0.19 [23]. The thicknesses of the palladium layer and the structural layer of the cantilever are a_1 and a_2, respectively. The Young's modulus of the palladium layer and the structural layer of the cantilever are E_1 and E_2, respectively. K is Sieverts's constant for the prediction of solubility of gases in metals [24]. For the case of hydrogen dissolving into palladium, K is 49 [22]. Note that Eq. 3.1 is only a valid approximation for hydrogen partial pressures less than 30 Torr.

Figure 3.2 shows the deflection of a cantilever tip due to the absorption of hydrogen when we assume a 100 μm long, 750 nm thick silicon nitride cantilever coated with a 50 nm layer of palladium. It can be seen from this figure that the ability to sense nanometer deflections of the cantilever tip gives sub-milli-Torr sensitivity of the hydrogen partial pressure. The requirement of milli-Torr sensitivity is particularly important for hydrogen sensors working in the atmosphere, as the typical partial pressure of

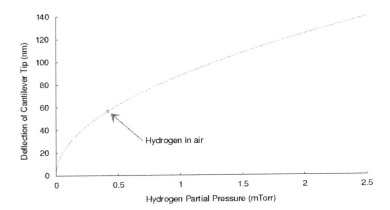

Figure 3.2 Deflection at the tip of a 100 μm long palladium/silicon nitride cantilever due to hydrogen absorption.

hydrogen in the atmosphere is 0.42 mTorr. This causes a cantilever tip deflection of 60 nm. The ability to measure deviations from the 0.42 mTorr norm is often desirable. Therefore, to use static mode cantilevers effectively for this example, it is clear that a technique to measure the movements of the cantilever tip to at least nanometer-scale precision is necessary.

3.1.4 Chapter Overview

Critical to the operation of this type of MEMS sensor is the method of detecting, or reading out, the height change (for static mode) or motion (for dynamic mode) of the MEMS beam to determine whether a detection event has occurred. Less critical, but still desirable, is the ability to address large numbers of MEMS beams, giving the aforementioned benefits.

This chapter looks at the MEMS position readout techniques that exist today and introduces a novel, integrated optical readout technique that has been developed at the University of Western Australia. A realization of the design using common silicon and MEMS fabrication technologies will be presented. A noise analysis of this technique will be performed and used to determine the minimum amount of MEMS movement that the technique is capable of measuring. It is found that the readout technique is sensitive enough to detect the thermal-mechanical Brownian motion of a cantilever tip at room temperature and pressure.

3.2 Current Techniques for MEMS Position Readout and Their Limitations

This section will look at the techniques available for determining the height position of the MEMS sensor beam.

A large number of MEMS sensor readout techniques have been demonstrated over the past 20 years. These can be classed as being either optical or electronic techniques. Generally speaking, optical techniques have far higher resolution than electronic techniques, yet electronic techniques are capable of addressing far larger numbers of cantilevers than optical techniques. Some optical techniques have the additional benefit of being able to operate in fluidic environments.

In 1986, Binning, Quate, and Gerber [25] announced the invention of the atomic force microscope (AFM), a feat for which they were awarded the Nobel Prize. This device is essentially a microcantilever with a sharp point on the tip, which builds up the profile of a surface by moving the cantilever over a surface of interest and watching the way in which the tip of the microcantilever responds to that surface. Therefore, it is unsurprising that when readout techniques were required for microcantilever sensors, the first techniques examined were those that had previously been invented for the AFM.

3.2.1 Optical Readout Techniques

Several optical techniques have now been designed for use as readouts for MEMS sensors. Some, like optical beam deflection (OBD), are adaptations of AFM-like readout techniques [26]. Newer techniques have been designed with integrated addressing of large arrays of sensors in mind [27, 28].

The OBD technique involves shining an external laser onto the top of a cantilever. The light from the laser is deflected from the tip of the cantilever to a distant quadrant photodetector that determines the movement of the cantilever from the movement of the laser beam. OBD is extremely precise, but due to difficulties in aligning external lasers the technique has only been extended to small arrays of eight cantilevers [29].

The most sensitive of the traditional optical readout techniques developed for AFM is the use of an external interferometer to determine the motion of the cantilever. Whilst the interferometric technique has the advantage of being extremely sensitive, it suffers from the disadvantage that it is extremely difficult to align the measurement laser to the tip of the cantilever.

Stievater et al. [30] used a microcavity interferometric technique to measure the movements of a small array of four MEMS beams in an arrangement the group named a photonic harp. This arrangement involved firing a laser through a fiber optic cable, which was aligned above four MEMS doubly clamped beams of different lengths, which were, in turn, fabricated above a reflective substrate. This arrangement created a resonant optical microcavity between the substrate and the MEMS beams. When the MEMS beams moved, this modulated the light, which, in turn, provided a sensitive measurement of the movement of the beams. This result was significant in that it led to a slight increase in the number of sensors that could be read out using interferometry. However, it still suffered from the difficulties inherent to aligning the laser directly above the MEMS beams.

Although traditional optical techniques are able to determine sensitivity with extremely high precision, to date, they have been limited in the number of MEMS devices that they can address simultaneously. To address this issue, later optical techniques involve the use of integrated microcavities. These are yet to achieve the high sensitivity of traditional, external optical techniques. Preussner et al. [24] demonstrated the use of an in-plane microcavity by etching a distributed Bragg reflector (DBR) into a silicon waveguide running to a microbeam. The actuation of the microbeam either shortens or lengthens the DBR cavity and provides a sensitive measurement of the movement of that beam.

Eichenfield et al. [25] created a zipper cavity from nanobeams. Two nanobeams are fabricated extremely close to each other. The close proximity of these nanobeams creates an optical cavity, and so light travelling through the nanobeams is modulated as these beams move.

One of the more promising modern optical techniques is the use of the cantilever as a waveguide [31]. Here a MEMS cantilever is aligned with a silicon photonics output waveguide. As the cantilever moves in and out of the plane of the waveguide, different proportions of the light traveling through the cantilever are coupled into the output waveguide. This technique allows for large numbers of cantilever sensors on a single chip. However, it has a very small dynamic range, as movement of the cantilever beyond a certain range results in no light entering the output waveguide.

3.2.2 Electronic Readout Techniques

Electronic techniques have been shown to be eminently suitable for reading the position of large arrays of MEMS devices. Chips containing up to 1000 cantilevers have been fabricated, and multiple applications can benefit from the ability to address this number of cantilevers on a single chip, even if the positional resolution is lower than that achievable by optical methods. In addition, electronic interrogation is cost effective and well established. However, electronic techniques cannot be used in areas of strong EM fields or in hazardous environments where there are ignition risks. In aqueous/electrolyte environments, ions in the solution tend to cause parasitic currents that can overwhelm the electric signal. The three main electronic techniques used are those based on piezoresistance, piezoelectricity, and capacitance.

Structures made from piezoresistive materials change their electrical resistance when the structure is deformed. By measuring this resistance change, the extent of the bending of a MEMS cantilever can be determined. In contrast to piezoresistivity, structures made from piezoelectric materials, such as zinc oxide, generate transient charge currents when the structure is deformed. Measuring these charges allows knowledge regarding the flexing of a MEMS cantilever to be determined. Finally, capacitance-based techniques rely on the change of capacitance that occurs when the distance between two conducting plates changes. Measuring this capacitance can be used to determine the distance between a MEMS cantilever and a substrate. Large parasitic capacitances can make this measurement difficult to perform. Piezoresistive techniques are currently the most common of the electronic techniques used to measure the movement of MEMS devices.

3.3 Integrated Gratings: A New Technique for Cantilever Readout

To take MEMS sensors out of the laboratory and into real-world conditions, a readout technique is required that is robust, has high precision, and can be extended to address multiple cantilevers on a single device. This section presents and analyzes a novel readout technique that provides these requirements. Furthermore, this technique can operate in various environmental conditions and is relatively easy to fabricate using silicon and complementary metal–oxide semiconductor (CMOS)-compatible technologies. In later sections of this chapter, the results obtained when an implementation of the technique was fabricated and tested will be presented. This novel approach has been pioneered by the authors at the University of Western Australia.

The technique we present and demonstrate in this chapter integrates silicon photonics technology with MEMS and is illustrated in Fig. 3.3. In sensing applications, the cantilever will change either its height or its mechanical resonance frequency in response to an adsorbed analyte. To sense such changes, we create an optically resonant cavity by suspending a micromachined beam with a reflective undersurface above a nanostructured diffraction grating etched into a waveguide. The diffraction grating will be designed to be efficient for light in the midinfrared region. Very effective waveguides for 1550 nm light can be fabricated using a silicon-on-insulator (SOI) wafer. Lasers at this wavelength are available and cheap due to their ubiquitous use in optical telecommunications.

When infrared light travels through the silicon waveguide, the grating will diffract some of the light out of the waveguide toward the micromachined beam. The mirror on the micromachined beam will reflect the light back toward the grating. The recombination of the remaining light in the waveguide with the reflected light

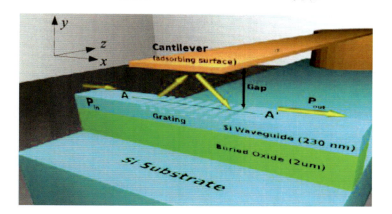

Figure 3.3 Isometric view of the interrogating grating structure that is fabricated and tested (not to scale). © [2012] IEEE. Reprinted, with permission, from Ref. [32].

leads to constructive and destructive interference in the light output from the waveguide. It acts as an interferometer. As a result, the intensity of the light travelling through the waveguide is amplitude-modulated by the movement of the micromachined beam due to the path length change in the interferometer. This entire optomechanical interaction occurs over the volume defined by the waveguide and the cantilever. Assuming 50 μm long, 10 um wide cantilevers that are a height of 2 μm above the substrate, this is a volume of 1000 μm^3. Over a sensor area of 1 cm^2, and assuming a fill factor of 50%, this technique can readily be extended to the interrogation of 10^5 microcantilever sensors. Subsequently, wavelength, time, or spatial multiplexing of these signals could allow them to be coupled into a single-output optical fiber. This will also allow the signals to be transmitted over exceptionally long distances [32]. Figure 3.4 shows an example of how such a multiplexed system might work. An on-chip wavelength division multiplexer (WDM) could be used to split a broadband laser into several wavelength components, with each wavelength component sent along a different waveguide. The light in each waveguide could then be used to address cantilevers via an interrogating grating. At the end of each of these waveguides, a de-multiplexer could combine the light and

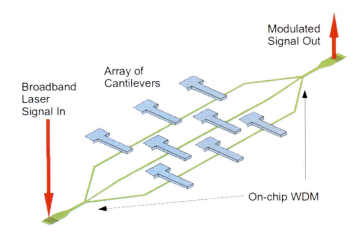

Figure 3.4 Schematic of a proposed system to address large arrays of microcantilevers.

an output grating could be used to provide the output power to the fibre optic.

Figure 3.5 shows a cross section of a full detection unit of a device through the line A'A indicated in Fig. 3.3. Light is launched into the silicon waveguide via an input grating coupler (not shown). The output light is modulated due to interference and is coupled out

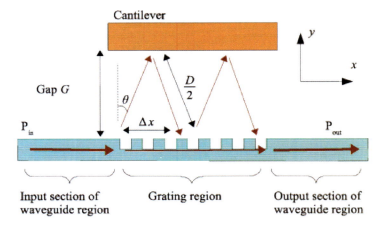

Figure 3.5 Cross section of the full device through section A'A from Fig. 3.3.

by an output grating coupler. The grating couplers were designed to be broadband and have optimized coupling efficiency for light at a wavelength of 1550 nm. These gratings have the same physical specifications as the grating designed and analyzed by Taillaert et al. [33]. By detecting the optical power at the output, a sensitive measure of the beam deflection can be obtained.

The transmission of an optical signal through the waveguide will now be analyzed to understand how modulation of the transmitted optical power is induced by a deflecting microcantilever. In the approach illustrated in Fig. 3.3, some of the optical power (P_{in}) of the waveguide input signal is coupled out of the waveguide by a diffraction grating positioned directly below a microcantilever. Fabry–Perot cavities are a type of optical resonator typically made of two parallel mirrors. For specific wavelengths, the distance between the two mirrors creates a standing wave. Optical cavities such as these are used as a component in lasers to control the lasing wavelength, in optical spectrometers to measure the optical wavelength of radiation emissions, and in many other applications. The reflective underside of the cantilever and the air–silicon waveguide grating form a resonant optical cavity in which the cantilever acts as a movable high-reflectivity mirror, while the grating acts as an angle and wavelength-dependent mirror, creating a structure similar to an angled Fabry–Pérot cavity [34]. As a result of the resonance effects in the cavity, the amount of input light (P_{in}) coupled into the output section (P_{out}) of the waveguide is a sensitive function of the separation between the grating and the cantilever.

3.3.1 *Optical Modeling of the Structure*

Optical considerations of the design were analyzed by undertaking 2D and 3D electromagnetic (EM) modeling of the structure using finite-difference time domain (FDTD) modeling. The model was based on an SOI platform for the optical waveguide/grating structure, which consisted of a 120 nm epitaxial silicon layer for the waveguide, a 2.0 micron thick buried oxide (BOX) for the bottom cladding layer, and a silicon handle wafer as the base. The waveguides are designed to be single mode in the y direction, which is perpendicular to the plane of the substrate. The waveguides are

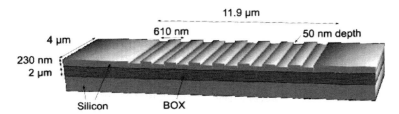

Figure 3.6 Isometric diagram of the modeled diffraction grating implemented in a SOI wafer (not to scale). The SOI wafer is made up of a 230 nm thick epitaxial silicon layer, a 2 μm thick BOX layer, and a silicon handle layer. The grating will be etched into the epitaxial silicon and has a pitch of 610 nm, depth 50 nm, length 11.9 μm, and width 4 μm.

multimode in the z direction (x, y, and z directions are defined in Fig. 3.3). SOI photonic structures have the advantage of being a relatively well-developed technology. Further, silicon provides very strong optical guiding so that minimal evanescent field coupling will occur. This strong guiding is useful as it reduces crosstalk and leakage, allowing the approach to be utilized with large sensor arrays where waveguides need to be closely spaced. The grating utilized is a square-wave nanostructured grating of 610 nm pitch, 50 nm depth, and 11.9 μm length and, in the absence of the cantilever structure, is an efficient waveguide output coupler with a coupling loss of approximately 6 dB. This reference grating is shown in Fig. 3.6. The bottom surface of the suspended cantilever is assumed to be a perfect reflector at the wavelength of interest (1550 nm) and to extend 1 μm beyond the interrogating grating on all sides.

The optical FDTD model works by taking the device to be modeled, numerically breaking it up into smaller volumes, and solving Maxwell's equations for EM radiation for a specified time period. This gives a simulation of the EM fields propagating through the device. The structure from Fig. 3.3 is implemented in the FDTD model, and a light source modeled as a transverse electric (TE)-polarized Gaussian beam was launched into the waveguide. The diffraction grating was placed a sufficient distance away (8 μm) from the input light source so that a stable propagating optical mode was incident on the grating section of the waveguide. The cross section used to determine the optical power in the output waveguide only

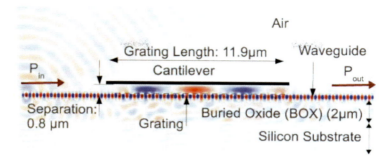

Figure 3.7 Modeled results at λ = 1550 nm for a cantilever with a perfect reflector over a SOI waveguide 230 nm thick. The grating has pitch 630 nm and is 11.9 μm long. The blue/red shading represents the calculated TE field distributions through section A′A in Fig. 3.5 when the cantilever–grating separation is 0.8 μm. This separation gives the maximum transmitted power. © [2012] IEEE. Reprinted, with permission, from Ref. [32].

contains that waveguide, so substrate modes and small evanescent field contributions are not included in the power calculations.

Figure 3.7 shows the optical field strength when the cantilever arm is at a height required for constructive interference (i.e., 0.8 μm) for an input wavelength of 1550 nm. It can be seen that most of the optical power stays within the waveguide and that a large amount of power is diffracted into the cavity between the cantilever and the grating.

Figure 3.8 shows the optical field strength when the cantilever arm is at a height required for destructive interference (i.e., 1.2 μm). When compared to Fig. 3.7, it can be seen that for the case of Fig. 3.8, most of the light dissipates into the substrate, so by the end of the grating, there is very little light left traveling through the waveguide.

Figure 3.9 shows the output power predicted by the FDTD simulations as a function of the separation between the grating and the cantilever. As this is an interferometric effect, it is not monotonic but rather periodic. It can be seen from Fig. 3.9 that this periodicity is 800 nm, and measuring only the static optical power using a single-waveguide structure under the cantilever will only provide unambiguous transmission values for deflections over a range of 400 nm. From these results, it is clear that the amplitude-

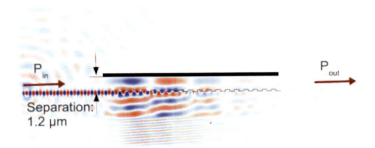

Figure 3.8 Modeled results at $\lambda = 1550$ nm for a cantilever with a perfect reflector over a SOI waveguide 230 nm thick. The grating has pitch 630 nm and is 11.9 μm long. The blue/red shading represents the calculated TE field distribution with a separation 1.2 μm (minimum in transmitted power). A significant portion of the energy is coupled into the substrate rather than the output waveguide. © [2012] IEEE. Reprinted, with permission, from Ref. [32].

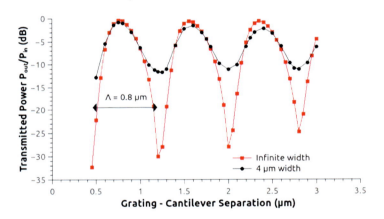

Figure 3.9 Modeled results at $\lambda = 1550$ nm for a cantilever with a perfect reflector over a SOI waveguide 230 nm thick. Power transmitted as a function of cantilever–grating separation for a diffraction grating of both 4 μm width and an infinite width (2D) approximation.

modulated optical power leaving the output waveguide can be used to determine the height position of the cantilever.

The extinction of the system can be defined as the difference between the maximum and minimum transmitted optical power. It can be seen in Fig. 3.9 that a 10–12 dB extinction is achieved as the cantilever arm deflects over the 800 nm range of periodicity. The comparison in Fig. 3.9 of the 4 μm grating width simulation to that of the "infinitely" wide grating shows that as the width of the grating is increased, the total extinction increases. This is due to fringing effects becoming less important as grating width increases. Nevertheless, the comparison indicates that a 4 μm wide grating achieves almost the same performance from 0–10 dB as an infinite grating. In most instances, the grating will be operated at the peak or at the 3 dB point, suggesting that a 4 μm wide grating is adequate for our positional readout needs and achieves optimum performance.

For the device to create a strong interference pattern, and achieve such large extinction ranges, it is important that the grating be effective at coupling light in and out at the operating wavelength. Through modeling, the grating was found to have a loss parameter, α, of 0.11 μm^{-1}. This value results in only 8% transmission for an 11 μm grating length when no cantilever was present, meaning that most of the light in the waveguide will pass through the grating–cantilever cavity when the cantilever is present.

An alternative design would be for multiple waveguides to be placed under a single cantilever at different distances from the cantilever anchor, allowing the bend profile along the length of the deflected cantilever to be determined. An example of a scheme that might implement this is shown in Fig. 3.10. Due to the repeating

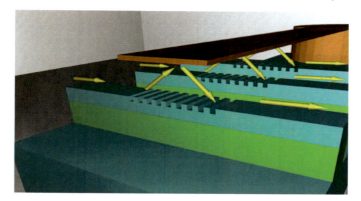

Figure 3.10 Isometric view of a proposed multiple interrogating grating structure.

spectral characteristics, the transmission spectra of the resonant structure allows operation over a 400 nm range in any of the linear regions shown in Fig. 3.9.

3.4 Integrated Grating Readout Technique Demonstration

3.4.1 *Device Fabrication*

To demonstrate this position readout technique, it was necessary to build a silicon photonic circuit containing interrogating gratings and then build MEMS microcantilevers above the gratings. The minimum feature size of the interrogating gratings was 315 nm, requiring deep ultraviolet (DUV) photolithography. The fabrication of these components was outsourced to Laboratoire d'électronique et de technologie de l'information (LETI), where the standard passive process of the ePIXfab silicon photonics platform was used [35]. The pertinent steps in this fabrication process are an initial 70 nm deep etch into the epitaxial silicon of an SOI wafer to form grating pits and a 220 nm etch of the epitaxial silicon, followed by a deposition of silicon dioxide that is chemomechanically polished to create a 100 nm flat layer above the epitaxial silicon. This process is shown in Fig. 3.11.

The design and fabrication of the MEMS structures for the device was almost entirely de-coupled from that of the photonic circuit. These MEMS structures were fabricated at the University of Western Australia using a multistep surface micromachining process. This process is shown in Fig. 3.12 and involves depositing very thin films of material, patterning those films using photolithography, and then removing the unwanted portions to create freestanding suspended structures. Matching the stress in subsequent films is important to create devices that will remain in the desired shape after release occurs.

The first step is to deposit the wiring and pads that will be used for electrostatic actuation of the MEMS structures. The second step is to deposit a sacrificial layer of a thickness that will become the

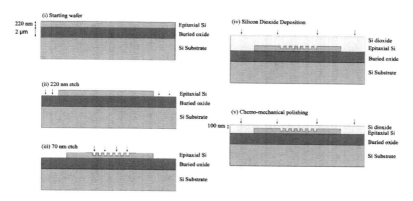

Figure 3.11 LETI process flow.

(i) Starting with an SOI wafer chosen with an epitaxial silicon thickness able to operate as a waveguide for infrared light (220 nm) and a SiO_2 thickness (2 μm) chosen to support the operation of the Si waveguide and grating couplers.

(ii) A 220 nm silicon etch performed to remove the parts of the epitaxial silicon that are not going to be needed for the photonic circuit. This forms the waveguides and adiabatic tapers.

(iii) Subsequently, a 70 nm silicon etch performed to define the diffraction gratings.

(iv) A layer of SiO_2 deposited.

(v) The layer of SiO_2 chemomechanically polished down to a height of 100 nm above the top of the epitaxial silicon. This step provides a flat planarized surface for the fabrication of the overlying MEMS structures.

height of the suspended MEMS device. Next, holes are etched into the sacrificial layer—these holes will become the supporting legs of the MEMS devices. Following this, the mirror material is deposited, and patterned to create mirrors in locations that will become the bottom mirror layer of the microcantilever. The structural layer is then deposited and patterned to the same geometry of the mirror material, and finally the release process is performed.

To keep the fabrication process simple, reduce the layer thickness, and remove multilayer stress balancing issues, the use of dielectric mirrors was not considered. Instead a thin layer of gold

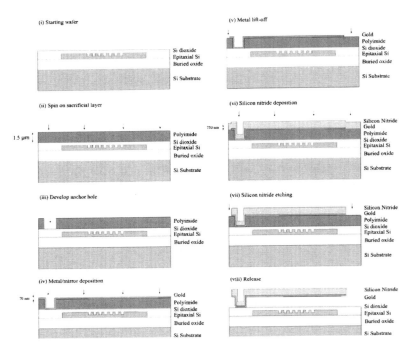

Figure 3.12 MEMS process flow. A MEMS cantilever is built by depositing and patterning several layers of various thin films. This figure does not include the steps for the deposition of the electrostatic pads and wiring.

was chosen to be the mirror. Gold is a particularly strong reflector of infrared radiation, giving 98%–99% reflectivity through the infrared [36]. A gold layer of 50 nm was considered sufficient to provide extremely good reflectivity at 1550 nm.

The structural layer for the MEMS devices was chosen to be nonstoichiometric silicon nitride (SiN_x). SiN_x is a chemically inert, mechanically strong ceramic with a Young's modulus typically between 120 and 315 GPa. SiN_x can be deposited using a plasma-enhanced chemical vapor deposition (PECVD) technique by combining the gases silane and ammonia [37]. The deposition rate can be extremely well controlled—the recipe used had a deposition rate of 28 nm/s, and the PECVD instrument used PC control to time the process to an uncertainty of less than a second.

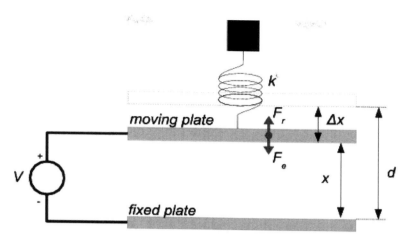

Figure 3.13 Electrostatic actuation of a cantilever modeled as two charged plates, one of which is movable on a simple spring. At rest, the two plates are separated by a distance d. When a voltage V is applied, the generated electrostatic force, F_e, draws the movable plate a distance Δx toward the fixed plated until F_e is balanced by the spring restoring force, F_r. If F_e is large enough that it can overwhelm F_r, then destructive snap-down can occur.

3.4.2 Electrostatic Actuation

Wiring for electrostatic actuation was deposited on these samples. To understand how the MEMS structures will move in this situation, the forces involved were modeled by considering two charged plates, one fixed and one movable on a spring with a spring constant k. This is schematically depicted in Fig. 3.13. When modeled like this, the force balance equation is $F_e = F_r$, where F_r is the restoring spring force and F_e is the electrostatic force. Assuming that the plate area, A, is much greater than the separation, x, between the plates, the electrostatic force between the substrate and the cantilever can be given by [38]

$$F_e = \frac{A\varepsilon V^2}{2x^2} \qquad (3.2)$$

where V is the applied voltage and ε is the permittivity of the medium between the plates. For air, the permittivity is 8.85×10^{-12} F/m [39].

The restoring spring force can be written as

$$F_r = k\Delta x = kd - kx \qquad (3.3)$$

where d is the initial starting separation between the plates, k is the spring constant, and x is the current separation between the plates. As can be seen from these equations, the electrostatic force, F_e, scales in relation to the inverse square of x, while the spring restoring force, F_r, scales directly in relation to x. Therefore, as the voltage is increased, and the plates approach each other (i.e., x becomes smaller), there will be a point where F_e overwhelms F_r. If this occurs, then the top plate will *snap down* and make contact with the bottom plate. In the case of surface micromachined MEMS, the two deposited plates will be extremely flat, meaning that when the plates make contact, van der Waals intermolecular forces will become dominant, bonding the two plates together [40]. This phenomenon is called *stiction* and is a potential cause of failure of the MEMS device.

It can be shown that if the spring constant k is indeed constant, then the beam can be deflected by up to one-third of the initial plate separation (i.e., $d/3$) before snap-down will occur. This is generally true for microcantilevers. However, due to effects such as strain stiffening, k is not constant, and it has been observed that doubly clamped beams can be deflected by up to one-half of the initial plate separation ($d/2$) without snap-down.

3.4.3 Fabricated Microcantilevers

A scanning electron micrograph (SEM) of a sample microcantilever fabricated by this process is shown in Fig. 3.14. The cantilever is not perfectly flat but is deflected upward from the anchor to the tip due to the relief of residual stresses after release. When the cantilever is at rest, the tip of the cantilever beam is 11.5 μm higher than the region of the beam near the anchor. The resonant frequency of the cantilever was measured using a laser Doppler vibrometer to be 13.2 kHz.

For the investigated cantilever (shown in Fig. 3.14), the grating is placed underneath the midpoint of the cantilever beam (rather than underneath the tip). Therefore, all cantilever position and

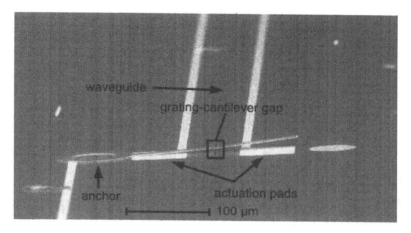

Figure 3.14 SEM image of a microcantilever. Note that the optical waveguide does not appear in an SEM image as it is below the SiO_2 planarization layer. The dashed line is drawn on the image to indicate the position of the optical waveguide.

movement measurements from this point on will refer to the region above the grating unless otherwise specified. When actuated at its resonant frequency (using the electrostatic actuation pads), the gap between the grating and the reflective underside was measured to range from 4.3 to 6.5 μm. Figure 3.15 shows the cantilever response to actuation at its resonant frequency as a function of actuation voltage.

The measured transmitted optical power at a wavelength of 1550 nm is shown in Fig. 3.16. A very strong amplitude modulation due to gap change is evident. As the modulation effect is interferometric in nature, the amplitude does not monotonically increase but rather can be seen to be periodic with respect to the gap distance, with maxima and minima separated by 400 nm. Figure 3.16 includes an overlay of a 2D FDTD simulation of the expected outputs of the structure. The measured results show good agreement with the simulated results.

One systematic difference between the modeling and the experimental measurements is the peak amplitude roll-off seen in Fig. 3.16, which only occurs in the experimental measurements. The main cause of this difference is that as the cantilever tilts upward,

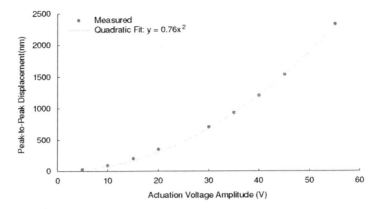

Figure 3.15 Measured cantilever peak-to-peak displacement amplitude as a function of sinusoidal wave actuation voltage at the resonant frequency of the microcantilever.

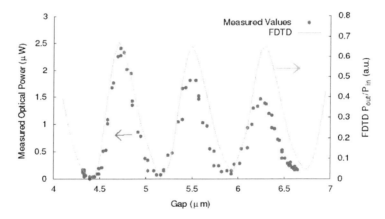

Figure 3.16 Measured and FDTD-simulated optical output of the device for a 1550 nm laser vs. cantilever–grating gap.

more light is reflected out of the area of the diffraction grating and so not coupled back into the waveguide. This concept is shown in Fig. 3.17. Two-dimensional FDTD simulations are not able to model this situation. By extending the FDTD simulations into the third dimension, this effect could be modeled as the tilt of the cantilever, and the width of the waveguide would then be taken into effect.

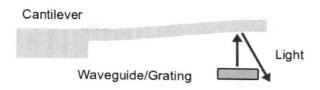

Figure 3.17 Cantilever deflecting light out of the waveguide region.

3.5 Grating Technique Noise and Limits of Detection Analysis

In this section, the transmission of the optical signal through the waveguide is analyzed to study the modulation of the transmitted optical power induced by the deflecting microcantilever. The results will be used to estimate the theoretical noise inherent in this technique when applied to measurement of the deflection of a microcantilever. This noise analysis will give an understanding of the smallest motion of the cantilever that we can measure with the readout technique.

3.5.1 Theoretical Noise Analysis

The main noise components in this system are those that arise from various thermal, electrical, and optical effects. These thermal, electrical, and optical noise components will now be calculated in order to determine the deflection noise density (DND) and minimum detectable deflection (MDD) for this readout method. The existing expressions for typical microcantilever behavior are used to calculate the thermal noise components, and new expressions tailored to this readout technique are derived to calculate the electrical and optical noise components.

The transmission efficiency through the device from input to output waveguide, η, is first defined as a function of cantilever height, z, as

$$\eta(z) = P_{out}(z)/P_{in}(z) \tag{3.4}$$

where $P_{out}(z)$ is the power in the output waveguide as a function of the cantilever–grating separation, z, and P_{in} is the power in the

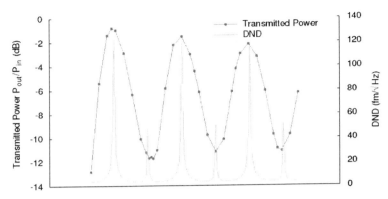

Figure 3.18 3D FDTD simulation of power transmitted as a function of cantilever–grating separation for a diffraction grating 4 μm in width. The shot-noise-limited DND, DND_{sn}, calculated from Eq. 3.11 over this separation range is also shown. The region where DND values are less than 25 fm/$\sqrt{Hz}$ is shaded, showing the operating ranges where DND can be kept below this level.

input waveguide entering the interrogating grating underneath the cantilever.

A measure of sensitivity, S, in units m^{-1} can then be defined as [40]

$$S = \frac{\delta \eta}{\delta z} = \frac{1}{P_{in}} \frac{\delta P_{out}}{\delta z} \qquad (3.5)$$

Figure 3.18 shows the 3D FDTD modeled transmitted power as a function of the cantilever–grating separation for a grating of 4 μm in width. Three-dimensional FDTD simulations were performed as the 2D FDTD simulations only considered the length and height of the grating, and a third dimension is required to consider the width of the grating. Greatest sensitivity will occur when operating in the regions of greatest slope of the transmitted power curve in this figure. One of these operating points is at a cantilever–grating separation of $z = 1$ μm (being the midpoint between the first maximum and minimum). When operating around this height, sensitivity can be numerically calculated from the simulation data to be $S = 3.0 \, \mu m^{-1}$.

The MDD will be limited by the shot noise of the photodetector, Johnson noise of the load resistor, noise in the measurement system, cantilever vibration due to thermal noise, and noise from the laser source. With the exception of the case for mechanical thermal noise, all DND components will be calculated independently of the microcantilever properties. All MDD components, and the DND component for mechanical thermal noise, will be calculated on the basis of the properties of a reference 50 μm long, 10 μm wide, 1 μm thick silicon nitride microcantilever.

MDD is defined as the case when the signal-to-noise ratio (SNR) is equal to 1, and so the MDD can be expressed by [41]

$$\text{MDD} = \frac{1}{\sqrt{\text{SNR}}} \tag{3.6}$$

and DND is generally calculated by [30]

$$\text{DND} = \frac{\text{MDD}}{\sqrt{\Delta f}} \tag{3.7}$$

where Δf is the measurement bandwidth.

Optical feed-forward techniques can significantly reduce laser relative intensity noise (RIN) [42], and measurement system noise can be filtered or compensated using synchronous detection techniques, and so are not included in this analysis.

3.5.1.1 Thermomechanical noise

Cantilever thermal noise is independent of the readout method, as it varies depending on the dimensions and material properties of the cantilever. For the purpose of this analysis it is assumed that a silicon nitride cantilever beam has been fabricated using the surface micromachining techniques described in Section 3.4.1. The MDD component due to thermomechanical Brownian motion, MDD$_{br}$, of such a cantilever can be estimated by [43]

$$\text{MDD}_{br} = \sqrt{\frac{2k_b T \Delta f}{\pi Q k f_0}} \tag{3.8}$$

where k_b is Boltzman's constant, T is temperature, Δf is the electrical bandwidth in Hertz, Q is the quality factor of the cantilever, k is the spring constant of the cantilever, and f_0 is the resonance frequency of the cantilever. The DND for thermal mechanical noise, DND$_{br}$, is then defined by

$$\text{DND}_{br} = \frac{\text{MDD}_{br}}{\sqrt{\Delta f}} = \sqrt{\frac{2k_b T \Delta f}{\pi Q k f_0}}. \quad (3.9)$$

A surface micromachined cantilever fabricated from typical PECVD silicon nitride will have a Young's modulus around 120 GPa and a density of 3184 kg/m^3 [44]. For a cantilever of length 50 μm, width 10 μm, and thickness 1 μm made from this material, we can estimate a spring constant $k = 2.3$ N/m and a resonant frequency $f_0 = 400$ kHz.

For the purposes of this analysis, a quality factor, Q, of 100 is chosen for the cantilever, as this is a typical room-pressure-limited value for microcantilevers [45]. Assuming an ambient room temperature of 293 K gives a DND$_{br}$ of 5.2 fm/$\sqrt{\text{Hz}}$. For the cantilever, using an electrical bandwidth matched to the mechanical bandwidth such that $\Delta f = 2f_0/Q = 8$ kHz, the thermomechanical MDD component, MDD$_{br}$, will be 460 fm. It is worth noting that increasing the length of the cantilever will also increase this DND component, while increasing the width and thickness will decrease the DND. This means that for sensors where the thermomechanical noise is an issue, shorter, wider, and thicker cantilevers are preferred.

3.5.1.2 Shot noise

The signal-to-shot-noise-limited MDD, MDD$_{sn}$, is defined by [30]

$$\text{MDD}_{sn} = \frac{1}{\sqrt{\text{SNR}_{sn}}} = \sqrt{\frac{2e\eta \Delta f}{S^2 P_{in} \gamma}}. \quad (3.10)$$

This leads to a shot-noise-limited DND, DND$_{sn}$, given by

$$\text{DND}_{sn} = \frac{\text{MDD}_{sn}}{\sqrt{\Delta f}} = \sqrt{\frac{2e\eta}{S^2 P_{in} \gamma}}. \quad (3.11)$$

At optimum sensitivity, on the basis of the FDTD simulations, an input power P_{in} of 1 mW at a wavelength of 1550 nm coupled into the input waveguide is assumed. If an InGaAs PIN detector with a photodetector responsivity γ of 1 A/W is used, the optimal shot-noise-limited DND for the cantilever is 4.1 fm/$\sqrt{\text{Hz}}$. For the same bandwidth, Δf of 8 kHz, the shot-noise-limited MDD will be

370 fm. Note that since η and, correspondingly, S are defined to be independent of P_in, both MDD_sn and DND_sn scale in relation to $1/\sqrt{P_\text{in}}$.

The shot-noise-limited DND over the gap range up to 3 μm is plotted in Fig. 3.18. It can be seen that the shot-noise-limited DND remains below 25 fm/$\sqrt{\text{Hz}}$ for most of this gap range.

3.5.1.3 Johnson noise

Johnson noise current is the thermal current in the load resistor of the photodetector, i_jn, and is defined by [46]

$$i_\text{jn} = \sqrt{\frac{4k_b T \Delta f}{R}} \qquad (3.12)$$

where R is the load resistance. The Johnson-noise-limited MDD, MDD_jn, is then defined as

$$\text{MDD}_\text{jn} = \frac{1}{\sqrt{\text{SNR}_\text{jn}}} = \sqrt{\frac{4k_b T \Delta f}{R S^2 P_\text{in}^2 \gamma^2}} \qquad (3.13)$$

and the Johnson-noise-limited DND, DND_jn, will be

$$\text{DND}_\text{jn} = \frac{\text{MDD}_\text{jn}}{\sqrt{\Delta f}} = \sqrt{\frac{4k_b T}{R S^2 P_\text{in}^2 \gamma^2}}. \qquad (3.14)$$

At optimum sensitivity the Johnson-noise-limited DND will be 1.3 fm/$\sqrt{\text{Hz}}$. This uses the same InGaAs PIN detector and power as for the shot noise analysis above, a photodetector responsivity γ of 1 A/W, and a load resistance of 1 kΩ at room temperature. Using the same bandwidth of $\Delta f = 8$ kHz as above, the Johnson-noise-limited MDD will be 120 fm.

3.5.1.4 Total noise

The total noise is the square root of the sum of the squares of all noise contributions, and so when taking the MDD components from shot noise, Johnson noise, and thermal mechanical noise, the final MDD is 600 fm. The total DND is similarly calculated to be 6.8 fm/$\sqrt{\text{Hz}}$.

This is an impressive result, as it predicts that this grating readout technique can be capable of subpicometer resolution. As the shot noise limit is lower than the thermal mechanical noise limit, the readout technique can also be used the study the Brownian motion of microcantilevers.

3.5.2 Experimental Limits of Detection

In this section, the MDD and DND equations will be applied to an optical measurement of a cantilever structure that was fabricated. The shot noise limit of this technology is low enough for the measurement system to be able to detect the thermomechanical motion of the cantilever beam (induced from room-temperature and pressure variations). In this section, the theoretical Brownian noise density of the cantilever will be calculated and compared to values measured by the system when the cantilever actuation signal is grounded.

Due to interest in characterizing MEMS cantilevers for use in atomic force microscopes (AFMs), substantial work in the literature has been performed on the topic of predicting Brownian motion for a MEMS cantilever. The z direction component of the Brownian noise density, $n_{zb}(f)$, in units of $m/\sqrt{Hz}$, of the tip of a MEMS cantilever around its resonant frequency (mode 1) can be predicted by [47]

$$n_{zb}(f) = \sqrt{\frac{2k_b T}{\pi Q k f_0} \frac{1}{\left(1 - \left[\left\{\frac{f}{f_0}\right\}^2 + \frac{f}{f_0}Q\right]\right)^2}}, \quad (3.15)$$

where k_b is Boltzmann's constant, T is temperature (K), Q is the quality factor of the cantilever, k is the spring constant of the cantilever, f_0 is the resonant mechanical frequency of the cantilever, and f is the frequency of interest. The values adopted for the cantilever are a temperature of 293 K, a quality factor of 7.2, and a resonant mechanical frequency of 13.2 kHz.

An accurate spring constant k for the cantilever that takes into account the medium that it is moving in can be calculated using the Sader method [48] to be 6.06 mN/m. The Sader method was designed to calculate parameters for AFMs and is known to be extremely precise.

The region measured by the grating is not at the tip of the microcantilever but rather at the midpoint. This region will only

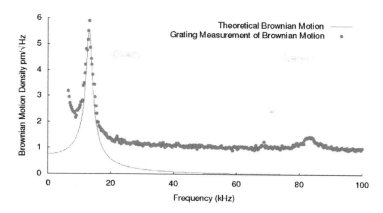

Figure 3.19 Predicted Brownian noise envelope compared to measured optical power modulation from a readout device.

move 34% the distance that the tip moves, so the Brownian noise deflection density at the midpoint above the interrogating grating, $n_{\text{zbm}}(f)$, can be estimated by

$$n_{\text{zbm}}(f) = 0.34 n_{\text{zb}}(f) \qquad (3.16)$$

This function is plotted in Fig. 3.19 (solid line).

Measurements for the Brownian motion were performed in an open laboratory environment, and Fig. 3.19 presents the power transmitted through the device as a function of frequency. Two peaks can be seen in the measured spectrum, one at the fundamental resonant frequency of the cantilever at 13.2 kHz and one at the first harmonic frequency of 83 kHz.

It can be seen that around the resonance frequency the measured values strongly follow the envelope predicted by Eq. 3.16, showing excellent agreement, and that this readout technique is sensitive enough to detect Brownian motion at the midpoint of the cantilever beam. The magnitude of the noise density measured at the fundamental resonant frequency peak is slightly greater than the theoretically predicted Brownian noise density. This is likely because of the additional acoustic noise present in the laboratory environment adding additional excitations to the cantilever. The noise floor when using this laser can be seen from Fig. 3.19 to be around 1 pm/$\sqrt{\text{Hz}}$.

The ability to use an integrated interrogating diffraction grating to determine the position of a MEMS cantilever with this level of sensitivity is an excellent result. Groups such as Nieradka et al. [19] have recently performed work using an external optics-based real-time Brownian noise extraction technique to measure the movement of microcantilever biosensors in environments where the external excitation of vibrations is undesirable. The integrated optical technique described in this chapter is sensitive enough to also be capable of this feat, and since this technique can be optical-fiber-fed, it eliminates the need for the alignment of large external optics.

3.6 Conclusions

MEMS-based gas sensors are a new technology with the potential to provide extremely sensitive chemical gas-sensing capabilities. For these sensors to be adopted commercially, a readout technique is required that is capable of measuring ultrasmall, out-of-plane movements of MEMS devices. It is desirable that such a technique have the ability to address large arrays of devices, while maintaining subnanometer position resolution.

This chapter has presented a position-sensing element that meets these requirements by using a nanostructured silicon photonics grating to create a resonant cavity beneath a suspended MEMS mechanical beam. The transmission of light through this cavity was measured, and found to give an extremely accurate measure of the position of the mechanical beam.

The technique was used to measure the Brownian motion of a MEMS cantilever at room temperature and pressure. The technique was shown to be sensitive enough to measure both first and second harmonic modes of the Brownian motion.

Acknowledgments

We acknowledge the support from the Australian Research Council, the Australia-India Strategic Research Fund, the Australian National

Fabrication Facility (Western Australian Node), and the Office of Science of the WA State Government.

References

1. Roylance, L., and Angell, J. A miniature integrated circuit accelerometer, in *Solid-State Circuits Conference. Digest of Technical Papers. 1978 IEEE International*, Vol. XXI, 1978, 220–221.
2. Terry, S. C., Jerman, J. H., and Angell, J. B. A gas chromatographic air analyzer fabricated on a silicon wafer, *IEEE Trans. Electron. Devices*, **26**(12), 1979, 1880–1886.
3. Ishihara, T., Suzuki, K., Suwazono, S., Hirata, M., and Tanigawa, H. CMOS integrated silicon pressure sensor, *IEEE J. Solid-State Circuits*, **22**(2), 1987, 151–156.
4. Bryzek, J., Mayer, R., and Barth, P. Disposable blood pressure sensors with digital on-chop laser trimming, in *Technical Digest of the IEEE Solid-State Sensor and Actuator Workshop, 1988*, 1988, 121–122.
5. Yalcinkaya, A. D., Urey, H., Brown, D., Montague, T., and Sprague, R. Two-axis electromagnetic microscanner for high resolution displays, *J. Microelectromech. Syst.*, **15**(4), 2006, 786–794.
6. Yang, Y. T., Callegari, C., Feng, X. L., and Roukes, M. L. Surface adsorbate fluctuations and noise in nanoelectromechanical systems, *Nano Lett.*, **11**(4), 2011, 1753–1759.
7. Boisen, A., and Thundat, T. Design & fabrication of cantilever array biosensors, *Mater. Today*, **12**(9), 2009, 32–38.
8. Norton, F. J. *Gas Analyzer*, US patent 230780012-Jan-1943.
9. Shaver, P. J. Bimetal strip hydrogen gas detectors, *Rev. Sci. Instrum.*, **40**(7), 1969, 901–905.
10. Greenwood, J. C. Etched silicon vibrating sensor, *J. Phys. E: Sci. Instrum.*, **17**(8), 1984, 650.
11. Howe, R. T., and Muller, R. S. Resonant-microbridge vapor sensor, *IEEE Trans. Electron Devices*, **33**(4), 1986, 499–506.
12. Howe, R. T. Polycrystalline silicon micromachining: a new technology for integrated sensors, *Annu. Biomed. Eng.*, **14**(2), 1986, 187–197.
13. Kalinina, S., Gliemann, López-García, H., M., Petershans, A., Auernheimer, J., Schimmel, T., Bruns, M., Schambony, A., Kessler, H., and Wedlich, D.

Isothiocyanate-functionalized RGD peptides for tailoring cell-adhesive surface patterns, *Biomaterials*, **29**(20), 2008, 3004–3013.

14. Lavrik, N. V., Tipple, C. A., Sepaniak, M. J., and Datskos, P. G. Gold nano-structures for transduction of biomolecular interactions into micrometer scale movements, *Biomed. Microdevices*, **3**(1), 2001, 35–44.

15. Kong, D., Mei, T., Tao, Y., Ni, L., Zhang, T., Lu, W., Zhang, Z., and Wang, R. A MEMS sensor array for explosive particle detection, in *Proceedings of the International Conference on Information Acquisition, 2004*, 2004, 278–281.

16. Alvarez, M., Calle, A., Tamayo, J., Lechuga, L. M., Abad, A., and Montoya, A. Development of nanomechanical biosensors for detection of the pesticide DDT, *Biosens. Bioelectron.*, **18**(5–6), 2003, 649–653.

17. Huber, F., Lang, H. P., Backmann, N., Rimoldi, D., and Gerber, C. Direct detection of a BRAF mutation in total RNA from melanoma cells using cantilever arrays, *Nat. Nanotechnol.*, **8**(2), 2013, 125–129.

18. Sader, J. E. Frequency response of cantilever beams immersed in viscous fluids with applications to the atomic force microscope, *J. Appl. Phys.*, **84**(1), 1998, 64–76.

19. Nieradka, K., Gotszalk, T. P., and Schroeder, G. A novel method for simultaneous readout of static bending and multimode resonance-frequency of microcantilever-based biochemical sensors, *Sens. Actuators, B*, **170**, 2012, 172–175.

20. Burg, T. P., Godin, M., Knudsen, S. M., Shen, W., Carlson, G., Foster, J. S., Babcock, K., and Manalis, S. R. Weighing of biomolecules, single cells and single nanoparticles in fluid, *Nature*, **446**(7139), 2007, 1066–1069.

21. Dufrêne, Y. F. Towards nanomicrobiology using atomic force microscopy, *Nat. Rev. Microbiol.*, **6**(9), 2008, 674–680.

22. Okuyama, S., Mitobe, Y., Okuyama, K., and Matsushita, K. Hydrogen gas sensing using a Pd-coated cantilever, *Jpn. J. Appl. Phys.*, **39**(Part 1, No. 6A), 2000, 3584–3590.

23. Salama, K., and Ko, C. R. Effect of hydrogen on the temperature dependence of the elastic constants of palladium single crystals, *J. Appl. Phys.*, **51**(12), 1980, 6202–6209.

24. Sieverts, A. Absorption of gases by metals, *Z. Metallkd.*, **21**, 1929, 37–46.

25. Binnig, G., Quate, C. F., and Gerber, C. Atomic force microscope, *Phys. Rev. Lett.*, **56**(9), 1986, 930–933.

26. Meyer, G., and Amer, N. M. Novel optical approach to atomic force microscopy, *Appl. Phys. Lett.*, **53**(12), 1988, 1045–1047.

27. Pruessner, M. W., Stievater, T. H., and Rabinovich, W. S. In-plane microelectromechanical resonator with integrated Fabry–Pérot cavity, *Appl. Phys. Lett.*, **92**(8), 2008, 081101–081101.
28. Eichenfield, M. A picogram- and nanometre-scale photonic-crystal optomechanical cavity, *Nature*, **459**(7246), 2009, 550–555.
29. Lang, H. P., Baller, M. K., Berger, R., Gerber, C., Gimzewski, J. K., Battiston, F. M., Fornaro, P., Ramseyer, J. P., Meyer, E., and Güntherodt, H. J. An artificial nose based on a micromechanical cantilever array, *Anal. Chim. Acta*, **393**(1–3), 1999, 59–65.
30. Stievater, T. H., Rabinovich, W. S., Ferraro, M. S., Papanicolaou, N. A., Bass, R., Boos, J. B., Stepnowski, J. L., and McGill, R. A. Photonic microharp chemical sensors, *Opt. Express*, **16**(4), 2008, 2423–2430.
31. Zinoviev, K., Dominguez, C., Plaza, J. A., Busto, V. J. C., and Lechuga, L. M. A novel optical waveguide microcantilever sensor for the detection of nanomechanical forces, *J. Lightwave Technol.*, **24**(5), 2006, 2132.
32. Putrino, G., Keating, A., Martyniuk, M., Faraone, L., and Dell, J. Model and analysis of a high sensitivity resonant optical read-out approach suitable for cantilever sensor arrays, *IEEE/OSA J. Lightwave Technol.*, **47**, 2012, 386–389.
33. Taillaert, D., F. Van Laere, Ayre, M., Bogaerts, W., D. Van Thourhout, Bienstman, P., and Baets, R. Grating couplers for coupling between optical fibers and nanophotonic waveguides, *Jpn. J. Appl. Phys.*, **45**(8A), 2006, 6071–6077.
34. Hernandez, G., *Fabry-Perot Interferometers*, Cambridge University Press, Cambridge; New York, 1986.
35. Dumon, P., Bogaerts, W., Baets, R., Fedeli, J.-M., and Fulbert, L. Towards foundry approach for silicon photonics: silicon photonics platform ePIXfab, *Electron. Lett.*, **45**(12), 2009, 581–582.
36. Bennett, J. M., and Ashley, E. J. Infrared reflectance and emittance of silver and gold evaporated in ultrahigh vacuum, *Appl. Opt.*, **4**(2), 1965, 221–224.
37. Huang, H., Winchester, K. J., Suvorova, A., Lawn, B. R., Liu, Y., Hu, X. Z., Dell, J. M., and Faraone, L. Effect of deposition conditions on mechanical properties of low-temperature PECVD silicon nitride films, *Mater. Sci. Eng. A*, **435–436**, 2006, 453–459.
38. Ladabaum, I., Jin, X., Soh, H. T., Atalar, A., and Khuri-Yakub, B. t. Surface micromachined capacitive ultrasonic transducers, *IEEE Trans. Ultrason. Ferroelectr. Freq. Control*, **45**(3), 1998, 678–690.

39. Mohr, P. J., Taylor, B. N., and Newell, D. B. CODATA recommended values of the fundamental physical constants: 2010, *Rev. Mod. Phys.*, **84**(4), 2012, 1527–1605.
40. Tas, N., Sonnenberg, T., Jansen, H., Legtenberg, R., and Elwenspoek, M. Stiction in surface micromachining, *J. Micromech. Microeng.*, **6**(4), 1996. 385.
41. Yaralioglu, G. G., Atalar, A., Manalis, S. R., and Quate, C. F. Analysis and design of an interdigital cantilever as a displacement sensor, *J. Appl. Phys.*, **83**(12), 1998, 7405–7415.
42. Fock, L. S., Kwan, A., and Tucker, R. Reduction of semiconductor laser intensity noise by feedforward compensation: experiment and theory, *J. Lightwave Technol.*, **10**(12), 1992, 1919–1925.
43. Kocabas, C., and Aydinli, A. Design and analysis of an integrated optical sensor for scanning force microscopies, *IEEE Sens. J.*, **5**(3), 2005, 411–418.
44. Riley, F. L. Silicon nitride and related materials, *J. Am. Ceram. Soc.*, **83**(2), 2000, 245–265.
45. Yasumura, K. Y., Stowe, T. D., Chow, E. M., Pfafman, T., Kenny, T. W., Stipe, B. C., and Rugar, D. Quality factors in micron- and submicron-thick cantilevers, *J. Microelectromech. Syst.*, **9**(1), 2000, 117–125.
46. Nyquist, H. Thermal agitation of electric charge in conductors, *Phys. Rev.*, **32**(1), 1928, 110–113.
47. Fukuma, T., Kimura, M., Kobayashi, K., Matsushige, K., and Yamada, H. Development of low noise cantilever deflection sensor for multienvironment frequency-modulation atomic force microscopy, *Rev. Sci. Instrum.*, **76**(5), 2005, 053704–053704-8.
48. Sader, J. E., Chon, J. W. M., and Mulvaney, P. Calibration of rectangular atomic force microscope cantilevers, *Rev. Sci. Instrum.*, **70**(10), 1999, 3967–3969.

Biography

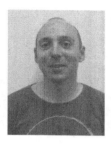

Gino Putrino was born in Perth, Australia, and is a researcher in the field of sensors based on optical microelectromechanical systems (MEMS). He received a BSc degree in computer science and a BE (Hons.) degree in electrical and electronic engineering from the University of Western Australia, Perth in 1999. He submitted a PhD thesis on research in the fields of silicon photonics and MEMS in mid-2013.

Putrino has worked in several IT and engineering roles in Australia and the U.S., in the cities of Perth, Sydney, Melbourne, San Francisco, Milwaukee and Portsmouth. He is currently a researcher at the University of Western Australia.

Chapter 4

Aluminum Gallium Nitride/Gallium Nitride Transistor-Based Biosensor

Anna Podolska, Gia Parish, and Brett Nener
School of Electrical, Electronic and Computer Engineering, University of Western Australia, 35 Stirling Highway, Crawley, WA 6009, Australia
anna.podolska@epfl.ch

Drug testing on live human cells is an expensive, time-consuming, and difficult process involving multiple specific assays with different formats and dynamic ranges. It also requires highly trained personnel to manipulate often dangerous chemicals for cell-labeling purposes. Therefore this research addresses an effort to develop an easy-to-use sensor device for label-free, real-time, live cell monitoring. An investigation into an AlGaN/GaN transistor-based sensor utilized for chemical and biological detection is presented. The biocompatibility, sensitivity, and optimized operational design are discussed in detail. Successful application of the sensor for drug testing is demonstrated. Results presented here demonstrate that an AlGaN-/GaN-based biosensor has potential to reveal the rich signaling texture of living cells that can be beneficial for development and testing of new drugs and treatment methods. This study concludes that further research and development of all solid-state sensor systems for biomedical applications is warranted.

Nanomaterials: Science and Applications
Edited by Deborah Kane, Adam Micolich, and Peter Roger
Copyright © 2016 Pan Stanford Publishing Pte. Ltd.
ISBN 978-981-4669-72-6 (Hardcover), 978-981-4669-73-3 (eBook)
www.panstanford.com

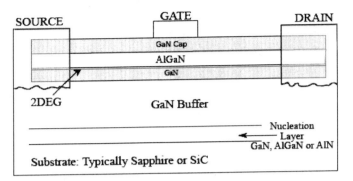

Figure 4.1 An example of an AlGaN/GaN heterostructure with multiple GaN and AlGaN layers grown on a crystalline substrate.

4.1 Introduction to Aluminum Gallium Nitride/Gallium Nitride Transistor-Based Biosensors

The AlGaN/GaN heterostructure is a very useful semiconductor material structure with multiple applications. This structure is created via metalorganic or molecular beam deposition of nanometer-scale crystalline films of GaN and AlGaN on crystalline substrates such as sapphire, SiC, Si, or bulk GaN. An example is shown in Fig. 4.1.

Within the last two decades, AlGaN/GaN developments have led to rapid progress in optoelectronic devices such as lasers and light-emitting diodes (LEDs), and high-electron-mobility transistors (HEMTs). Applications under development range from photonics and high-power electronics to chemical and biological sensors. These rely on AlGaN's/GaN's exceptional properties, as listed below:

- High physical and chemical stability [1, 2]
- A wide bandgap that allows operation at elevated temperatures (up to 600°C)
- High spontaneous and piezoelectric polarization, which is responsible for the creation of a high-electron-mobility and high-density two-dimensional electron gas (2DEG) channel for use in transistors, even in undoped structures
- Superior biological compatibility when compared to GaAs and even Si [3, 4]

- High sensitivity to surface charges [5]
- Optical transparency of AlGaN/GaN in the visible range, allowing simultaneous electronic and microscopic control of biosensing.

These properties determine the AlGaN/GaN heterostructure is an outstanding candidate material for the realization of biological and chemical sensors. The AlGaN/GaN field-effect transistor (FET) is the specific device that is implemented. The current between the source and drain of the FET is measured. High sensitivity to surface charges introduced to the active area (between source and drain) is a key property for detection of biological and/or chemical compounds of the gateless FET. This sensitivity is defined by properties of high electron mobility and a high-density 2DEG.

In the most general meaning of the term a "biosensor" is a device capable of detecting biological activity. Normally such devices consist of a bioreceptor and a transducer. A bioreceptor has properties that allow specific interaction with samples of interest, the analytes. Such interaction results in a biological and/or chemical signal that can be detected by a transducer. The transducer transforms the detected signal into an electrical or optical output that can be further processed and analyzed. Such a definition is schematically illustrated in Fig. 4.2.

AlGaN/GaN FETs are well suited for the construction of transducers. Depending on the application, enzymes, antibodies, DNA, or live cells can be used as bioreceptors. However, live cells are the major focus of this chapter. Thus, an AlGaN/GaN transducer, utilized for characterization of live cell electrical properties, will be discussed

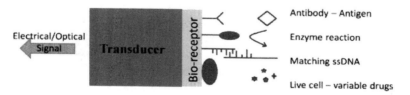

Figure 4.2 Functional principles of a biosensor illustrating four key types of bioreceptor modification and the resulting reaction with analytes of interest such as, from top to bottom of the image on the right, antibody–antigen, enzyme reaction, detection of matching ssDNA, and live cell drug detection.

further in more detail. Also, sensing utilizing this material system can be beneficial in terms of the possibility of monolithic integration with III-nitride optoelectronics for combined spectroscopic analysis, transistors for on-chip signal processing, and surface acoustic wave devices [6] for analog signal filtering.

One of the earliest approaches to the characterization of live cell electrical properties has been demonstrated by Hodgkin and Huxley in the early 50s. They studied single cells by transfixing the cellular membrane with glass microelectrodes and recording the intracellular signal of the neuronal cells [7]. The work of Abuse [8] in the mid-70s continued on from Hodgkin and Huxley's approach and led to the development of the patch-clamp technique, which is still widely used in pharmaceutical and physiological research. However, the patch-clamp procedure has a few major disadvantages. It is complicated and requires specially trained personnel. It is also invasive and always destroys the cell after measurement. During a patch-clamp measurement the cells are subjected to a high degree of stress, which makes an observation over several hours impossible. Moreover, the patch-clamp technique can be used to observe only a few cells at the same time.

At around the same time as development of the patch-clamp technique, the first planar microelectrode array for the recording of the extracellular signal of cells was designed by Thomas et al. [9]. In the early 80s this method was combined with the patch-clamp technique to simultaneously record intracellular and extracellular signals [10]. On the basis of these techniques studies on cultured cells were continued by numerous research groups examining many different cell types over the years [11–15]. Another device capable of extracellular signal recording was introduced in the early 90s by Fromherz et al. FETs were used for the measurement of extracellular signals from single cells [16], as well as the capacitive stimulation of neurons through a thin oxide layer [17]. FET devices do not exhibit any of the disadvantages mentioned above for the patch-clamp technique. An additional advantage of FETs is their ion sensitivity. Ion-sensitive field-effect transistors (ISFETs) have historically been based on silicon technology because of the cost-effective mass production that is available. However, long-term chemical stability of silicon ISFETs in liquids can only be achieved through sophisticated insulation [18]. AlGaN-/GaN-based ISFETs are an excellent alternative to Si ISFETs since they exhibit superior stability to the liquid phase [19–21]. In 2003 the first application of AlGaN-/GaN-based ISFETs for pH sensing was reported by Steinhoff et al. [20]. Two years later, the same authors reported the recording of an action potential from heart muscle cells and demonstrated the superior signal amplitude of AlGaN-/GaN-based FETs compared to similar devices based on silicon technologies [22].

4.2 Current Technological Challenges and Limitations

One major motivation is that AlGaN-/GaN-based live cell sensor technology can assist in drug development and low-cost diagnostics of disease for the broader community. To convert an AlGaN/GaN HEMT into an ISFET the gate electrode must be replaced with live cells. Electrical potential on the cell membrane will act as the gate electrode. Therefore any changes in the state of the cell due to membrane ion transport will be reflected in the change of charge on the AlGaN/GaN surface, which produces a signal that can be easily detected and amplified. However, there are some challenges in stabilization of short- and long-term drift of the sensor signal, improvement of the ion sensitivity to meet or exceed the 59 mV/pH benchmark set by glass electrodes, reliable packaging and encapsulation of sensor chips that can ensure viable conditions for live cells, and, last but not least, the need for all-solid-state reference electrodes. Commonly applied reference electrodes negate such advantages as sensor integrability and scalability to micro- and nanodimensions and make sensor operation as bulky as standard glass ion-sensitive electrodes (approx. 15–20 cm long). The following section describes an investigation into overcoming this particular drawback.

    The semiconductor interface with living cells must be separately addressed. In particular, compatibility between the semiconductor surface and the living cell, as well as attachment and morphology at the interface, must be understood for accurate interpretation of sensor signals.

4.2.1 Reference-Electrode-Free Operation

Ever since Bergveld [23] introduced the concept of an ISFET the field of solid-state-based sensing devices has been focused on material selection to improve the performance of ISFETs, both for pH and for specific ion-sensing applications. As discussed in the introduction, Si-based FETs were used for chemical sensing at first. The sensing was realized through conductivity modulations of the source–drain channel due to chemical responsiveness of the gate metal oxide layer. Unfortunately, Si-based devices suffered from chemical instability and drift in liquid solutions and therefore are not suitable for live cell–based sensors. Also, optimally designed Si-based devices are normally off. Thus, it is crucial to apply a reference electrode in order to bias the gate of the transistor beyond the threshold voltage to allow minority carriers to travel through the conductive channel. Although Si-based transistors can operate without a reference electrode when fabricated on heavily doped Si wafers (normally-on devices), such heavy doping results in decreased device performance (e.g., poor electron mobility) and increased manufacturing costs. Therefore most Si-based ISFETs utilize a reference electrode as part of the sensor, which introduces bulkiness and fragility to the system. An average size of a standard reference electrode is approximately 15–20 cm long, while the biggest AlGaN/GaN sensor tested in this work is only 3 × 3 mm). On-chip miniaturized Ag/AgCl reference electrodes have been designed and tested, but their fabrication is typically complex. An electrode leakage solution remains a serious issue compromising sensor accuracy and device lifetime [24]. Another approach has been to bias the transistor with an on-chip noble metal electrode, for example, gold, deposited on the gate area. This addition on its own is not found to be adequate. The metal/electrolyte interface potential is rendered unstable. To account for such instability a reference field-effect transistor (REFET) with a chemically passivated gate surface can be used in conjunction with the unpassivated ISFET device [25]. However, despite many attempts, this method also suffers from chemical instability and drift [26].

In contrast to the Si-based transistor sensors, conventionally grown AlGaN/GaN HEMTs are normally on and therefore are an excellent alternative. They have higher device transconductance, vastly improved chemical stability, and diminished charging effects [20]. It has been shown that both ultrathin (below 10 nm thick layers) AlGaN/GaN structures and traditional AlGaN/GaN structure devices (20–30 nm thick layers) can maintain high sensitivity even when used without a reference electrode. The transconductance can be very high when the gate–drain voltage is near zero [22, 27]. This concept is now extended to AlGaN/GaN biosensor devices. The results show that a reference electrode is not required for selective ion detection.

The key difference between systems operated with and without a reference electrode is the way in which the sensor response is measured. In both cases, the device current is kept constant using a feedback loop during sensor measurements. For any ISFET operated with a reference electrode, the source–drain voltage also remains constant, while the gate voltage (liquid-gated via the reference electrode) is varied. In this case the change in the surface potential is attributed to the varying potential applied to the reference electrode and Nernstian behavior (the linear shift in gate voltage, 59 mV per unit of pH) is expected. In the reference-electrode-free setup, the conductivity of the conducting channel is being probed directly, as the effective gate bias changes with exposure to different ion concentrations. Thus, any variations in surface potential result in changing channel conductivity. At the same time the source–drain voltage is varied to maintain a constant device current. In this case, gate voltage (V_G) is not measured directly. However, even without a reference electrode, near-Nernstian behavior can be demonstrated through calculations using measured drain-to-source current or voltage (I_{SD} or V_{SD}) to obtain V_G.

The behavior of FETs operated in the nonsaturated (triode) regime can be described by Eq. 4.1 [28]:

$$I_D = \mu C \frac{W}{L} V_{SD} (V_G - V_T) - \frac{1}{2} V_{SD} \tag{4.1}$$

where I_D is the drain current, μ is the channel electron mobility, C is the capacitance per unit area of the gate, W is the channel width, L is the channel length, V_{SD} is the source-to-drain voltage, V_G is the gate voltage, and V_T is the threshold voltage. For very small drain voltages ($V_{SD} << V_G - V_T$) Eq. 4.1 can be approximated as a linear equation

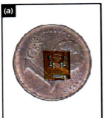 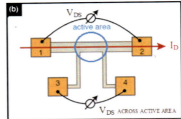

Figure 4.3 Photograph of ungated AlGaN/GaN heterostructure-based devices (a) and measurement configuration for Kelvin probe measurements (b). Yellow (squares 1–4) areas: 20/50/300 nm Al/Cr/Au ohmic contacts. Gray area: mesa etched structure.

(Eq. 4.2) [28]:

$$I_D = \mu C \frac{W}{L} V_{SD}(V_G - V_T) \quad I_D = \mu C \frac{W}{L} V_{SD}(V_G - V_T) \quad (4.2)$$

In the case of precisely known parameters (through design and measurement) the variable gate voltage V_G can be obtained from the above equation.

4.2.2 Device Design, Fabrication, and Packaging

The AlGaN/GaN ISFET devices discussed in this chapter were designed for reference-electrode-free measurements. Device design was based on a four-point probe measurement configuration (Kelvin probe or four-terminal sensing) to provide more accurate measurements than traditional two-terminal sensing (Fig. 4.3). Not only is this design more accurate but the sheet resistance of the device can be measured, if necessary. The separation of current and voltage electrodes in four-terminal measurement eliminates the impedance contribution of the wiring and contact resistances. Therefore the effects of any differences in ohmic contacts that can occur during processing and differences in sensor wiring are eliminated.

During measurements the source–drain potential V_{SD} was adjusted using a feedback loop to keep I_D constant (Fig. 4.3) when the effective gate bias changes with exposure to different ion concentrations. The change in V_{SD} due to changes in the charge on the exposed active area were logged as a function of time and therefore changes in channel conductivity can be calculated according to Eq. 4.3 and used for further calculations to obtain changes in gate potential referred to the source contact, if necessary (Eq. 4.4). Furthermore, the current I_D was selected such that the device was operating in the linear region.

The conductivity of the reference-electrode-free sensor can be calculated according to the equations below, where V_{DS-34} refers to voltage across the active area:

$$6 = \frac{I_D}{V_{DS-34}} \qquad (4.3)$$

$$6 = \frac{(V_G - V_T)\mu C W}{L} \qquad (4.4)$$

where capacitance per unit area of the dielectric layer (i.e., AlGaN and the GaN cap) is given by Eq. 4.5 below (by combining C_{AlGaN} and $C_{GaN\ cap}$ in series to give the total C), with the dielectric constant for the AlGaN layer empirically related to the Al mole fraction (x) by the relationship given in Eq. 4.6.

$$C = \frac{\varepsilon_0 \varepsilon_{material}}{d} \qquad (4.5)$$

$$\varepsilon_{material}(x) = -0.5x + 9.5 \qquad (4.6)$$

The channel width and length are defined during device fabrication and can easily be accounted for in calculations described above.

All devices discussed in this chapter were processed according to standard in-house processes at the Western Australian Node of the Australian National Fabrication Facility. Prior to any technological steps, the wafers were cleaned using standard cleaning procedures. Optical microscopy was used for material and sensor characterization during the technological steps. To realize the ISFET sensor for this project standard UV photolithography was used for pattern definition. Mesa etching of AlGaN/GaN wafers was performed in an Oxford 100 inductively coupled plasma reactive ion etching (ICP RIE) system using a Cl_2-based etch process. After defining the active area with etching, the 20/50/300 nm Al/Cr/Au ohmic contacts to the 2DEG channel were realized through thermal metal evaporation and annealing in a rapid thermal annealing (RTA) system.

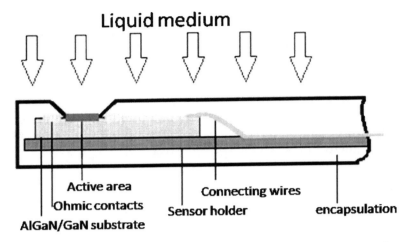

Figure 4.4 Absorption and penetration of the moisture through the encapsulation of ISFET sensor chip.

It is crucial to achieve stability and reproducibility of the device in aggressive liquid environments. The possibility of electrochemical reaction (as well as short circuiting) between metal contacts and liquid must be eliminated. Therefore, passivation and encapsulation of the device is normally used to physically separate metal contacts from liquids, while the sensitive gate area should be left open to the solution (Fig. 4.4) [29].

Moreover, encapsulation should provide the possibility for general sensor cleaning and sensor replacement, if necessary, as well as be compatible with mass production techniques, preferably at the wafer stage [30]. It should also allow for robust sterilization for biological, pharmaceutical, and medical applications. The biocompatibility of materials used for encapsulation is another challenge that needs to be addressed. There are numerous methods reported in the literature, such as photolithographic structuring or curing [31], sealing around the chemically sensitive gate area with elastomeric material, capillary fill, embedding of chips by means of a male mold, and encapsulation with prefabricated housing [29, 30, 32, 33]. Although numerous materials such as glass [34], epoxy resin [35, 36], polyimide [37], and SiN [38] have been used for

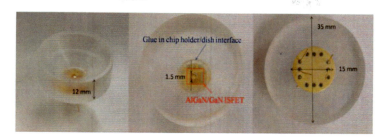

Figure 4.5 Petri dish–packaged AlGaN/GaN ISFET device on TO-8 12-pin transistor outline packages for live cell measurements (side, top, and bottom views).

encapsulation, none of these materials can completely meet all the requirements outlined above.

The active area of all devices used in this study was defined by an AZ2035 negative photoresist that was hard-baked for 1 hour at 200°C. The baked photoresist was resistant to acids and bases in the pH range from 2 to 12. After this passivation step, the wafer was cut using a diamond saw in order to separate single-sensor devices, which were individually characterized.

For the experiments where cells are coupled to the sensor, devices were further encapsulated using printed circuit board (PCB) holders with Cu metallization or a standard chip holder (TO-8 12-pin transistor outline package), glue, silicon rubber, and custom-machined Petri dishes (see Fig. 4.5 below). Individual devices were glued onto holders and bonded to the photomask-defined PCB metal tracks with silver epoxy or wire bonded to a chip holder with gold wire. Silicone rubber was configured as an o-ring around the sensitive area of the device to protect it from the glue used on the rest of the chip for Petri dish attachment. The Petri dish was machined in a conic shape with a 1.5 mm hole in the center to decrease the capillary effect at the sensor/dish interface. Passivated and encapsulated devices for cell measurements can be seen in Fig. 4.5.

This type of encapsulation was based on available resources and was cost effective, easy, and quick to realize. The sensor surface could be easily washed and sterilized. Also, devices could be recovered and repackaged, if necessary.

4.3 Investigation into Improved Biocompatibility

The high bond strength of AlGaN/GaN semiconductor material makes it extremely resistant to chemical attacks. This, when combined with the surface charge sensitivity of the high-electron-mobility and high-electron-density 2DEG, allows very sensitive but robust sensors for biomedical applications to be created [22, 39, 40]. However, the biocompatibility of this material system must be thoroughly investigated.

Prior to this work, some short-term studies have been published on the biocompatibility between AlGaN/GaN HEMT structures and human embryonic kidney (HEK) and other cells [3, 4, 22, 41]. However, no long-term investigations have been reported on AlGaN/GaN HEMTs and live cell biocompatibility. In this work, the biocompatibility was investigated using methods and techniques that are both comprehensive and complementary.

It is well known that silicon can be easily attacked by biological agents, in particular by cell growth media [4]. Although adequate cell growth can be achieved on an oxidized silicon surface, the adhesion and growth of living cells on AlGaN/GaN were demonstrated to be superior to silicon, independent of device processing steps [4]. Cimalla et al. also reported that rat fibroblast cells (3T3 cells) demonstrated good proliferation and adhesion to the group III nitrides. This was independent of the aluminum concentration in the $Al_xGa_{1-x}N$ alloy ($x = 0$, 0.22, or 1). Also, slightly improved behavior after pretreatment by oxidation was observed. However, to obtain quantitative data they used a manual device called a Neubauer counter that is prone to human error due to manual counting of cells [5]. When exposed to toxic materials the HEK cell line demonstrated a greater increase in cell mortality than did the rat fibroblast cell line in the work of Cimalla et al. This indicates HEK cells are more sensitive to toxic effects. Therefore this cell line was chosen to perform all biocompatibility experiments described in herein. Also, the instrumentation used for quantitative analysis of mortality was more sensitive and accurate than the manual counting using a Neubauer counter glass slide.

Despite the apparently strong advantages of AlGaN over silicon, it is still important to acquire accurate long-term and quantitative

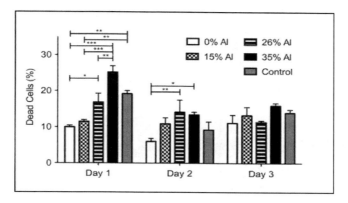

Figure 4.6 Flow cytometry results for mortality of HEK cells grown on $Al_xGa_{1-x}N$/GaN heterostructures with a different percentage of Al (x) and in the control well. Note that x = 0% corresponds to an AlGaN/GaN structure with a thin GaN cap. *p <0.05; **p <0.01; ***p <0.001.

data for cell viability on AlGaN structures as the aluminum mole fraction is varied. Such variation is needed for the optimization of the electrical properties of the sensor. Detailed information on the assessment of biocompatibility starting with simple optical investigations and finishing with sophisticated flow cytometry and electron microscopy methods can be found in the paper published by authors of this chapter [42]. The main results are presented below to highlight key discoveries. To distinguish between different mortality mechanisms of cells the biocompatibility experiment included the flow cytometry analysis (Fig. 4.6) as well as an optical investigation (Fig. 4.7). Additionally cell attachment is demonstrated here on a nanoscale level of electron microscopy images.

The bar diagram shown in Fig. 4.6 represent the flow cytometry results. It can be seen that the concentration of cells at the beginning of the experiment on a 26% Al and 35% Al AlGaN surface is about half of that on the GaN-capped (0% Al) sample and the control well. Therefore there is an average 10% increase in cell mortality with an increase in the Al mole fraction from zero to 35%. However, there are only 4% more dead cells on the control surface than on the AlGaN/GaN wafers with a 35% Al mole fraction.

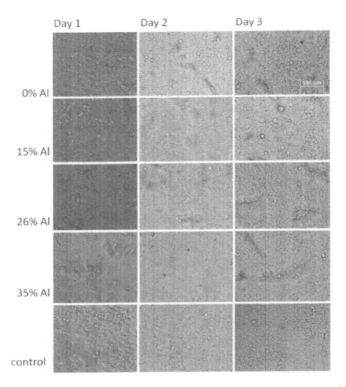

Figure 4.7 Optical micrograph of HEK cells grown on $Al_xGa_{1-x}N/GaN$ heterostructures with a different percentage of Al (x) and in the control well. Note that $x = 0\%$ corresponds to an AlGaN/GaN structure with a thin GaN cap. The calibration bar is shown in the top right image.

There are two mechanisms for cell mortality that may affect flow cytometry results. The first is any type of toxic effect that will decrease cell proliferation and attachment, and the second is the natural mortality of cells in an overcrowded well. Once cells are confluent, they cover the well. As they become overconfluent some cells will detach, die, and float in the medium. These dead cells are not a reflection of toxicity. Paradoxically, this means that more dead cells may be counted in wells that have the best surface for cell growth, because in these wells, initially more cells will have grown, leading to more rapid overcrowding. This is the likely reason why the

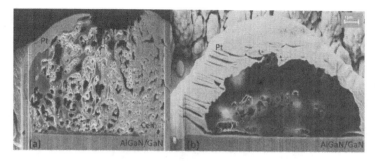

Figure 4.8 FIB/SEM cross sections of liquid-nitrogen-fixed (a) and chemically fixed (b) HEK cell on AlGaN/GaN. Beam voltage = 5 kV. Scale = 1 μm.

control well shows a relatively high percentage of dead cells. It can also be seen that in wells with AlGaN/GaN samples, the number of dead cells increases with the Al concentration. However, in all cases there were still populations of live cells after three days (Fig. 4.7). The number of optical micrographs of HEK cells growing on AlGaN heterostructures presented in Fig. 4.7 demonstrates gradual proliferation and consistent attachment of cells to all experimental types of AlGaN/GaN surfaces used in this experiment. Overall these results indicate that there is good potential for combining HEK cells and the AlGaN/GaN heterostructure for biosensor applications, especially with GaN-capped structures.

The interface between a sensor surface and a live cell is of major interest for interpretation of measured signals. Some insight into cell attachment on the micro- and nanoscale was achieved with scanning electron microscopy (SEM) and transmission electron microscopy (TEM) methods. Results of the SEM and TEM study for the AlGaN/GaN semiconductor/cell interface can be found in the literature [42]. The demonstration of interface attachment of the cell to the AlGaN/GaN surface obtained with a focused ion beam (FIB)/SEM can be found in Fig. 4.8.

The TEM section of AlGaN/GaN and HEK cells obtained in this work is unique in the application of FIB cutting to section the semiconductor/cell interface and provides detailed information about morphology of the interface (Fig. 4.9).

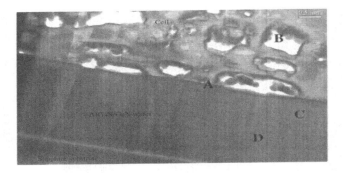

Figure 4.9 Cross-sectional TEM image of HEK cell on AlGaN/GaN. A: cell/semiconductor interface; B: cavities in the cytosol resulting from the FIB preparation technique; C: regions of GaN near the AlGaN layer where strain defects can be seen; D: threading dislocations in the bulk of the GaN. Beam voltage = 200 kV. Scale = 0.5 μm.

4.4 Drug Testing

In the last decade, cell-based AlGaN/GaN FET sensors have been demonstrated for the measurement of cell action potentials, noninvasive cell electrophysiological measurements, and electrical stimulation of cell cultures [22, 43, 44]. However, the strength of the recorded signal was only in the range of tens to hundreds of microvolts [43–45]. Moreover, all of the above-reported work employed a reference electrode as part of the measurement setup and most lacked clear control experiments. This work reports on the development and optimization of AlGaN-/GaN-based biosensors that can successfully operate without a reference electrode. These demonstrate that a high-amplitude (millivolts) signal can be recorded during stimulation of live cells with various chemicals. Chemicals include ionomycin and KCl, which trigger membrane depolarization of living cells, and $CaCl_2$, which influences calcium transport through the cell membrane. The influences of various calcium channel inhibitors and an activator have been also investigated.

All measurements included below were performed on Petri-dish-packaged, four-point bar-shaped, 10 nm $Al_{0.3}Ga_{0.7}N$- and 2 nm GaN-capped devices. Time-dependent recordings of voltage across the

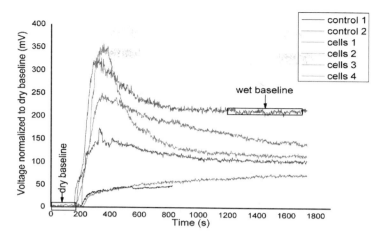

Figure 4.10 Time-dependent voltage response of an AlGaN/GaN sensor to cells suspended in Hank's balanced salt solution (HBSS) and HBSS-only controls. Multiple experiments were performed on the same device with different batches of cells and control solution. These have been normalized to the sensor response in the air (dry baseline).

sensitive area were taken under constant current of 100 µA using a DT82E DataTaker.

Preliminary measurements, using HEK cells from Invitrogen, were undertaken to develop and confirm measurement protocols. The results of the initial investigations to determine reproducibility and baseline behavior of the sensors are given in Fig. 4.10. Multiple runs were performed on the same device with different batches of cells and control solution. For the devices with cells in Hank's balanced salt solution (HBSS), a peak in voltage can be seen immediately after cell seeding. This voltage drops back down to a stable lower voltage 15–20 minutes later. This time approximately corresponds to that for the cells to settle on the surface of the device. No such behavior was observed for the control devices, where HBSS with no cells was present. From Fig. 4.10, two baselines can also be seen: the dry baseline (before the device is exposed to any liquid) and the wet baseline (after exposure to HBSS or cells in HBSS). Stabilization of the wet baseline is essential for correct assignment of responses occurring as the result of further exposure

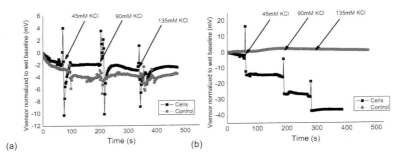

Figure 4.11 Response of AlGaN/GaN sensor with and without cells (labeled as cells and control, respectively) recorded during exposure to 45 mM, 90 mM, and 135 mM of KCl (final concentration) without buffering with HEPES (a) or after buffering with 30 mM HEPES (b). Arrows show the time points at which KCl is added.

to the chemical compounds. For the remainder of the section, device response will be represented as a change in voltage relative to the dry baseline.

To further optimize the sensor, a temperature-controlled environmental chamber with glove-box access was constructed to enable experimental operation/measurement of the sensor, whilst maintaining the required physiological conditions for live cells. Measurements, performed inside this chamber under constant temperature (37°C) and constant light conditions, are further discussed below.

Cell activity was assessed by membrane depolarization after exposure to KCl and compared to the control sample where KCl was added to HBSS solution without cells. Cell depolarization is a rapid change in the cell membrane potential due to exposure to very high concentration of potassium and chlorine ions. This rapid change in the membrane potential can be easily detected by the AlGaN/GaN sensor. However, the sensor itself is sensitive to the concentration of anions in the solution. This can be clearly seen from the response of the control device (Fig. 4.11a), which would only be due to the sensitivity of the device to anion concentration. The response from the device with cells is similar, indicating that even with cells present, the dominant influence is the sensitivity of the device to the change in solution composition. Therefore 4-(2-hydroxyethyl)-

1-piperazineethanesulfonic acid (HEPES) was added to the HBSS to buffer ions. Consequently the addition of KCl will have less effect on anion concentration, allowing changes in sensor surface potential due to the biological activity of the cells to be detected. Thus, a clear difference between devices with cells and the control devices can be observed in the presence of HEPES (Fig. 4.11b).

4.4.1 Sensing Human Coronary Artery Endothelial Cells

The main focus of the study presented here is to confirm measurement of biological activity by the biosensors through stimulation of human coronary artery endothelial cells (HCAEC) with chemicals such as $CaCl_2$ and a number of inhibitors and activators that influence calcium transport through the cell membrane.

Calcium-dosing experiments were performed with HCAE cells obtained from Dr. Livia Hool's laboratory (School of Anatomy, Physiology and Human Biology, University of Western Australia). HCAE cells were isolated from normal human coronary arteries. The cells were then seeded in calcium-free HBSS on the device-sensitive area. For measurements, HBSS solution was buffered with 30 mM HEPES. After wet baseline stabilization, $CaCl_2$ solution was added to HBSS by titration. The concentration of $CaCl_2$ was slowly stepped through the following concentrations (in mM): 0, 0.1, 0.2, 0.3, 0.4, 0.5, 0.8, 1.1, 2.1, 3.1, 5.1, and 10.1. Time for response stabilization was allowed between additions. Figure 4.12 demonstrates results of $CaCl_2$ titration on the packaged sensor with HCAE cells suspended in HBSS and the control device in HBSS with no cells. The observed substantial difference between the response of devices with cells and the control device was repeated in multiple measurements, with saturation of cell response occurring in each instance at a concentration of around 2.5–3 mM $CaCl_2$. This saturation level correlates well with normal physiological calcium intake measured with conventional methods [46].

To further prove detection of calcium channel activity of HCAE cells, Mibefradil, Nisoldipine, and HC-030031 inhibitors and BayK(-) 8644 activator for calcium ion channels were purchased from Sigma Aldrich. In all experiments, 1 µM of the drug (either inhibitor or activator) was added to HBSS after wet baseline stabilization and the

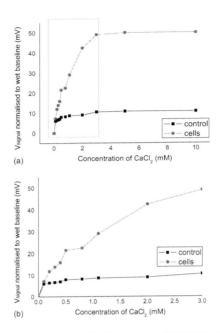

Figure 4.12 Response of AlGaN/GaN sensor in HEPES-buffered HBSS with and without HCAE cells (labeled as cells and control, respectively) recorded for calcium dosing under slow titration conditions (a). Enlargement of graph to show response for low concentrations (dotted area) is given in (b).

system was incubated for a further 10 minutes. After incubation, a calcium-dosing experiment was performed by slow calcium titration with the same protocol as the calcium-dosing experiment described above. Drug-free calcium dosing was used as the control for inhibitor and activator experiments along with the cell-free control.

Incubation of cells in the presence of inhibitors or activators is expected to result in decreased or increased response to calcium dosing, respectively. Incubation is necessary to provide time for the reaction between the chemical and the cell.

The measured results have been normalized to the calcium dosing response without any drug treatment, in addition to being compared to the response for control devices with no cells (Fig. 4.13). It can be seen that the presence of the calcium channel activator S-BayK 8644 increased the measured response and the

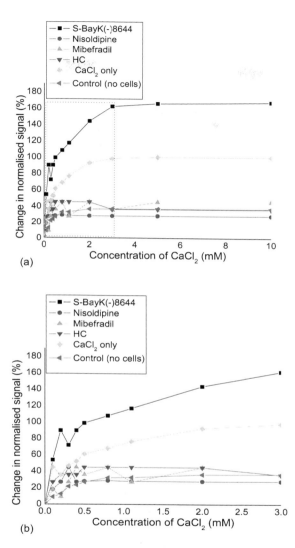

Figure 4.13 Response of AlGaN/GaN sensor in HEPES-buffered HBSS with and without HCAE cells in the presence of inhibitors (Mibefradil, Nisoldipine, HC-03001) and activator (S-BayK(−)8644), recorded for calcium dosing under slow titration conditions (a). Enlargement of dotted area in graph to show response at low concentrations (b). Signals are normalized to $CaCl_2$ titration curve in the absence of inhibitor or activator ($CaCl_2$ only).

presence of the inhibitors decreased the measured response, almost to the level of the control device with no cells. This provides a clear demonstration of the utility of this biosensor to assess both activators and inhibitors of calcium channels.

The results obtained from the cellular calcium intake experiments, presented in Figs. 4.12 and 4.13, demonstrate the capabilities of AlGaN/GaN live cell–based biosensors for label-free detection of physiological cellular events. The device exhibited sensitivity to changes in live cell membrane potential due to increasing concentration of active ions as well as to activation and inhibition of ion channels in the cell membrane. Detection of cellular ion transport signaling provides great insight into overall cellular response. Such a sensor could be very beneficial for pharmacological research dealing with pluridimensional therapeutic targets. This requires a fully matured AlGaN/GaN live cell–based biosensor that can be used as one integrated assay for label-free, real-time, cell-based monitoring replacing multiple specific assays with different formats and dynamic ranges [47].

4.5 Conclusions

In this chapter, AlGaN/GaN heterostructures are investigated as the transducer element for biological sensing. A number of optimizations were introduced. Firstly, the biological sensor was thoroughly investigated for interaction between the semiconductor surface and the living cells attached. The TEM section of AlGaN/GaN and HEK cells obtained in this work is unique in the application of FIB to section the semiconductor/cell interface. Secondly, the sensor design has focused on reference-electrode-free operation. Reference-electrode-free device design is crucial for sensor miniaturization and integration, and this work is the first significant attempt to investigate such an approach. The reference-electrode-free device was fabricated and successfully revealed the rich signaling texture of living cells, providing potential for a comprehensive readout for drug activity. In terms of future work, the first and the most approachable step from an engineering point of view would be a miniaturization and array arrangement of sensors to perform measurements with higher resolution. This step should be followed by appropriate packaging and passivation to ensure overall reliable operation of the chip. TEM and SEM images of the cell/semiconductor interface were obtained and are consistent with the cells being attached. However, there is still much to understand about the nature of cell attachment and about the distribution and functioning of ion channels in the attached cell membrane. Further research in this direction can significantly contribute to the analysis of data obtained with AlGaN/GaN biosensors. Additional TEM imaging of multiple sections of one attached cell can provide 3D information about membrane morphology at the cell/semiconductor interface.

This study has demonstrated that AlGaN-/GaN-based biosensors have tremendous potential to reveal the rich signaling texture of living cells and can provide a comprehensive readout of drug activity.

Acknowledgments

The authors acknowledge partial funding of the work by the Australian Research Council (ARC) Discovery Project scheme (DP0988241) and the ARC Future Fellowships of LCH (FT100100 756) and KDGP (FT100100271). AP received the William and Marlene Schrader Postgraduate Scholarship for Biomedical Engineering. We also acknowledge the scientific and technical assistance of the Centre for Microscopy, Characterisation & Analysis at UWA. This work was performed in part at the Western Australian Node of the Australian National Fabrication Facility.

References

1. Pearton, S. J., Zolper, J. C., Shul, R. J., and Ren, F. GaN: processing, defects, and devices, *J. Appl. Phys.*, **86**(1), 1999, 1–78.
2. Ren, F., and Pearton, S. J. *Semiconductor Device-Based Sensors for Gas, Chemical, and Biomedical Applications*. CRC Press, 2011.
3. Young, T.-H., and Chen, C.-R. Assessment of GaN chips for culturing cerebellar granule neurons, *Biomaterials*, **27**(18), 2006, 3361–3367.

4. Cimalla, I., et al. AlGaN/GaN biosensor: effect of device processing steps on the surface properties and biocompatibility, *Sens. Actuators, B*, **123**(2), 2007, 740–748.

5. Neuberger, R., Müller, G., Ambacher, O., and Stutzmann, M. High-electron-mobility AlGaN/GaN transistors (HEMTs) for fluid monitoring applications, *Phys. Status Solidi A*, **185**(1), 2001, 85–89.

6. Wong, K.-Y., Tang, W., Lau, K. M., and Chen, K. J. Surface acoustic wave device on AlGaN/GaN heterostructure using two-dimensional electron gas interdigital transducers, *Appl. Phys. Lett.*, **90**(21), 2007, 213506.

7. Hodgkin, A. L., and Huxley, A. F. A quantitative description of membrane current and its application to conduction and excitation in nerve, *J. Physiol.*, **117**(4), 1952, 500–544.

8. Abuse, A., Woodson, A. P. B. J., Traynor, M. E., Schlapfer, W. T., and Barondes, S. H., Single-channel currents recorded from membrane of denervated frog muscle fibres, *Nature*, **260**, 1976, 799–802.

9. Thomas, Jr., C. A., Springer, P. A., Loeb, G. E., Berwald-Netter, Y., and Okun, L. M. A miniature microelectrode array to monitor the bioelectric activity of cultured cells, *Exp. Cell Res.*, **74**(1), 1972, 61–66.

10. Pine, J. Recording action potentials from cultured neurons with extracellular microcircuit electrodes, *J. Neurosci. Methods*, **2**(1), 1980, 19–31.

11. Novak, J. L., and Wheeler, B. C. Multisite hippocampal slice recording and stimulation using a 32 element microelectrode array, *J. Neurosci. Methods*, **23**(2), 1988, 149–159.

12. Borkholder, D. Cell based biosensors using microelectrodes [Online], 1998. Available at https://ritdml.rit.edu/handle/1850/5746 (accessed-Sep. 21,2012).

13. Martinoia, S., Bove, M., Carlini, G., Ciccarelli, C., Grattarola, M., Storment, C., and Kovacs, G. A general-purpose system for long-term recording from a microelectrode array coupled to excitable cells, *J. Neurosci. Methods*, **48**(1–2), 1993, 115–121.

14. Droge, M. H., Gross, G. W., Hightower, M. H., and Czisny, L. E. Multielectrode analysis of coordinated, multisite, rhythmic bursting in cultured CNS monolayer networks, *J. Neurosci.*, **6**(6), 1986, 1583–1592.

15. Eggers, M. D., Astolfi, D. K., Liu, S., Zeuli, H. E., Doeleman, S. S., McKay, R., Khuon, T. S., and Ehrlich, D. J. Electronically wired petri dish: amicrofabricated interface to the biological neuronal network, *J. Vac. Sci. Technol. B Microelectron. Nanometer Struct.*, **8**(6), 1990, 1392–1398.

16. Schätzthauer, R., and Fromherz, P. Neuron–silicon junction with voltage-gated ionic currents, *Eur. J. Neurosci.*, **10**(6), 1998, 1956–1962.
17. Fromherz, P., and Stett, A. Silicon-neuron junction: capacitive stimulation of an individual neuron on asilicon chip, *Phys. Rev. Lett.*, **75**(8), 1995, 1670–1673.
18. Schöning, M., Tsarouchas, D., Beckers, L., Schubert, J., Zander, W., Kordoš, P., and Lüth, H. A highly long-term stable silicon-based pH sensor fabricated by pulsed laser deposition technique, *Sens. Actuators, B*, **35**(1–3), 1996, 228–233.
19. Eickhoff, M., Schalwig, J., Steinhoff, G., Weidemann, O., Görgens, L., Neuberger, R., Hermann, M., Baur, B., Müller, G., Ambacher, O., and Stutzmann, M. Electronics and sensors based on pyroelectric AlGaN/GaNheterostructures: part B; sensor applications, *Phys. Status Solidi C*, **0**(6), 2003, 1908–1918.
20. Steinhoff, G., Hermann, M., Schaff, W. J., Eastman, L. F., Stutzmann, M., and Eickhoff, M. pH response of GaN surfaces and its application for pH-sensitive field-effect transistors, *Appl. Phys. Lett.*, **83**(1), 2003, 177–179.
21. Stutzmann, M., Steinhoff, G., Eickhoff, M., Ambacher, O., Nebel, C. E., Schalwig, J., Neuberger, R., and Müller, G. GaN-based heterostructures for sensor applications, *Diam. Relat. Mater.*, **11**(3–6), 2002, 886–891.
22. Steinhoff, G., Baur, B., Wrobel, G., Ingebrandt, S., Offenhäusser, A., Dadgar, A., Krost, A., Stutzmann, M., and Eickhoff, M. Recording of cell action potentials with AlGaN/GaN field-effect transistors, *Appl. Phys. Lett.*, 86(3), 2005, 033901–033901-3.
23. Bergveld, P. Development of an ion-sensitive solid-state device for neurophysiological measurements, *IEEE Trans. Biomed. Eng.*, **BME-17**(1), 1970, 70–71.
24. Suzuki, H., Hirakawa, T., Sasaki, S., and Karube, I. Micromachined liquid-junction Ag/AgCl reference electrode, *Sens. Actuators, B*, **46**(2), 1998, 146–154.
25. Chang, K.-M., Chang, C.-T., Chao, K.-Y., and Chen, J.-L. Development of FET-type reference electrodes for pH-ISFET applications, *J. Electrochem. Soc.*, **157**(5), 2010, J143–J148.
26. Vonau, W., Oelßner, W., Guth, U., and Henze, J. An all-solid-state reference electrode, *Sens. Actuators, B*, **144**(2), 2010, 368–373.
27. Kang, B. S., Wang, H. T., Lele, T. P., Tseng, Y., Ren, F., Pearton, S. J., Johnson, J. W., Rajagopal, P., Roberts, J. C., Piner, E. L., and Linthicum, K. J. Prostate specific antigen detection using AlGaN/GaN high electron mobility transistors, *Appl. Phys. Lett.*, **91**(11), 2007, 112106–112106-3.

28. Bergveld, P. Thirty years of ISFETOLOGY: what happened in the past 30 years and what may happen in the next 30 years, *Sens. Actuators, B*, **88**(1), 2003, 1–20.
29. Oelßner, W., Zosel, J., Guth, U., Pechstein, T., Babel, W., Connery, J. G., Demuth, C., Grote Gansey, M., and Verburg, J. B. Encapsulation of ISFET sensor chips, *Sens. Actuators, B*, **105**(1), 2005, 104–117.
30. Shaw, J. E. Capillary fill encapsulation of ISFETs, *Sens. Actuators, A*, **37**, 1993, 74–76.
31. Moody, G. J., Slater, J. M., and Thomas, J. D. R. Membrane design and photocuring encapsulation of flatpack based ion-sensitive field effect transistors, *Analyst*, **113**(1), 1988, 103–108.
32. Lochhead, M. J., and Yager, P. *Multiple Patterned Structures on a Single Substrate Fabricated by Elastomeric Micro-Molding Techniques*, US patent 6039897, 2000.
33. Briand, D., Weber, P., and deRooij, N.-F. Silicon liquid flow sensor encapsulation using metal to glass anodic bonding, in *17th IEEE International Conference onMicro Electro Mechanical Systems, 2004 (MEMS)*, 2004, 649–652.
34. Decroux, M., Van den Vlekkert, H. H., and De Rooij, N. F. Glass encapsulation of CHEMFET's: a simultaneous solution for CHEMFET packaging and ion-selective membrane fixation, in *Proceedings of the 2nd International Meeting on Chemical Sensors*, 1986, 403–406.
35. Bratov, A., and Dominguez, C. Photocurable polymers applied as encapsulating materials for ISFET production, *Sens. Actuators, B*, **25**(1), 1995, 823–825.
36. Sibbald, A., Whalley, P. D., and Covington, A. K. A miniature flow-through cell with a four-function CHEMFET integrated circuit for simultaneous measurements of potassium, hydrogen, calcium and sodium ions, *Anal. Chim. Acta*, **159**, 1984, 47–62.
37. Ho, N. J., Kratochvil, J., Blackburn, G. F., and Janata, J. Encapsulation of polymeric membrane-based ion-selective field effect transistors, *Sens. Actuators*, **4**, 1983, 413–421.
38. Linkohr, S., Pletschen, W., Schwarz, S. U., Anzt, J., Cimalla, V., and Ambacher, O. CIP (cleaning-in-place) stability of AlGaN/GaN pH sensors, *J. Biotechnol.*, **163**(4), 2013, 354–361.
39. Kokawa, T., Sato, T., Hasegawa, H., and Hashizume, T. Liquid-phase sensors using open-gate AlGaN/GaN high electron mobility transistor structure, *J. Vac. Sci. Technol. B Microelectron. Nanometer Struct.*, **24**, 2006, 1972.

40. Alifragis, Y., Volosirakis, A., Chaniotakis, N. A., Konstantinidis, G., Iliopoulos, E., and Georgakilas, A. AlGaN/GaN high electron mobility transistor sensor sensitive to ammonium ions, *Phys. Status Solidi A*, **204**(6), 2007, 2059–2063.
41. Yu, J., Jha, S. K., Xiao, L., Liu, Q., Wang, P., Surya, C., and Yang, M. AlGaN/GaNheterostructures for non-invasive cell electrophysiological measurements, *Biosens.Bioelectron.*, **23**(4), 2007, 513–519.
42. Podolska, A., Tham, S., Hart, R. D., Seeber, R. M., Kocan, M., Kocan, M., Mishra, U. K., Pfleger, K. D. G., Parish, G., and Nener, B. D. Biocompatibility of semiconducting AlGaN/GaN material with living cells, *Sens. Actuators, B*, **169**(0), 2012, 401–406.
43. Yu, J., Jha, S. K., Xiao, L., Liu, Q., Wang, P., Surya, C., and Yang, M. AlGaN/GaNheterostructures for non-invasive cell electrophysiological measurements, *Biosens. Bioelectron.*, **23**(4), 2007, 513–519.
44. Witte, H., Warnke, C., Voigt, T., de Lima, A., Ivanov, I., Vidakovic-Koch, T. R., Sundmacher, K., and Krost, A. AlGaN/GaN-based HEMTs for electrical stimulation of neuronal cell cultures, *J. Phys. Appl. Phys.*, **44**, 2011, 355501.
45. Steinhoff, G., Baur, B., Wrobel, G., Ingebrandt, S., Offenhäusser, A., Dadgar, A., Krost, A., Stutzmann, M., and M. Eickhoff. Recording of cell action potentials with AlGaN/ GaN field-effect transistors, *Appl. Phys. Lett.*, **86**, 2005, 033901.
46. Sperelakis, N. Cell physiology sourcebook, *Recherche*, **67**, 2001, 02.
47. Peters, M. F., Vaillancourt, F., Heroux, M., Valiquette, M., and Scott, C. W. Comparing label-free biosensors for pharmacological screening with cell-based functional assays, *Assay Drug Dev. Technol.*, **8**(2), 2010, 219–227.

Biography

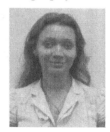

Anna Podolska received her BSE (Hons.) degree in physical and biomedical electronics from the National Technical University of Ukraine "Kiev Polytechnic Institute" in 2007. From 2010 till 2014 she worked toward her PhD degree at the University of Western Australia and was funded by the prestigious William and Marlene Schrader Postgraduate Scholarship (Biomedical Engineering). Right now her thesis is undergoing an examination process. Currently she is working as a research scientist at the Laboratory of Physics of Living Matter, EPFL University.

Podolska worked as a research associate with the Microelectronic Research Group at the University of Western Australia before commencing her PhD. She joined Curtin University in the second half of 2013 as a research fellow working on the development of physical sensors for deep exploration technology. Her main research interests are physical and biomedical all-solid-state sensors and electronic design.

Chapter 5

Understanding Melanin: A Nano-Based Material for the Future

A. B. Mostert,[a] P. Meredith,[a] B. J. Powell,[a] I. R. Gentle,[a,b] G. R. Hanson,[c] and F. L. Pratt[d]

[a]*Centre for Organic Photonics and Electronics, School of Mathematics and Physics, University of Queensland, St. Lucia, Brisbane, QLD 4072, Australia*
[b]*School of Chemistry and Molecular Biosciences, University of Queensland, St. Lucia, Brisbane, QLD 4072, Australia*
[c]*Centre for Advanced Imaging, University of Queensland, St. Lucia, Brisbane, QLD 4072, Australia*
[d]*ISIS Facility, Rutherford Appleton Laboratory, Chilton, Didcot OX11 0QX, UK*
a.mostert@uq.edu.au

Melanin, the human skin pigment, is an emerging bioelectronic material due to its unique electrical properties as well as being readily prepared in electronic grade thin films on the nanometer scale. These electrical properties include bistable electrical switching, broadband optical absorbance, Arrhenius-dependent conductivity, and an electron paramagnetic free-radical signal. Furthermore, melanin has other electrical properties, such as water-dependent conductivity and potential protonic conduction. However, to use melanin as a bioelectronic material, greater clarity is required on its charge transport behavior. Here we show that the current charge transport model for melanin, an amorphous semiconductor model,

---

Nanomaterials: Science and Applications
Edited by Deborah Kane, Adam Micolich, and Peter Roger
Copyright © 2016 Pan Stanford Publishing Pte. Ltd.
ISBN 978-981-4669-72-6 (Hardcover), 978-981-4669-73-3 (eBook)
www.panstanford.com

cannot describe melanin's hydration-dependent conductivity. We go on to show with a hydration-dependent muon spin resonance (μSR) experiment that melanin's charge transport properties are described by a comproportionation reaction, in which water self-dopes the system with extra charge carriers. This new understanding of melanin's charge transport properties opens up new avenues of exploration. We specifically see melanin as a candidate for nanoscale devices, which can act as transducers of ionic signals to electronic signals.

5.1 Introduction

5.1.1 *Melanin, the Nanobioelectronic Material*

In recent years, the discipline of bioelectronics has begun to re-emerge [1]. The field has grown, partly due to the need to interface biological systems to modern electronics to aid, for example, in diagnostics and observations for medical treatments [1]. The central problem within bioelectronics is the interfacing of biological systems to modern computer technology. The essential task is to transduce protonic/ionic signals in biological media to electronic signals in computers and vice versa.

To accomplish transduction an electronic device is used, preferably in a transistor configuration for signal amplification, utilizing a material that links the electronic and protonic/ionic signals within a common charge transport mechanism. This has been recently demonstrated via the use of hydrogenated palladium contacts in the first bioprotonic field-effect transistor [2]. However, the more common approach to transduction is to use an alternative transistor configuration, the organic electrochemical transistor (OECT), since they are well developed [3, 4]. To give an example of how transduction can work and how it relates to an OECT device, a schematic is presented in Fig. 5.1.

The OECT device is a transistor but operates by a different mechanism [1, 3, 4]: Cations in the biological solution are injected into an active channel of poly(3,4-ethylenedioxythriophene):poly(styrene sulfonate) (PEDOT:PSS) (see Fig. 5.2 for chemical structure) when a

Introduction

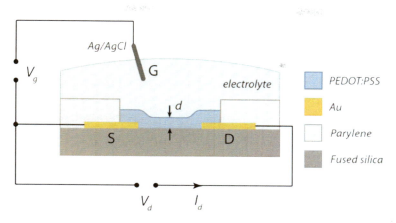

Figure 5.1 A cross-sectional schematic of an organic electrochemical transistor (OECT) [4]. An active layer (PEDOT:PSS) is spin-coated upon fused silica with source (S) and drain (D) contacts. The contacts are then insulated from the electrolyte by a parylene layer. Within the electrolyte an Ag/AgCl electrode is placed to act as the gate (G). V_g, V_d, and I_d refer to the gate voltage, drain voltage, and drain current, respectively. Reprinted with permission from Ref. [4]. Copyright © 2013 WILEY-VCH.

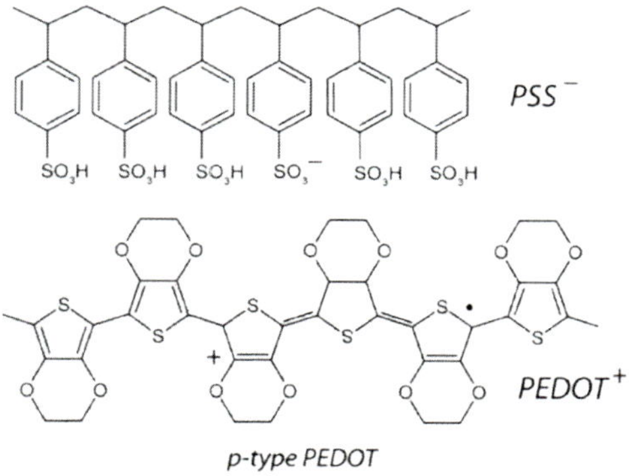

Figure 5.2 A chemical diagram for a PEDOT:PSS polymer blend. PEDOT is a p-type polymer in which the positive charge is compensated by a negative charge on a sulfonate group. Reprinted with permission from Ref. [1]. Copyright 2014 American Chemical Society.

positive bias is applied to the gate electrode. The cations compensate the sulfonate groups in the PSS, which in turn de-dopes the PEDOT, switching off the channel. In short, the cation signal changes the electronic signal due to the underlying, linked charge transport mechanism. Since the device is in a transistor configuration, one can get large amplification of the original ionic signal [3, 4].

Furthermore, and of importance in a book such as this on nanotechnology, the effectiveness of OECT devices can be enhanced to improve their ability to switch on and off by making nanometer-thick films [4]. The aim of improving switching speed (to $\sim$1 KHz) is to enable OECT devices to interface with neurons, which communicate in the 1 KHz range within the body. To obtain $\sim$1 KHz switching the active channel of an OECT device has to be made of thin films with thicknesses below 100 nm [4].

However, upon inspection of the recent literature on OECT devices, there are only two, deeply investigated transducing materials, PEDOT:PSS and polyaniline [3]. The preceding fact opens up a large area for investigating alternative materials to be used in OECT devices. In this chapter we introduce the reader to an additional material candidate for transduction: the skin pigment melanin.

We believe melanin can be used in a bioelectronics setting because:

- Melanin is biocompatible, since it is a naturally occurring pigment [5].
- Melanin is a conductive material with conductivies ranging from 10^{-8} S cm^{-1} to 10^{-4} S cm^{-1}, depending on the state of hydration [6, 7].
- Melanin can be made into device-quality thin films with thickness less than 100 nm, thus opening up device integration with neurons [8–13].
- Melanin is able to link electronic and protonic/ionic signals in a common mechanism with an equilibrium chemical reaction: the comproportionation reaction.

The first three points above have been well established in the literature, but it is the fourth point that is new and that enables melanin to be used as a viable transducing material. However, the task of demonstrating this mechanism will first require a discussion of what melanin is. This will be followed by an overview of the current charge transport model for melanin for the last 40 years, which is that melanin is an amorphous semiconductor. This discussion is important since our equilibrium reaction model essentially displaces the amorphous semiconductor model. We will then show experimental data that support a new model: the comproportionation reaction model. We will finish with the potential of melanin as a bioelectronic material.

5.1.2 What Is Melanin?

The melanins are nature's pigments and are found throughout the biosphere [14]. It is believed that melanin's main function is photoprotection [14, 15], since it is predominantly found in places where protection from ultraviolet (UV) radiation is necessary, such as the skin, hair, and eyes.

The most common form of melanin, the brown-black pigment, is referred to as eumelanin [16]; it is made from two primary building blocks (Fig. 5.3), 5,6-dihydroxyindole (DHI) and 5,6-dihydroxyindole-2-carboxylic acid (DHICA). These molecules belong to the highly reactive o-quinone chemical compounds [17]. The high reactivity of DHI and DHICA leads to melanin being a polymer with no single clear and distinguishable chemical unit [14, 16]. It is therefore termed a chemical heterogenous polymer [16]. In this chapter, we will focus on eumelanin and refer to eumelanin as melanin.

Melanin has no crystal structure, indicating no long-range structure [19], though there do appear to be $\pi-\pi$ interactions (also

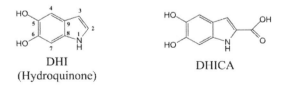

DHI
(Hydroquinone)

DHICA

Figure 5.3 The chemical precursors of eumelanin, 5,6-dihydroxyindole (DHI) and 5,6-dihydroxyindole-2-carboxylic acid (DHICA), with additional oxidative states. Reprinted with permission from Ref. [18]. Copyright 2010 American Chemical Society.

known as aromatic stacking) such as those seen in graphite [20–22]. On the basis of this secondary structure knowledge, it has been argued that the melanin polymer is made of stacked oligermers, in which small sheets of indolequinone units are stacked upon one another in small modules [16, 20–22], such as graphene sheets stacked within graphite.

Melanin has also exhibited other interesting properties such as bistable reversible switching [23–25], an observation that is the basis for the amorphous semiconductor model [26]; water-dependent conductivity behavior in the solid state [7, 16, 27]; a persistent and stable free radical [10, 16, 28–38]; an unusual broadband optical absorbance spectrum [6, 16, 39] (Fig. 5.4); and an ability to chelate large amounts of metal ions [40]. All of these properties impact melanin's potential bioelectronic capabilities.

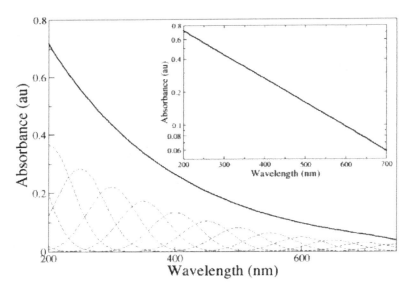

Figure 5.4 The optical absorbance spectrum for melanin. The spectrum exhibits a broadband, exponential decaying spectrum (see inset for log-linear axes). The peaks under the spectrum indicate individual absorbance peaks for modeled chromophores within melanin. These combine to produce the broadband absorbance. Reproduced from Ref. [6], Copyright (2006), with permission of the Royal Society of Chemistry.

5.2 The Basics of Melanin Charge Transport

5.2.1 *The Current Model: Amorphous Semiconductor*

It is important to understand the current model for melanin, which is based on amorphous semiconductor theory, since it is the purpose of this chapter to introduce a new charge transport model for melanin. Melanin has been believed to be an amorphous semiconductor due to four key observations:

- Melanin exhibits Arrhenius temperature dependence on its conductivity like that of a semiconductor, that is, $\sigma = \sigma_0 \exp(E_a/2k_B T)$ [7, 8, 16, 27].
- Melanin has bistable switching behavior [23–25].
- Melanin has broadband optical absorbance (Fig. 5.4) [41].
- Melanin has a stable free radical, which has been interpreted as that unpaired electrons reside at the Fermi energy level of the melanin [25].

The second point can be understood by reference to the density of states/energy level diagram for an amorphous semiconductor (Fig. 5.5). Within an amorphous semiconductor, most of the energy states around the Fermi energy (E_F) are localized electronic states. The result is the conductivity of the material is quite low. However, if one applies a large enough electric field, one is able to promote some electrons (holes) with enough energy to E_c (E_v), which corresponds to the *mobility edge*. At this energy level the electrons become delocalized and the conductivity of the material increases dramatically. Essentially, a switch is made between two different but stable conductivity regimes. The third point can also be explained by Fig. 5.5. Unlike crystalline materials that exhibit a clear cutoff energy in optical absorbance, amorphous semiconductors have a "tail" that is indicative of excitations from localized states to mobile states.

However, there are two main critiques to the amorphous semiconductor model as applied to melanin. The first is that melanin's broadband absorbance spectrum has an alternative explanation coupled with the underlying oligermer structure that does not need an amorphous semiconductor model. Instead, the spectrum is a convolution of multiple individual chemical choromophores [6, 16,

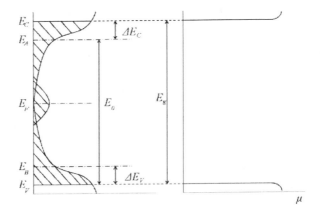

Figure 5.5 (Left) The density of states for an amorphous semiconductor such as amorphous silicon. There are several energy levels. E_V (E_C) is the valence (conduction) mobility edge, E_B (E_A) is the valence (conduction) level, E_F is the Fermi energy, E_0 is the optical gap, ΔE_V (ΔE_C) is the energy gap between the valence (conduction) level and mobility edges, and E_g is the mobility gap. (Right) The energy is plotted against the mobility, μ. Above (top) and below (bottom) the mobility edges are high-mobility states. Reprinted from Ref. [42]. © IOP Publishing. Reproduced with permission. All rights reserved.

43]. This may potentially explain the localized states within melanin, but to get delocalized electronic states, one needs large 2D sheets of melanin. Such sheets appear to be excluded since the oligermers discussed above tend to be small (Section 5.1.2). The second critique is that the actual experimental observation of the bistable switching behavior was only achieved when the melanin material was wetted. The switching behavior has never been observed in dry melanin. This would make melanin the only amorphous semiconductor that switches on the basis of its hydration state. This observation is so significant that the original experimenters attempted to rationalize these observations by modifying the basic conductivity equation for semiconductors to [23, 24]

$$\sigma = \sigma_0 \exp\left(\frac{E_D}{2k_B T}\right) \exp\left(\frac{e^2}{2k_B T r}\left(\frac{1}{\kappa} - \frac{1}{\kappa'}\right)\right) \quad (5.1)$$

where σ is the conductivity, σ_0 is the dry conductivity in the infinite temperature limit, E_D is the energy gap of dry melanin, T is the temperature, r is the screening length, κ' is the dielectric constant of dry melanin, and κ is the effective dielectric constant of melanin due to the presence of absorbed water. Essentially, the first term of the equation is the usual semiconductor Arrhenius term, but the second term is a modification that changes the effective bandgap. As melanin is hydrated (changing κ), the energy gap E_D decreases, thus enabling electron (hole) promotion to the mobility edge in a bistable switching experiment. Furthermore, Eq. 5.1 has the advantage of explaining the aforementioned (Section 5.1.2) hydration-dependent conductivity.

However, to date no systematic work has been done to test Eq. 5.1. It will be our aim to demonstrate that Eq. 5.1 does not describe melanin's charge transport. Instead, our data, as will become clear, favor a chemical equilibrium reaction interpretation.

5.2.2 Investigating Melanin Charge Transport

We will first introduce a water adsorption isotherm, which will be used to normalize all data sets. The normalization is important since it quantifies the water content of melanin as a function of water vapor pressure, the key experimental variable for the study. Hydration conductivity work will then be presented to show Eq. 5.1 does not describe melanin's conductivity. A proposal for an alternative charge transport model will then be presented on the basis of an unusual technique: muon spin resonance (μSR). After introducing this new model, its ramifications for ionic/electronic transduction in a bioelectronics setting will be discussed. If the reader is interested in the basics of the actual experimental methodology, the last section can be consulted.

5.3 How Wet Is Melanin?

Melanin's conductivity is dependent on its hydration state [7, 16, 23, 27, 44, 45]. Therefore, it is critical to first determine what the water content is of a sample of melanin.

To achieve this we first synthesized melanin from auto-oxidation from dl-Dopa, as reported in previously published methodologies

[46]. Circular pellets were then pressed from the powder under 10 tons, to a thickness of 1 mm. We selected pellets since this is the most common morphology that has been used in charge transport properties in the past. Therefore, to make meaningful comparisons, we conducted our studies on pellets as well.

The water content of melanin was determined by the use of a vacuum-capable microbalance with an external computer control unit, which was attached to a vapor delivery system [18]. Essentially, water vapor (freeze-thawed-pumped three times) was let into the microbalance at a desired pressure (monitored via an MKS Baratron pressure transducer) and the mass of the sample recorded. The equilibrium time for water unto melanin adsorption was about 45 minutes for each new pressure.

The water–melanin adsorption isotherm (water content vs. pressure data) that was obtained can be seen in Fig. 5.6. The data indicate that there is a large physical interaction between melanin and water vapor, with a large weight gain at low relative pressure, for example, the mass had increased by 10% at a relative pressure

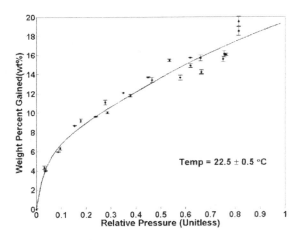

Figure 5.6 Equilibrium adsorption isotherm for melanin pellets in the presence of water vapor, denoted as a relative pressure. Here relative pressure is the vapor pressure of water divided by the saturation vapor pressure of water. Reprinted with permission from Ref. [18]. Copyright 2010 American Chemical Society.

of 0.3 and then up to a maximum of 20% at high vapor pressures. The water uptake depends somewhat on morphology. For example, we see depressed uptake in our pressed powder pellets compared to the powders used by Powell and Rosenberg [27], due to a reduced surface area. In conclusion, we've presented the first water–melanin adsorption isotherm for pressed powder melanin pellets, and the data indicate a very strong presence of water within melanin's structure.

5.4 Determining the Hydration-Dependent Conductivity Data

5.4.1 The Importance of Different Contact Geometries

To test Eq. 5.1 we obtained conductivity data as a function of the water content of melanin [47]. For our first experiment we contacted the pellet using the sandwich geometry (Fig. 5.7, inset) since there are two previous reports of hydration-dependent conductivity on melanin [7, 27] utilizing the same geometry, which allows for easy comparison. Contacting was by gold deposition followed by copper wiring attachment via silver epoxy. This left an active channel of about 0.08 cm. The sample was placed within an aluminum (to reduce electrical noise) vacuum chamber attached to a vapor delivery system similar to the adsorption isotherm system described in Section 5.3, though the gauge we used was a BOC-Edwards GK series 0–50 mbar. The sample was hydrated in the same manner as for the adsorption isotherm, which enabled us to determine the water content of the sample with Fig. 5.6.

Under a constant applied voltage (15 V) from a Keithley 2400 the current was monitored before, during, and after illumination from a white-light light-emitting diode (LED). The LED light source was powered such that the sample was exposed to the minimum light that still gave a discernible photoconductivity in the dry state. The dark conductivity results for the sandwich geometry were extracted from the photoconductivity data, where the dark conductivity value was taken as the point before light illumination.

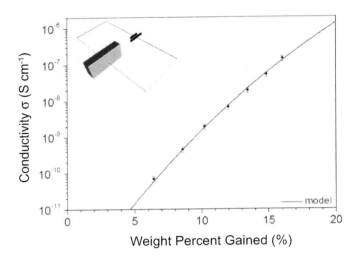

Figure 5.7 Melanin dark conductivity vs. water content utilizing the sandwich geometry. The solid line (model) is the predicted curve using Eq. 5.1. Reprinted with permission from Ref. [47]. Copyright 2012, AIP Publishing LLC.

Figure 5.7 shows the hydration-dependent dark conductivity of the sandwich-configured melanin sample. The qualitative behavior is very similar to that reported previously [7, 27], albeit with lower error and higher signal-to-noise (S/N) ratio the conductivity increases by orders of magnitude in a subexponential manner. Critically, the data appear to fit the hydration-dependent conductivity model, as exhibited by Eq. 5.1, thus apparently confirming the amorphous semiconductor model, though we noted that the fitting parameters were wholly unrealistic (see Mostert et al. [47]).

However, our adsorption studies (Section 5.3) caused us to consider the potential problem of the sandwich sample not being at equilibrium with the water vapor atmosphere, since the surface area available was reduced by the presence of the contacts. This problem forced us to consider an alternative, open-contact arrangement, called the van der Pauw geometry (Fig. 5.8, inset). Essentially, this four-contact geometry has the advantage of exposing more surface area of the sample to the environment (∼71%) when compared to the sandwich configuration (∼37%). Melanin samples were contacted in a similar manner as for the sandwich sample, though leaving a 2 mm active channel and a sample thickness of about 1 mm. We used these samples in two different experimental setups. The first setup utilized the same equipment employed for the sandwich-configured sample. Dark conductivity curves were obtained using the van der Pauw methodology, obtaining current–voltage sweeps for voltages from 0–5 V. Photoconductivity data were also obtained in a similar manner as for the sandwich-configured data. As for the hydration procedure, it remained the same as for the adsorption isotherm, again allowing one to determine the water content of melanin using Fig. 5.6. The second setup was based on glassware and conceptually similar to one of the previously reported studies [27], resulting in a lower S/N ratio. For further details, see Mostert et al. [47].

When we compared the data sets obtained from the van der Pauw geometry (Fig. 5.8) to the sandwich geometry (Fig. 5.7), an

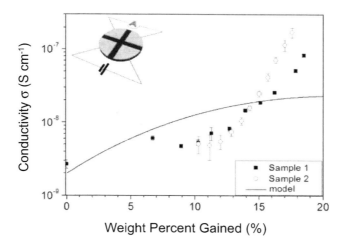

Figure 5.8 Melanin dark conductivity vs. water content utilizing the van der Pauw geometry. The solid line (model) is the predicted curve using Eq. 5.1. The two sets of data represent different experimental setups. Sample 1 was done in a system that acted as a Faraday cage. Sample 2 was done in a glass-based chamber, similar to previous literature studies [27] for comparison. Reprinted with permission from Ref. [47]. Copyright 2012, AIP Publishing LLC.

irreconcilable difference emerged. From the van der Pauw geometry one can infer three distinct regimes in the conductivity isotherm: an initial sharp increase up to ~6.5 wt%, a plateau up to ~11 wt%, and superexponential behavior up to maximum hydration. This is seen in both aluminum and glass chamber experimental setups, albeit with values below 10% weight gain unavailable for the glass setup due to electrical noise. These data cannot be rationalized when compared to the literature [7, 27] or in terms of the amorphous semiconductor model irrespective of fitting parameters, as demonstrated by the fit. Clearly, an open-contact geometry, which mimics closest the conditions under which the adsorption isotherm was obtained, is at equilibrium, but not the sandwich configuration. The data clearly presents a major flaw in the current amorphous semiconductor model.

5.4.2 Photoconductivity Data

The photoconductivity data we obtained from our experiments we present in Fig. 5.9. We present only the data on the sandwich geometry for brevity and greater clarity, though qualitatively similar results were obtained for the van der Pauw geometry.

In Fig. 5.9, a stable current level is attained after the initial application of a voltage. Illumination induces a photocurrent response that reaches a maximum value with a time constant of the order of seconds. When the illumination is removed, the photocurrent dissipates with a time constant again of the order of a few seconds, and finally a new, lower (of up to 2%) equilibrium dark conductivity is re-established.

What is noticeable at higher water content is the decrease of the photoconductivity after it reached a peak. This, coupled with the observed increasing dark conductivity at higher water content, suggests strongly that heating from nonradiative coupling of white light into the melanin sample [39, 48] causes water to evaporate and thus decreases the current. These effects are more pronounced at higher water content as expected from melanin's water-binding capacity [18, 27]. Therefore, we have further evidence that water plays a key role in the underlying charge transport mechanism.

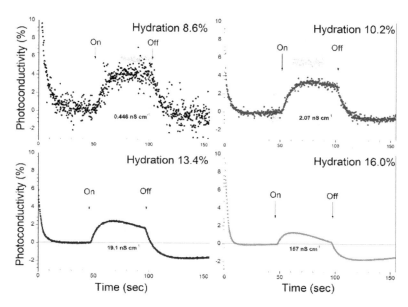

Figure 5.9 Plots of photoconductivity vs. time for four different hydration levels, (top left) 8.6%, (top right) 10.2%, (bottom left) 13.4%, and (bottom right) 16.0%, under a sequence where the sample is in the dark for 50 s, illuminated for 50 s, and in the dark for 50 s. The dark conductivity (initial equilibrium value pre-illumination), hydration level, and the light on/off points are indicated. Reprinted with permission from Ref. [47]. Copyright 2012, AIP Publishing LLC.

This heating and subsequent water desorption that produces an apparent negative conductivity conflict with previous observations. In the past negative conductivity results have been used to justify and strengthen the case for an amorphous semiconductor model [49]. The argument was that the negative conductivity after illumination was due to trap states in the photobandgap of melanin— a feature seen in amorphous semiconductors. In brief, trapped electrons left in the photobandgap after illumination are unable to contribute to the previous level of conductivity. In contrast our simpler explanation of heating induced water desorption emerges under careful environmental control. Thus, the data indicate that the amorphous semiconductor model is not applicable to melanin.

5.5 Muon Spin Resonance: Evidence for an Alternative Transport Model

5.5.1 Introducing the Concepts behind Muon Spin Resonance

To further elucidate the charge transport properties of melanin, we decided to employ a magnetic resonance technique called μSR [50, 51]. We turned to μSR for several reasons.

- μSR is a magnetic resonance technique, which allows one to discount electrical effects other than bulk the conductivity due to electrical contacts.
- μSR probes the local environment of a material. This complements the macroscopic electrical measurements we discussed in Section 5.4.1.
- The probe, the positive muon, behaves chemically like a proton [50]. However, the muon weighs one-ninth the mass of a proton and is distinguishable from other protons in a sample [50]. This allows one to utilize the kinetic isotope effect to determine the mobility behavior of protons in a sample [50].
- The positive muon can also magnetically couple to free radicals (unpaired electrons) within a sample. This allows us to determine the chemical environment as well as the number density of the free radicals [52, 53]. This is of interest since melanin is known to have several, stable free radicals present (consult Mostert et al. [35] for more information).

From the μSR we will demonstrate that charge transport in melanin is determined by an equilibrium reaction.

5.5.2 µSR Relaxation Parameters

There are three key parameters in the μSR data we present. The first is the muon mobility v, which measures the hopping rate of muons through a sample. Since the positive muons behaves chemically like a light proton, the muon's hopping rate is used to infer the proton mobility within a sample [54]. The second variable is the spin lattice relaxation (λ) rate (of the order 10^{-6} Hz) for muons coupled to free radicals. The important thing to note is that the rate λ results in the muon being depolarized due to the number of free-radical magnetic centers in the sample. As a consequence, λ can be written as proportional to the free-radical spin density [52]. The final variable accounts for the muon relaxation due to nuclear magnetic moments. Since there are many nuclear magnetic moments in a sample in the form of protons, the nuclear magnetic background is treated statistically as a Gaussian distribution. The mean of this distribution is taken as the externally applied magnetic field while the variance is expressed as Δ^2/γ^2, where γ is the gyromagnetic ratio for the muon and Δ is the third and final fitting parameter of interest, called the diamagnetic relaxation rate. Essentially, Δ reflects changes in the random nuclear background [54].

5.5.2.1 μSR experiment

The μSR data were obtained from a controlled, water-dependent μSR experiment conducted on the EMU spectrometer at the ISIS facility, Didcot UK. Melanin pellet samples were mounted on a silver plate background and placed within a standard liquid sample holder (4K-Closed Cycle Refrigerator-Cell [CCR]) with vacuum capability, to which a vacuum line was attached. The vacuum line acted as a vapor delivery line and was built on the same principles as for the conductivity experiment (Section 5.4.1). Hydration and water content determination was achieved as for the adsorption and conductivity experiments. The muons were produced by a proton beam collision on a graphite target via a pion decay [50, 51]. The 100% spin-polarized muon beam was then directed into the sample where it was allowed to precess. After a mean lifetime of 2.19 μs the muon itself undergoes a decay as follows:

$$\mu^+ \rightarrow e^+ + \nu_e + \overline{\nu_\mu} \tag{5.2}$$

where μ^+ is the positive muon, e^+ is a positron, ν_e the electron neutrino, and $\bar{\nu}_\mu$ the muon antineutrinos. This decay is emitted preferentially along the direction of the muon spin. This allows one to infer the muon spin polarization upon decay by use of the asymmetry [50, 51]

$$A(t) = \frac{N_F(t) - N_B(t)}{N_F(t) + N_B(t)} \qquad (5.3)$$

where $A(t)$ is the muon asymmetry, t is time, and $N_F(t) - N_B(t)$ is the number count of positrons in the forward (backward) detectors, which are set around the sample. For a more detailed view of the experimental setup, Blundell [50] and Cox [51] are highly recommended. Finally, at each hydration level a longitudinal repolarization experiment was performed by running a 10 Mev (million events) spectrum at 0 gauss, followed by a series of 5 Mev runs for magnetic fields ranging from 1 to 4500 gauss.

The μSR asymmetry data were then analyzed using a program called Wimda [55] to the following model:

$$A_T(t, B) = A_D(0, B)K(t, B, \Delta, \nu) + A_P(0, B)e^{-\lambda t} + A_{Ag} \qquad (5.4)$$

where $A_T(t, B)$ is the total asymmetry (as a function of time and magnetic field), $A_D(0, B)$ is the initial asymmetry fraction due to dipolar muons, $A_P(0, B)$ is the initial asymmetry fraction for muons coupled to free radicals and A_{Ag} is the asymmetry fraction from the silver backplate. The other entities are the function labeled K [54], which is essential for inferring ν and Δ, both of which are explained above (Section 5.5.2).

5.5.2.2 μSR results

The relaxation data for the variables λ, ν and Δ as a function of melanin's hydration content are presented in Fig. 5.10. Upon analysis, we found that the muon hopping rate ν, the proxy for proton mobility in melanin (refer to Section 5.5.2), remained constant throughout the hydration range of melanin. Since the muon mobility remained constant, we concluded that the proton mobility did not change either. Therefore, the conductivity isotherm presented in Fig. 5.8 cannot be explained by any mobility changes of protons in melanin.

However, when one inspects the behavior of Δ and λ in Fig. 5.10, one sees qualitative changes in their behavior that mirrors the conductivity data obtained in Fig. 5.8. To understand why that is so, our first observation was to note that λ is proportional to the

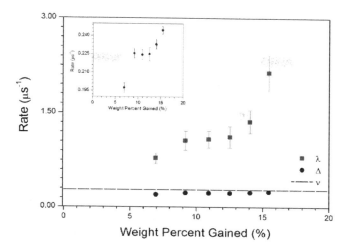

Figure 5.10 The μSR relaxation data obtained on hydrated melanin pellets. Note the significant correlation between the relaxation parameters' behavior and the conductivity behavior in Fig. 5.8. However, the parameter ν was found to be constant at 0.277 ± 0.032 μs^{-1}, indicating that changes in muon mobility, and hence proton mobility, do not explain the conductivity of hydrated melanin. Data reproduced from Mostert et al. [35] with permission of the authors and PNAS.

free-radical density in a sample. Therefore, the unpaired electrons within melanin increase in number as one hydrates the sample, concomitantly with the conductivity. This strongly suggests that changes in free-radical density may explain the conductivity of melanin.

We believe, when one investigates the studies on melanin's free-radical behavior using electron paramagnetic resonance [6, 34, 35, 46], there appears to be only one candidate that can explain both the conductivity and μSR behavior: an equilibrium reaction called the comproportionation reaction (Fig. 5.11).

This reaction can be understood very simply. Initially, two chemical entities within melanin exist at different oxidative states. A reaction then occurs between these entities involving water. The end products are hydronium and free radicals, called semiquinones, which are at an intermediate oxidative state. Our proposed model is very simple: As one adds water to melanin, an imbalance between

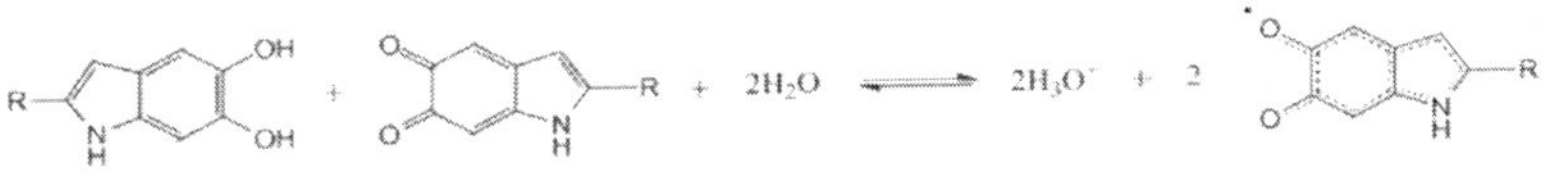

Figure 5.11 The comproportionation reaction as envisaged for melanin. Hydroquinone and quinone species (left) react together to form an intermediate redox state, the semiquinone (right). Water molecules in the environment take up protons released from the reaction.

reactants and products results. Therefore, by le Chatelier's principle, the reaction will offset the imbalance by generating more products. This leads to an increase in semiquinone free radicals. Furthermore, the dipolar relaxation Δ can be accounted for by the generation of hydronium. The formation of hydronium repositions hydrogen atoms within hydrated melanin, which changes the nuclear magnetic background. In essence, the μSR data indicate that our solid-state experiment is a solid-state titration curve. This behavior has additional support from solution-based electron paramagnetic resonance (EPR) studies (Fig. 5.12 and Refs. [32, 34]).[a] In these EPR studies, a base is added, which results in a titration curve that looks remarkably similar to both the μSR and conductivity data. The addition of a base will have the same effect as adding water.

With this evidence in mind, we propose that the conductivity behavior as seen in Section 5.4.1 can be explained by an increase in charge carrier density, both protonic as well as electronic. This is achieved by an underlying mechanism that links the two charge entities, making melanin an ideal transducing element for OECT devices. We call this mechanism *self-doping*.

5.5.3 The Origin of Charge Transport in Melanin: The Comproportionation Reaction

One may now ask whether self-doping via the comproportionation reaction can explain the literature data. First, the generation of carriers as a result of a local chemical reaction at the oxygen–hydrogen (alcohol) sites (Fig. 5.11) would lead to the electro-

---

[a]There is a subtlety in melanin electron paramagnetic studies, especially in the solid state. Melanin has two major populations of free radicals, the charged semiquinone and an uncharged carbon-centered radical, which does not appear to be part of charge transport. See Mostert et al. [35].

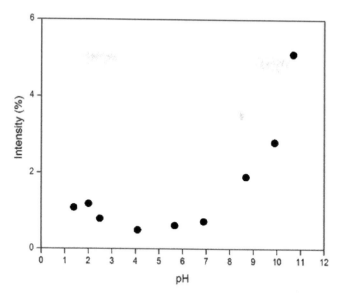

Figure 5.12 A pH-dependent titration EPR study for colloidal suspensions of melanin. We have previously reported these data [34], which show that the EPR signal intensity (a proxy for the free-radical density) varies in a similar manner to the electrical conductivity. Data reproduced from Mostert et al. [36] with permission of the authors and PNAS.

chemical evolution of hydrogen [27]. Electrical signatures such as nonohmic blocking behavior, long resistance-capacitance (RC) time constants, and dielectric hopping [7, 27, 49, 56, 57] are all characteristics of ionic systems, not just localized electrons. The apparent Arrhenius temperature behavior of the conductivity [7, 8, 27, 58] (Section 5.2.1), which has been used to support the amorphous semiconductor model, can also be explained with the new model, since a chemical equilibrium reaction is also described by an Arrhenius factor. Finally, we return to why McGinness et al. and others [23, 24] observed bistable electrical switching. An examination of the experimental geometry, a melanin powder sandwiched between metal contacts, reveals a simple explanation: the sample was acting as a parallel plate capacitor with unblocking of contacts at high electric fields. This phenomenon would lead to hysteresis in the resistance as a function of applied voltage and is characteristic of ionic systems with electrically blocking contacts.

This effect also explains why the switching only occurred in hydrated material—no significant free-carrier density exists in dry melanin. Hence, it would appear that a transport model based upon self-doping via the comproportionation equilibrium is consistent with many of the major electrical and electrochemical measurements made on melanin over the past 40 years. This insight stimulates a range of new fundamental questions such as:

- What is the kinetic mechanism for the proton transfer reaction—there have been suggestions of excited-state proton transfer-mediating nonradiative relaxation in melanin [59, 60]?
- Can one manipulate the comproportionation equilibrium and hence control the doping using metal ion chelation or the addition of other cationic species [34, 38, 46]?

These are questions for a new era of melanin bioelectronic materials.

5.6 Melanin: The Potential Ionic-to-Electronic Transducing Material

We have started this chapter asking the question as to whether there are alternative ionic-to-electronic transducing materials to PEDOT:PSS for use in OECTs. We then demonstrated, via electrical and magnetic resonance studies, that the skin pigment melanin is such a material. The fundamental reason for our conclusion is that melanin links ionic and electronic entities together in a common mechanism, which is the pre-eminent requirement for use in an OECT device.

Another standout reason to consider melanin is that it can be spin-coated to sub-100 nm thin films [8–13]—a nanotechnological requirement that is needed for a high-frequency response (Section 5.1.1). Furthermore, melanin is a skin pigment and thus is inherently biocompatible. Finally, as our data indicate, the material is conductive, even though we have used a low-conductivity morphology, which is the pressed powder pellet.

However, we wish to raise an additional advantage, which is that melanin can be an ion-specific detector. Since the work and conclusions we have presented here are new, our discussion as to why melanin can be ion specific will not be based on new experimental work but on previous literature results.

To understand melanin's ion-selective capability the comproportionation reaction should be considered again (Fig. 5.11). The chemical entities involved in the reaction belong to a class of compounds called quinones. In the reaction, a hydroquinone reacts with a quinone and water to produce hydronium and semiquinones. The key to melanin's ion selectivity is that the quinone group of materials has a strong affinity for transition metal ions [16, 46]. In the case of melanin, reports indicate a special affinity for iron (Fe^{3+}) and copper (Cu^{2+}), with about 8% weight gained in metal ion at saturation levels [40]. Furthermore, from the EPR literature on melanin–metal ion interactions, it appears that iron and copper ions have an affinity for the semiquinone in particular [46]. This appears to result in the removal of a semiquinone from the comproportionation reaction since the semiquinone is complexed. This in turns lead to the production of more hydronium and semiquinones via Le Chatelier's principle. However, even though the semiquinone that is bound to metal ions is not partaking in the comproportionation reaction, the free radical on the semiquinone remains in existence [46]. In other words, melanin may be generating additional charge carriers in the presence of copper and iron metal ions.

Therefore, it is our conclusion that melanin shows a great deal of promise as a potential ion-to-electron transducing material with a targeting capability for iron and copper metal ions.

5.7 Conclusions

The field of bioelectronics is emerging as a major field of study [1]. This could be attributed to the maturing of OECT technology via fabrication and miniaturization down to nanometer length scales [1, 3, 4]. However, the OECT concept has been limited to only a few materials. We have addressed this issue by introducing charge transport and magnetic resonance measurements on the skin pigment melanin. We have demonstrated that melanin's charge transport mechanism links ionic and electronic signals in a common chemical equilibrium reaction: the comproportionation reaction. Furthermore, we have highlighted that melanin has metal ion–binding capabilities that should also modulate the comproportionation reaction. Therefore, we believe melanin is a unique transducing material since it can select certain kinds of cations. Furthermore, due to melanin's sensitive dependence on the environment, one can envisage an all solid-state OECT device that requires no electrolyte to function. Our hope is that the work presented here will give impetus to research on melanin as a nanotechnological material in an OECT setting. As for the future, work should commence on characterizing melanin thin-film behavior in an OECT device configuration to demonstrate that such devices are viable and confirm melanin's bioelectronic potential.

Acknowledgments

We acknowledge the contribution of Johannes de Boor to preliminary conductivity measurements, Chris Noble in assistance with EPR experiments, and Karl Davy and Jeremy Ruggles in assisting with the adsorption isotherm work. The work was funded in part by the Australian Research Council (ARC) Discovery Program (DP0879944). BJP was supported by an ARC QEII Fellowship (DP0877875) and PM was supported by a Queensland Smart State Senior Fellowship and University of Queensland Vice Chancellor's Senior Research Fellowship. ABM was funded by the Australian Postgraduate Award scheme. The μSR measurements and access to the ISIS facility were made possible through the Australian Nuclear Science and Technology Organisation (ANSTO) and the Access to Major Research Facilities Programme (AMRFP). Finally, the authors wish to acknowledge the profound contribution of Dr. John McGinness to this field. He sadly passed away in September 2010, and we respectfully dedicate this work to his memory.

References

1. Rivnay, J., Owens. R. M., and Malliaras, G. G. The rise of organic bioelectronics, *Chem. Mater.*, **26**, 2014, 679–685.

2. Zhong, C., et al. A polysaccharide bioprotonic field-effect transistor, *Nat. Commun.*, **2**, 2011, 476.
3. Lin, P., and Yan, F. Organic thin-film transistors for chemical and biological sensing, *Adv. Mater.*, **24**, 2012, 34–51.
4. Rivnay, J., et al. Organic electrochemical transistors with maximum transconductance at zero gate bias, *Adv. Mater.*, **25**, 2013, 7010–7014.
5. Gray-Schopfer, V., Wellbrock, C., and Marais, R. Melanoma biology and new targeted therapy, *Nature*, **445**, 2007, 851–857.
6. Meredith, P., et al. Towards structure–property–function relationships for eumelanin, *Soft Matter*, **2**, 2006, 37–44.
7. Jastrzebska, M., et al. Electrical conductivity and synthetic DOPA-melanin polymer for different hydration states and temperatures, *J. Biomater. Sci. Polym. Ed.*, **7**, 1995, 577–586.
8. Abbas, M., et al. Structural, electrical, electronic and optical properties of melanin films, *Eur. Phys. J. E*, **28**, 2009, 285–291.
9. Bothma, J., et al. Device-quality electrically conducting melanin thin films, *Adv. Mater.*, **20**, 2008, 3539–3542.
10. Goncalves, P. J., Filho, O. B., and Graeff, C. F. O. Effects of hydrogen on the electronic properties of synthetic melanin, *J. Appl. Phys.*, **99**, 2006, 104701.
11. Lee, H., et al. Mussel-inspired surface chemistry for multifunctional coatings, *Science*, **318**, 2007, 426–430.
12. Lee, H., Lee, B. P., and Messersmith, P. B. A reversible wet/dry adhesive inspired by musselsand geckos, *Nature*, **448**, 2007, 338–342.
13. Wünsche, J., et al. Eumelanin thin films: solution-processing, growth, and charge transport properties, *J. Mater. Chem. B*, **1**, 2013, 3836–3842.
14. Prota, G. *Melanins and Melanogenesis*, Academic Press, San Diego, CA, 1992.
15. Barnes, G., and Gentle, I. *Interfacial Science: An Introduction*, Oxford University Press, Oxford, UK, 2005.
16. Meredith, P., and Sarna, T. The physical and chemical properties of eumelanin, *Pigm. Cell Res.*, **19**, 2006, 572–594.
17. Ito, S. A chemist's view of melanogenesis, *Pigm. Cell Res.*, **16**, 2003, 230–236.
18. Mostert, A. B., et al. Gaseous adsorption in melanins: hydrophilic biomacromolecules with high electrical conductivities, *Lagmuir*, **26**, 2010, 412–416.

19. Thathachari, Y. T., and Blois, M. S. Physical studies on melanins, *Biophys. J.*, **9**, 1969, 78–89.
20. Watt, A. A. R., Bothma, J. P., and Meredith, P. The supramolecular structure of melanin, *Soft Matter*, **5**, 2009, 3754–3760.
21. Zajac, G. W., et al. The fundamental unit of synthetic melanin: a verification by tunneling microscopy of X-ray scattering results, *Biochim. Biophys. Acta*, **1199**, 1994, 271–278.
22. Stark, K. B., et al. Spectroscopic study and simulation from recent structural models for eumelanin: II: oligomers, *J. Phys. Chem. B*, **107**, 2003, 11558–11562.
23. McGinness, J., Corry, P., and Proctor, P. Amorphous semiconductor switching in melanins, *Science*, **183**, 1974, 853–855.
24. Culp, C. H., Eckels, D. E., and Sidles, P. H. Threshold switching in melanin, *J. Appl. Phys.*, **46**, 1975, 3658–3660.
25. Filatovs, J., McGinness, J. E., and Proctor, P. H. Thermal and electronic contributions to switching in melanins, *Biopolymers*, **15**, 1976, 2309–2312.
26. Mott, N. F., and Davis, E. A. *Electronic Processes in Non-Crystalline Materials*, Clarendon Press, 1979.
27. Powell, M. R., and Rosenberg, B. The nature of the charge carriers in solvated biomacromolecules, *Bioenergetics*, **1**, 1970, 493–509.
28. Blois, M. S. The melanins: their synthesis and structure, *Photochem. Photobiol. Rev.*, **3**, 1978, 115–135.
29. Blois, M. S., Zahlan, A. B., and Maling, J. E. Electron spin resonance studies on melanin, *Biophys. J.*, **4**, 1964, 471–490.
30. Chio, S., Hyde, J. S., and Sealy, R. C. Temperature-dependent paramagnetism in melanin polymers, *Arch. Biochem. Biophys.*, **199**, 1980, 133–139.
31. Chio, S., Hyde, J. S., and Sealy, R. C. Paramagnetism in melanins: pH dependence, *Arch. Biochem. Biophys.*, **215**, 1982, 100–106.
32. Cope, F. W., Sever, R. J., and Polis, B. D. Reversible free radical generation in the melanin granules of the eye by visible light, *Arch. Biochem. Biophys.*, **100**, 1963, 171–177.
33. Felix, C. C., et al. Melanin photoreactions in aerated media: electron spin resonance evidence for production of superoxide and hydrogen peroxide, *Biochem. Biophys. Res. Commun.*, **84**, 1978, 335–341.
34. Froncisz, W., Sarna, T., and Hyde, J. S. Cu_2^+ Probe of metal-ion binding sites in melanin using electron paramagnetic resonance spectroscopy: I. Synthetic melanins, *Arch. Biochem. Biophys.*, **202**, 1980, 289–303.

35. Mostert, A. B., et al. Hydration-controlled X-band EPR spectroscopy: a tool for unravelling the complexities of the solid-state free radical in eumelanin, *J. Phys. Chem. B*, **117**, 2013, 4965–4972.
36. Mostert, A. B., et al. Role of semiconductivity and ion transport in the electrical conduction of melanin, *Proc. Natl. Acad. Sci. U. S. A.*, **109**, 2012, 8943–8947.
37. Sarna, T., Hyde, J. S., and Swartz, H. M. Ion-exchange in melanin: an electron spin resonance study with lanthanide probes, *Science*, **192**, 1976, 1132–1134.
38. Sarna, T., Froncisz, W., and Hyde, J. S. Cu_2^+ Probe of metal-ion binding sites in melanin using electron paramagnetic resonance spectroscopy: 2. Natural melanin, *Arch. Biochem. Biophys.*, **202**, 1980, 304–313.
39. Meredith, P., and Riesz, J. Radiative relaxation quantum yields for synthetic eumelanin, *Photochem. Photobiol.*, **79**, 2004, 211–216.
40. Hong, L., and Simon, J. D. Current understanding of the binding sites, capacity, affnity, and biological significance of metals in melanin, *J. Phys. Chem. B*, **111**, 2007, 7938–7947.
41. McGinness, J. Mobility gaps: a mechanism for band gaps in melanins, *Science*, **177**, 1972, 896–897.
42. Meredith, P., et al. Electronic and optoelectronic materials and devices inspired by nature, *Rep. Prog. Phys.*, **76**, 2013, 034501.
43. Tran, M. L., Powell, B. J., and Meredith, P. Chemical and structural disorder in eumelanins: a possible explanation for broadband absorbance, *Biophys. J.*, **90**, 2006, 743–752.
44. Baraldi, P., et al. Electrical charactersitics and electret behaviour of melanin, *J. Electrochem. Soc.*, **126**, 1979, 1207–1212.
45. Bridelli, M., Capelletti, R., and Crippa, P. R. Electret state and hydrated structure of melanin, *Bioelectrochem. Bioenerg.*, **8**, 1981, 555–567.
46. Felix, C. C., et al. Interactions of melanin with metal ions. Electron spin resonance evidence for chelate complexes of metal ions with free radicals, *J. Am. Chem. Soc.*, **100**, 1978, 3922–3926.
47. Mostert, A. B., et al. On the origin of electrical conductivity in the bioelectronic material melanin, *Appl. Phys. Lett.*, **100**, 2012, 093701.
48. Nighswander-Rempel, S. P., et al. A quantum yield map for synthetic eumelanin, *J. Chem. Phys.*, **123**, 2005, 194901.
49. Crippa, P. R., Cristofoletti, V., and Romeo, N. A band model for melanin deduced from optical absorption and photoconductivity experiments, *Biochim. Biophys. Acta*, **538**, 1978, 164–170.

50. Blundell, S. J. Spin-polarized muons in condensed matter physics, *Contemp.Phys.*, **40**, 1999, 175–192.
51. Cox, S. F. J. Implanted muon studies in condensed matter science, *J. Phys. C: Solid-State Phys.*, **20**, 1987, 3187–3319.
52. Pratt, F. L. Muon spin relaxation as a probe of electron motion in conducting polymers, *J. Phys.: Condens. Matter*, **16**, 2004, 4779–4796.
53. Roduner, E. Radical reorientation dynamics studied by positive-muon avoided level crossing resonance, *Hyperfine Interact.*, **65**, 1990, 857–872.
54. Hayano, R. S., et al. Zero- and low-field spin relaxation studied by positive muons, *Phys. Rev. B*, **20**, 1979, 850–859.
55. Pratt, F. WIMDA: a muon data analysis program for the Windows PC, *Physica B*, **289–290**, 2000, 710.
56. Jastrzebska, M., Jussila, S., and Isotalo, H. Dielectric response and a.c. conductivity of synthetic dopa-melanin polymer, *J. Mater. Sci.*, **33**, 1998, 4023–4028.
57. Jastrzebska, M., et al. Dielectric studies on charge hopping in melanin polymer, *J. Mol. Struct.*, **606**, 2002, 205–210.
58. Strzelecka, T. Semiconductor properties of natural melanins, *Physiol. Chem. Phys.*, **14**, 1982, 223–231.
59. Olsen, S., et al. Convergent proton transfer photocyles violate mirror image symmetry in a key melanin monomer, *J. Am. Chem. Soc.*, **129**, 2007, 6672–6673.
60. Meng, S., and Kaxiras, E. Mechanism for ultrafast nonradiative relaxation in electronically excited eumelanin constituents, *Biophys. J.*, **95**, 2008, 4396–4402.

Biography

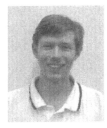

Bernard Mostert obtained his PhD in physics from the University of Queensland working on bioelectronic materials. He then spent time as a research fellow under the Marie Curie program at the University of Lancaster, UK, working on molecular electronic materials. He has since returned to the University of Queensland to continue research in the area of bioelectronics as a postdoctoral research associate working with Prof. Paul Meredith.

Chapter 6

Phase Transition in CdSe Quantum Dots and Deposition of CdSe Quantum Dots on Graphene Sheets

Fehmida K. Kanodarwala and John A. Stride
School of Chemistry, University of New South Wales, Sydney, NSW 2052, Australia
f.kanodarwala@unsw.edu.au

To date, quantum dots (QDs) have been synthesized through a number of different processes ranging from colloidal synthesis and electrochemical methods to chemical vapor deposition (CVD). This chapter focuses on the synthesis of high-quality CdSe nanocrystals through a bench-top colloidal synthesis, paying particular attention to the effects on the size and crystallinity of the QDs of varying the reaction temperature and reagent concentrations. Powder X-ray diffraction (PXRD) analysis and high-resolution transmission electron microscopy (HRTEM) have been used to highlight a transition of the crystallite phases obtained, from cubic zinc blende to hexagonal wurtzite and back again to the cubic phase as a function of reaction time. The nature of this phase shift is believed to be due to the rapid growth along the {111} crystallite facets, with the facial facets then "catching up," to restore the cubic symmetry.

Nanomaterials: Science and Applications
Edited by Deborah Kane, Adam Micolich, and Peter Roger
Copyright © 2016 Pan Stanford Publishing Pte. Ltd.
ISBN 978-981-4669-72-6 (Hardcover), 978-981-4669-73-3 (eBook)
www.panstanford.com

High-quality trioctylphosphine/trioctylphosphine oxide (TOP/TOPO)-capped CdSe QDs displaying a narrow emission band were then grafted onto graphene nanosheets through a simple wet-chemical procedure. A significant red shift of both the broad absorption and the narrow emission spectrum of the QDs was observed upon attachment to graphene, as determined by UV-Vis absorption and photoluminescence spectroscopies, whilst HRTEM data clearly show the successful decoration of the graphene sheets with CdSe QDs. This type of nanocomposite may have potential applications in the fields of optics, biological imaging, and sensing.

6.1 Introduction: Colorful World of Quantum Dots

Quantum dots (QDs), also known as nanocrystals, qdots, or even artificial atoms, are typically crystalline semiconductor nanoparticles containing elements from groups of II–VI, III–V, or IV–VI of the periodic table. QDs are composed of only several hundred to a few thousands of atoms. The small size of QDs, typically around 2 to 10 nm, bestows unique properties. On this small length scale, materials behave differently, granting them novel electronic and optical properties attributed to a phenomenon known as quantum confinement [1].

In bulk semiconductor materials, the lower-level *valence band* (VB) is almost completely filled with electrons and the upper-level *conduction band* (CB) remains nearly empty. Electrons can jump from the VB to the CB by crossing the energy barrier, or *bandgap*, E_g, by the acquisition of sufficient energy. However, under normal conditions in which $kT \ll E_g$, most of the electrons do not possess sufficient energy to cross into the CB. An electron can jump across this energy gap, driven by the energy provided through an applied voltage, photon flux, or heat. A positively charged *hole* is left behind in the VB when this occurs.

As oppositely charged entities, the excited electron and the positively charged hole are bound to each other by electrostatic Coulombic forces, giving rise to an electrically neutral quasiparticle known as an *exciton*. The physical separation between the electron and the hole is known as the exciton Bohr radius, which is analogous to that of atoms and is material dependent. In bulk semiconductors the size of the crystal is much larger than the exciton Bohr radius, leading to unrestricted motion of the excitons with respect to the crystal. However, when the size of the semiconductor crystal becomes sufficiently small that it approaches the length of the exciton Bohr radius, the motion of the exciton is confined, leading to the phenomenon known as *quantum confinement*. In QDs the exciton is confined in all the three spatial dimensions.

The effects of confinement on the electronic energy levels of a semiconductor material are significant. Figure 6.1 shows the energy

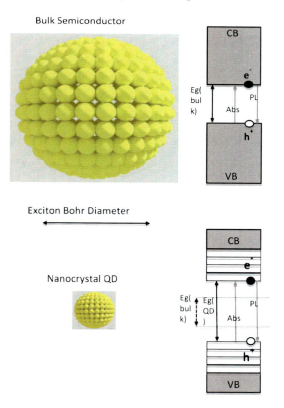

Figure 6.1 Schematic representation of a typical bulk semiconductor and a nanocrystal QD and their associated electron energy levels. E_g is the energy bandgap.

levels of a bulk semiconductor and of a QD of the same material. In a bulk semiconductor, the energy levels within the VB and CB are so close that they can be treated as being continuous bands. Electrons excited to the CB do not stay there permanently, rapidly relaxing back to the VB, with the resultant emission of a photon of a wavelength corresponding to the energy loss. As the bandgap of a bulk semiconductor is fixed, this transition leads to fixed emission frequencies. In the case of QDs, the same processes of the formation of the exciton and its recombination exist; however, there is a major difference in the densities of states due to the finite particle size. With decreasing size of the particle, there is a corresponding increase in exciton confinement. This increased confinement makes the energy levels, which were formerly continuous to become discrete, implying that there exists small and finite separation between the energy levels. This implies that smaller crystals will have larger bandgaps. This is known as quantum confinement and the crystals exhibiting it are known as QDs.

The emission frequency of QDs is bandgap dependent, enabling precise control over the output wavelength; small QDs produce light with short wavelengths (toward blue if in the visible spectrum) and large QDs longer wavelengths (toward red).

QDs can be fabricated through many different methods, including molecular beam epitaxy (MBE), electron beam lithography (EBL), metal organic chemical vapor deposition (MOCVD), and colloidal synthesis. We will be focusing on colloidal synthesis as this the method used to synthesize QDs in the current chapter.

In the colloidal synthesis of QDs, a seed molecular cluster is placed in a solvent in the presence of other precursors to initiate particle growth. The molecular cluster used as the seed mostly consists of the same elements as those required in the subsequent QD, or different elements that are not required in the final QDs but that facilitate the seeding process. Some precursors may not be present at the beginning of the reaction process: however, as the reaction proceeds and as the temperature is increased, additional amounts of precursors are periodically added to the reaction either dropwise as a solution or as a solid. The formation of nanoparticles from the precursor has to be carried out under controlled conditions to ensure that the monodispersity of the cluster compound is maintained throughout nanoparticle growth in order to obtain a monodisperse population of nanoparticles. As at this stage some clusters grow at the expense of others due to Ostwald ripening, leading to particles of varying size.

The organometallic precursor route for the synthesis of CdSe QDs can address this issue quite efficiently. It involves high-temperature decomposition of an organometallic precursor such as dimethylcadmium ($Cd(CH_3)_2$) in a coordinating solvent consisting of a mixture of trioctylphoshine (TOP) and trioctylphoshine oxide (TOPO) [2]. TOP not only acts as a solvent of the Cd precursor, but it also serves as the source of surface ligands for the resulting QDs. CdSe QDs with a narrow size distribution can be produced by separating the nucleating and growth stages. Even though this route produces high-quality QDs it still possesses a few shortcomings; for instance, ($Cd(CH_3)_2$) is extremely hazardous, expensive, and air sensitive and is a pyrophoric material; it may even be explosive because of the release of gas during the reaction, and this route needs complicated glove-box techniques. Peng's group proposed the replacement of ($Cd(CH_3)_2$) with other Cd source compounds such as CdO [3, 4] or other cadmium salts that possess an anion of a weak acid (such as cadmium carbonate [5] and cadmium acetate). All of these synthetic routes were carried out in the coordinating solvent TOPO and TOP. The QDs in this work followed a similar approach, as detailed in Section 6.2.

Recently there has been interest in synthesizing QDs that emit in the infrared (IR) or near-IR region, as this is believed to improve the optoelectronic properties of QDs and may make them of use in optical signal processing [6]. There are many proposed methods to achieve this shift to longer wavelengths, such as making core–shell QDs [7] or QDs with a small direct-bandgap semiconductors like CdP [8]. By combining the electronic properties of graphene with those of QDs in graphene–QD nanocomposites, it may be possible to shift the emission of QDs to longer wavelengths in a controlled manner. There have been recent reports of the decoration CdSe QDs on graphene sheets and the effect on the optoelectronic properties of the QDs was investigated [9, 10]. Wang et al. synthesized CdSe

QDs in situ of deposition onto graphene and were able to tune the fluorescence of the QDs by controlling the size of the QDs by limiting the growth (reaction) time.

Graphene consists of carbon atoms that are arranged on a 2D honeycomb structure made up of hexagons—a molecular-scale *chicken wire* [11]. Although the existence of graphene had been hypothesized for a long time, it was only recently (2004) isolated in its free form by Geim et al. [12]. The structural rigidity of graphene is reflected in its electronic properties. The valence electrons on each carbon centre may be thought of as being sp^2 hybridized, in which the $2s$ and two $2p$ orbitals mix, leading to a trigonal planar geometry about the nucleus; as such there exist σ-bonds between adjacent carbon atoms, separated in graphene by 1.42 Å. According to Pauli's exclusion principle, the bands formed by the propagation of σ-bonding throughout the 2D lattice are half filled, forming a deep VB. The third $2p$ orbital on each carbon atom lies perpendicular to the planar structure and forms covalent π-interactions with neighboring carbons. As each p-orbital is half filled, this π-band also remains half filled. This unique band structure of graphene grants it an unusual semimetallic behavior [13].

Due to its unique electrical [14], mechanical [15], optical, and thermal properties [16], graphene can be tailored both structurally and chemically in a number of different ways for a variety of applications. It is conceivably of use as a transparent electrode material [17] for sensors, displays, and solar cells, in lithium ion batteries [18], or in polymer composites [19]. To enhance the properties and widen the scope of applications of graphene, research is being carried out on the surface modification of the material. Metal atoms [20], or molecules [21], have been deposited on the surface and there has been some decoration of the surface with QDs such as metal oxides [22], metals [23] and magnetite [24].

We have successfully uniformly deposited our preformed CdSe QDs on graphene sheets, achieving a shift to longer wavelengths, a red shift, in both the optical absorption and the emission of the QDs; details are discussed in Section 6.3.

6.2 Phase Transition in CdSe Quantum Dots

CdSe exists in two crystalline phases, namely the hexagonal wurtzite (WZ) and the cubic zinc-blende (ZB) structures. Most synthetic techniques currently employed usually produce QDs having the WZ structure. Very recently, ZB–CdSe QDs have been successfully obtained [25, 26] but there is a lack of systematic or comparative studies in relation to the more conventional WZ system.

This chapter studies the transition of the crystallite phases of mixed-phase QDs from predominantly cubic ZB to hexagonal WZ and back again to the cubic ZB phase simply by changing the reaction time.

CdSe QDs were synthesized in a colloidal synthetic route using Schlenk line methods. The CdSe QDs were synthesized in a similar manner to two previously reported methods of Yu et al. [27] and Murray et al. [2]. These methods were combined and modified in order to study the various factors leading to QD synthesis. All samples were dispersed in toluene.

The selenium precursor (TOPSe) was prepared as follows: 0.25 mmol (0.197 g) of selenium powder was dissolved in 2 mL of tri-*n*-octylphosphine (TOP) and 2 mL of toluene in a sample tube under an inert atmosphere. The mixture was then sonicated for 10 min at room temperature, until the entire amount of selenium had dissolved in TOP, giving rise to a colorless solution.

In a typical procedure, 0.125 mmol (0.160 g) of CdO was mixed with 2 g lauric acid in a 50 mL three-necked round-bottom flask and degassed for 30 min and then heated to 130°C under a nitrogen flow, with constant stirring, until all of the mixture became optically clear. The system was allowed to cool to room temperature, and then 2 g of TOPO was added. The flask was resealed and reheated up to 320°C under a nitrogen flow. The pre-prepared TOPSe was then quickly injected into the reaction flask containing the Cd solution. The temperature of the reaction mixture decreased to 280°C upon the injection of TOPSe and it was maintained at this temperature for the growth period of the QDs.

Aliquots of the reaction solution were removed at regular intervals at 30, 60, 120, 300, and 600 s and then cooled. This series of samples are referred to as QD-30S, QD-60S, QD-120S, QD-300S, and QD-600S for 30, 60, 120, 300, and 600 s samples, respectively in all future discussions.

The rapid cooling of the particles was found to be essential in order to avoid additional growth of the particles; this was achieved by cooling the sample tubes in an ice bath. This effective method of terminating the growth of the QDs yielded samples of near-monodisperse particle size that did not require additional size-selective precipitation.

When the QDs reached 60°C, slightly above the melting point of TOPO, 20 mL of anhydrous methanol was added to the aliquot, resulting in the reversible flocculation of the crystallites, but this also aided the removal of excess TOP and TOPO. The flocculate was separated from the supernatant by centrifugation. The precipitate thus obtained was washed thrice with acetone (centrifuged at 3000 rpm for 10 min in each cycle). Subsequent vacuum drying of the precipitate at 60°C produced freeflowing TOP/TOPOcapped CdSe QDs as a solid sample.

The CdSe QDs were stored in either solid form in sealed sample tubes in the dark or by redispersing them in toluene. Storing them as a dispersion was preferable, as this was found to avoid particle aggregation and oxidation over time. A schematic representation of the synthesis is illustrated in Fig. 6.2.

The QDs that were synthesized in this work were characterized using a number of different analysis techniques. Electron microscopy was used to analyze the structure of the QDs, ultraviolet-

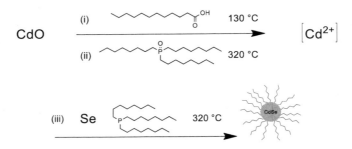

Figure 6.2 Schematic representation of synthesis of CdSe QDs through reaction of CdO in the presence of (i) lauric acid, (ii) TOPO, and (iii) TOP at 320°C.

visible (UV-Vis) spectroscopy to determine the absorption characteristics, photoluminescence (PL) spectroscopy to give the emission characteristics, dynamic light scattering (DLS) to determine the size, X-ray photoelectron spectroscopy (XPS) for elemental characterization, nuclear magnetic resonance (NMR) spectroscopy to acquire more information about the interaction of the capping agent with the core and powder X-ray diffraction (PXRD) for phase identification of the QDs. A detailed description of each of them is mentioned in the subsequent sections.

A Philips CM200 field emission transmission electron microscope operating at an accelerating voltage of 200 kV, with a Bruker silicon drift detector (SDD) EDAX system, was used for TEM. The microscope was also equipped with an SIS charge-coupled device (CCD) camera, which enabled high-resolution digital imaging.

A Cary 100 UV-Vis spectrophotometer was used to carry out absorption spectra in the 200–900 nm wavelength range. PL spectra were measured on a custom-built microscope coupled to an Acton 2300 spectrometer. Fourier transform infrared spectroscopy (FTIR) was performed using an Avatar 320 FTIR spectrometer. DLS measurements were carried out on a Malvern Zetasizer Nano ZS.

PXRD measurements of the samples were performed using a Philips X'pert Multipurpose X-ray Diffraction System (MPD) operating at 40 kV and 40 mA with a CuKα source ($\lambda = 0.154056$ nm). Complete Rietveld analysis was performed on the data to obtain phase compositions. Pair distribution function (PDF) analysis was performed using the 11ID-B beamline, located in sector 11 at the Advanced Photon Source at Argonne National Laboratory, Illinois by Dr. Katharine L. Page, a postdoctoral fellow with Dr. Thomas Proffen, NPDF instrument scientist at the Los Alamos National Laboratory, New Mexico. XPS was performed on an ESCALAB 220i XL instrument using a monochromated Al Kα X-ray source ($h\nu = 1486.6$ eV) operated at 10 kV and 12 mA.

The two crystalline forms of CdSe hexagonal WZ structure and the cubic ZB structure are shown in Fig. 6.3. WZ is a two-component analogue of a hexagonal diamond structure and is represented by a hexagonal lattice with bases 0 and

$$\frac{1}{3}\hat{a} + \frac{1}{3}\hat{b} + \frac{1}{3}\hat{c}$$

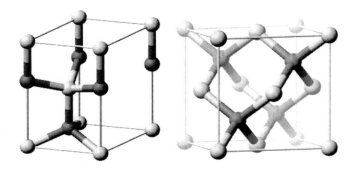

Figure 6.3 Crystal structures of CdSe: wurtzite (left) and zinc blende (right).

ZB is a two-component analogue to the diamond structure and is represented as facecentered cubic (FCC), with bases 0 and

$$\frac{1}{4}(\hat{x} + \hat{y} + \hat{z}).$$

In the case of CdSe, the parameters of these structures are $a = 0.4135$ nm and $c = 0.6749$ nm for WZ and $a = 0.608$ nm for ZB [28]. Mainly all the synthetic techniques currently employed usually produce QDs in the WZ structure. Very recently, ZB–CdSe QDs have been successfully obtained [25, 26] but there is a lack of any systematic or comparative study in relation to the conventional WZ system.

PXRD was employed to determine the crystalline phase structure of the CdSe QDs in the aliquots. The unique features of ZB–CdSe QDs with a CuKα source are a sharp (111) peak at $2\theta = 25.4°$, a deep valley between the (220) and (311) peaks, and a blunt (440) peak at $2\theta = 60.9°$. In contrast, for WZ–CdSe, there is a broad peak around $2\theta = 25°$ and a (103) peak at $2\theta = 45.6$ [29].

Figure 6.4 shows the PXRD patterns obtained for QD-30S, QD-60S, QD-300S, and QD-600S [30]. The highly crystalline nature of the QDs is evident from the sharpness of the diffraction peaks. Comparing the spectra in Fig. 6.4 a transition from ZB to WZ and back to ZB can be observed across the series. We performed Rietveld refinement on the PXRD spectra to obtain details of the percentage phase compositions and derive the sizes of the QDs using the Debye–Scherrer equation; these are listed in Table 6.1. It can be deduced

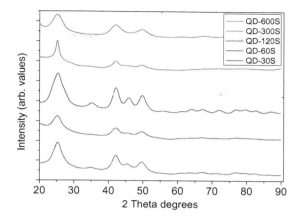

Figure 6.4 Combined powder X-ray diffraction spectrum of the aliquots taken at different time intervals. QD-30S, QD-60S, QD-300S, and QD-600S exhibit the cubic phase, whereas QD-120S exhibits the hexagonal phase. Reprinted from Ref. [30]. Copyright (2015), with permission from Elsevier.

Table 6.1 Size of the QDs deduced from PL, UV-Vis, DLS, and PXRD and percentage of the phases obtained from PXRD

Sample	PL λ(nm)	UV-Vis λ(nm)	UV-Vis Size (nm)	DLS Size (nm)	PXRD Size (nm)	PXRD Cubic %	PXRD Hexagonal %
QD-30S	622	561	3.28	5.708	3.87 ± 0.13	65.5	34.5
QD-60S	619	566	3.41	6.668	3.74 ± 0.11	73.3	26.7
QD-120S	629	591	4.21	10.648	3.91 ± 0.39	31.1	69.9
QD-300S	640	594	4.33	13.396	5.57 ± 2.21	85.5	14.5
QD-600S	644	602	4.67	15.554	2.67 ± 0.01	99.8	0.2

from these values that an increase in the percentage of the cubic phase and a subsequent decrease in the hexagonal phase occurs with increasing growth time except for 120 s, when the opposite was observed. As such, the samples QD-30S and QD-60S are more cubic in character, the QD-120S is more hexagonal and the QD-300S and QD-600S are once again more cubic.

We repeated the experiments three times and found the same results each time. We observe that the CdSe QDs in this series are a mixture of both the phases though, varying in the percentage of the two phases. Thus, we speculate that the growth of ZB–CdSe is

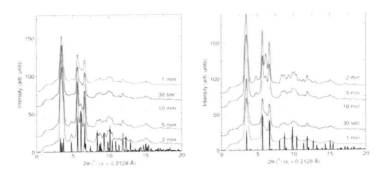

Figure 6.5 SXRD compared with simulated WZ diffraction pattern (black) (left) and with simulated ZB diffraction pattern (black) (right).

reinforced along the WZ (0 0 1) direction, whilst not absolutely in the WZ phase, but with some ZB lattice stacking faults. This WZ–ZB polytypism phenomenon in semiconductors is common, the structural difference between WZ and ZB is subtle, and the internal energy difference is small [31]. The transition between WZ and ZB is usually determined by synthetic parameters, and since WZ is a metastable phase, it requires vigorous conditions for its growth [32, 33].

PDF analysis is a powerful method that extracts structure-related information from powder diffraction data. Since it takes into account not only Bragg's law for ordered lattices but also diffuse scattering due to short-range ordering, it can be employed for structural elucidation of QDs [34]. PDF thus provides more detailed information regarding the phases as compared to PXRD data. Figure 6.5 shows the PDF data of CdSe QDs; they illustrate that the WZ (102) and (103) reflections are present in every sample, with the amount increasing in the order QD-60S, QD-30S, QD-600S, QD-300S, and QD-120S, whilst at the same time, the ZB character decreases, which is in agreement with the PXRD data.

Figure 6.6 shows the normalized UV-Vis absorption and PL emission spectra of the CdSe QDs. QD-30S, QD-60S, QD-120S, QD-300S, and QD-600S have absorption edges at the wavelengths 561, 566, 591, 594, and 602 nm respectively, and emission edges at the wavelengths 622, 619, 629, 640, and 644 nm, respectively. This progressive red shift indicates the increasing size of the QDs with

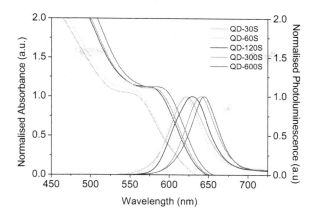

Figure 6.6 UV-Vis absorption and photoluminescence emission spectra of QD-30S, QD-60S, QD-120S, QD-300S, and QD-600S. Reprinted from Ref. [30]. Copyright (2015), with permission from Elsevier.

increasing duration of the reaction. The difference in the absorption edge and the emission peak relates to the energy gap, that is, a measure of energy loss upon absorption and re-emission.

The diameters of the QDs were calculated using the wavelength of the absorption edges using Eq. 3.1 reported by Xia et al. [29] (Table 6.1)

$$D = 1.6122 \times 10^{-9}\lambda^4 - 2.6575 \times 10^{-6}\lambda^3$$
$$+ 1.6242 \times 10^{-3}\lambda^2 - 0.4277\lambda + 41.57, \quad (6.1)$$

where D (nm) is the calculated diameter of CdSe and λ (nm) is the wavelength of first absorption peak. It was found that there was a subsequent increase in the size of the QDs across the series, in the range of 3.28 to 4.67 nm. We compared these sizes with those deduced from PXRD, which we found to lie in the range of 2.67 to 3.87 nm, and from this it can be concluded that both the sizes are in broad agreement with each other. It should be noted that the size of QD-600S deduced from PXRD is the smallest in the series, although it should be the largest; this can be attributed to the polycrystalline nature of the particle. The corresponding hydrodynamic sizes, that is, the size of the core and the capping agent TOP/TOPO obtained from DLS were typically a multiple of two to three of these values, lying in the range of 5.71 to 15.55 nm. Since DLS measures the

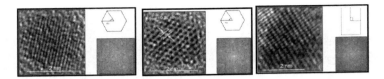

Figure 6.7 HRTEM image and FFT of QD-30S (left), QD-60S (center), and QD-120S (right). Reprinted from Ref. [30]. Copyright (2015), with permission from Elsevier.

hydrodynamic diameter in comparison to the PXRD or HRTEM, which only measure the core.

The HRTEM image of QD-30S in Fig. 6.7 (left) clearly shows spherical particles with the lattice fringes representing well-crystallized QDs. The measured lattice spacing $d = 0.36$ nm matches the calculated lattice spacing of (100) planes in ZB–CdSe. The fast Fourier transform (FFT) patterns are hexagonal and the angles between different crystal planes are all equal to 60°, consistent with the calculated ones for ZB–CdSe. As we proceed further with respect to the duration of reaction, we observe in the HRTEM of QD-60S as shown in Fig. 6.7 (center), that it has the lattice spacing $d = 0.36$ nm matching that of the ZB-CdSe, and even the FFT pattern is hexagonal with a 60° angle between the crystal planes.

While as we progress in the reaction we notice in the HRTEM of QD-120S, as shown in Fig. 6.7 (right), that it has a lattice spacing corresponding to the WZ–CdSe, that is, $d = 0.36$ nm, and the FFT pattern is rectangular with a 90° angle between the crystal planes.

As we further move on with the reaction we notice in the HRTEM image of the QD-300S as shown in Fig. 6.8 (left), the lattice spacing

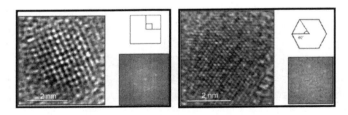

Figure 6.8 HRTEM image and FFT of QD-300S (left) and QD-600S (right). Reprinted from Ref. [30]. Copyright (2015), with permission from Elsevier.

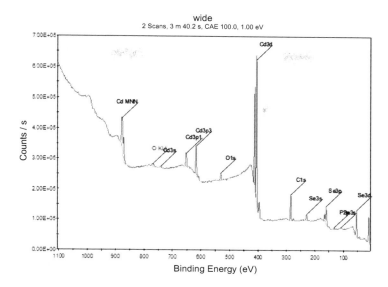

Figure 6.9 XPS spectrum of QD-30S.

$d = 0.36$ nm characteristic of ZB–CdSe and the FFT pattern is a square with a 90° angle between the crystal planes. The HRTEM of QD-600S, as shown in Fig. 6.8 (right), is similar to that of the ZB–CdSe with lattice spacing $d = 0.36$ nm and the FFT is hexagonal with 60° angle between the crystal planes.

To derive the compositional information of the synthesized CdSe QDs XPS was performed. Figure 6.9 shows the XPS spectrum of QD-30S. It can be seen from the spectra that it shows the presence of Cd, Se, and P from the QDs and their surfaces and C and O from the QDs surface and from absorbed gaseous molecules. There is no evidence of any *shake-up* peaks in the spectrum. These are photoemission peaks from species that get ionized prior to the observed photoemission process and they usually occur several electronvolts higher to the binding energy of the main peaks in the spectrum. The peak position for Cd3d is at 405.09 eV, Se3d at 54.06 eV, P3s at 133.7 eV, C1s at 285.05 eV, and O1s at 531.18 eV. In bulk CdSe the difference between the Cd and Se peak positions is 350.97 eV [35] whereas the observed difference between the Cd and Se peaks in our QDs is 351.03 eV. This difference could be due to the

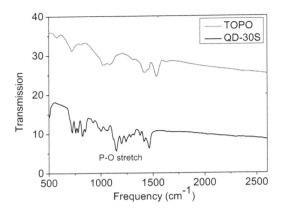

Figure 6.10 Plot of FTIR analysis of QD-30S.

fact that the bulk CdSe is referenced to the VB edge of CdSe. The peak position for phosphine oxides, sulfides, and selenides is at 132.2 eV [36] and our P3s peak is 1.5 eV higher.

Figure 6.10 shows the FTIR spectrum of the QD-30S. It was used to analyse the presence of TOPO on the surface of the QDs. The spectrum of the QDs has peaks matching to all of the TOPO peaks in intensity and frequency except the one for P-O stretch shifted lower by ~ 20 cm^{-1} relative to the bulk TOPO. This is in agreement with the IR measurements of triphenylphosphine oxides, which show P-O shifts of 20–60 cm^{-1} upon complexation with CdI_2 and other metal salts [37]. The FTIR of other samples showed a similar trend.

6.3 Deposition of CdSe Quantum Dots on Graphene Sheets

The procedure that was adopted herein for the synthesis is a modified form of a method first reported by Wang et al. [38]. Graphene sheets were synthesized by the solvothermal approach pioneered at UNSW by Stride and Choucair; the graphene samples used were prepared by Dr. Choucair [39]. In a typical CdSe deposition reaction, 10 mg (0.138 mmol) of graphene was dispersed into 6.3 mL of octadecene (ODE) under ultrasonication. Then 1 mL

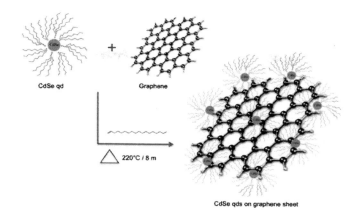

Figure 6.11 Schematic representation of synthesis of QD-G through reaction of CdSe QDs with graphene in the presence of ODE at 220°C for 8 min. Reprinted from Ref. [40]. Copyright (2014), with permission from Elsevier.

of CdSe QDs prepared by the method developed in X.3 was added into the ODE–graphene suspension and sonicated. The mixture thus obtained was placed in a 50 mL three-necked round-bottomed flask and heated to 240°C for 8 min under a nitrogen flow. After cooling to room temperature, the final product was isolated by centrifugation (1500 rpm for 5 min) to remove free CdSe QDs as a by-product. The samples were washed with ethanol several times and dried in a vacuum oven at 60°C. This sample is referred to as QD-G in all future discussions. To better understand the mechanism of attachment of CdSe QDs on the graphene sheets, to evaluate the role of dilution on the reaction of CdSe QDs with graphene and to rule out the possibility of an increase in the absorption wavelength being due to an increase in size of the CdSe QDs, several control reactions were performed. The sample of dilution study is referred to as diluted quantum dot heat-treated with graphene (DQD-G) and the one for sonication study is referred to as quantum dot sonicated with graphene (SQD-G) in all future discussions.

A schematic representation of the synthesis of CdSe QDs on graphene is shown in Fig. 6.11.

UV-Vis absorption spectroscopy was preformed on all samples. Figure 6.12 (left) gives a combined UV-Vis spectrum of the different

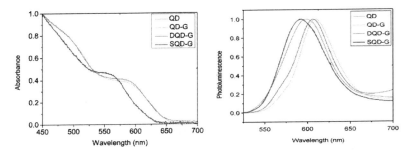

Figure 6.12 UV-Vis absorption spectrum (left) and photoluminescence spectrum (right) of QD (quantum dot), QD-G (quantum dot heat-treated with graphene), DQD-G (diluted quantum dot heat-treated with graphene), and SQD-G (quantum dot sonicated with graphene).

samples of CdSe QDs deposited on graphene, normalized to the absorption at 450 nm. The UV-Vis absorption for free QDs (labeled QD) is at 563 nm, while that for sonicated graphene with CdSe QDs (SQD-G) is also found at absorbance 563 nm. This suggests that the mean particle size is 3.34 nm in radius calculated from the absorbance at 563 nm [29] and in agreement with PXRD line-broadening measurements, which indicated this to be 2.79 ± 0.09 nm. Meanwhile, the diluted CdSe QDs heat-treated with graphene (sample DQD-G) were found to have an absorption edge of 593 nm, the same as that found for the heat-treated QDs with graphene (QD-G). The 30 nm shift in the QD absorption is therefore clearly independent of concentration effects; it cannot be the result of the particle–particle interactions on the surface. The UV-Vis absorption data implies that the mechanism by which the QDs are deposited onto the graphene is related to the heat treatment of the QDs rather than simple physisorption or any other physical adhesion phenomenon. The shift of 30 nm in the absorption of the CdSe QDs upon deposition onto graphene represents a significant difference, clearly related to a physical and presumably electronic interaction between the two, consistent with a relaxation in the confinement of the exciton pair, potentially as a result of quantum tunnelling between the QDs and graphene.

Having generated the exciton pairs in the broadband absorption of light, the emission characteristics are central to the nature of QDs; typically these have narrow wavelength dispersion. μ-PL measurements largely conform to the absorption behaviour obtained using UV-Vis spectroscopy. Figure 6.12 (right) gives a composite of PL spectra of the different samples of QDs deposited on graphene. The emission spectrum of free QDs has a narrow luminescence band peaking at 597 nm, whilst the emission in sample SQD-G was found to lie to a slightly shorter wavelength of 590 nm. Meanwhile, the sample DQD-G had a narrow emission band, peaking at 612 nm, whilst the QD-G sample emits at 615 nm. As such the wavelength corresponding to the peak in the emission band of the CdSe QDs was found to increase by 18 nm over the emission of the free particles upon deposition onto graphene and to not be quenched in any way by the interaction with the sheets.

HRTEM was used to evaluate the structure of the QDs deposited on graphene (Fig. 6.13) [40]. The images show free graphene

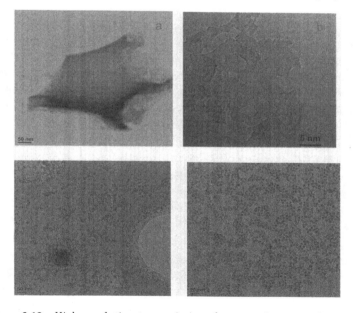

Figure 6.13 High-resolution transmission electron microscopy images of (a) graphene sheet, (b) SQD-G–quantum dot sonicated with graphene, (c) QD-G–quantum dot heat-treated with graphene, and (d) high-resolution image of (c). Reprinted from Ref. [40]. Copyright (2014), with permission from Elsevier.

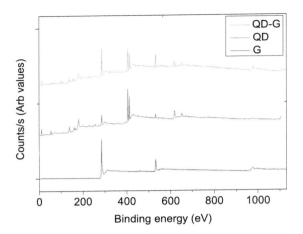

Figure 6.14 X-ray photoelectron spectroscopy of G (graphene sheet), QD, and QD-G (quantum dot heat-treated with graphene). Reprinted from Ref. [40]. Copyright (2014), with permission from Elsevier.

sheets (Fig. 6.13a); similarly the image obtained for SQD-G (Fig. 6.13b) shows only graphene sheets, without any QDs on the surface. However, the image of the QD-G sample, clearly shows QDs dispersed on graphene (Fig. 6.13c), with a regular distribution of the particles (Fig. 6.13d) of approximately 5 nm diameters, in perfect agreement with the size determinations by the analysis of the UV-Vis absorption edge and the line broadening in the PXRD. It is interesting to note that the QDs are deposited on the graphene sheet in largely hexagonal arrays, whilst still maintaining their spherical shape; this is consistent with a close-packed structure representing an energy minimum in the chemical potential between neighbouring QDs [41].

The elemental composition of the samples was determined with XPS (Fig. 6.14). One can observe that graphene gives two distinct peaks at 286 eV and 574 eV attributed to carbon and oxygen, respectively. The presence of an oxygen peak indicates the presence of defects in the carbon material and even some surface-bound water molecules from moisture in the air. These peaks are not present in a significant amount in the QD sample but are significantly enhanced in the QD-G sample, indicating the presence of graphene in the QDs, which gets bound to the graphene surface.

Table 6.2 XPS atomic percentage and peak binding energy (eV) of graphene, QD and QD-G (A–E refer to different carbon atoms in the XPS spectrum)

Elements	Atomic percentage			Peak BE (eV)
	Graphene	QD	QD-G	
C1s A	62.17	55.69	68.82	285.03
C1s B	12.72	3.24	1.23	286.65
C1s C	4.81	4.57	3.68	288.09
C1s D	5.81	0	0	288.93
C1s E	1.96	0	0	290.85
Ti2p3	0.5	0	0.2	459.36
O1s A	6.13	7.82	9.57	531.28
O1s B	5.89	0.92	4.3	533.13
Cd3d5	0	15.77	7.09	405.19
Se3d	0	9.66	3.76	53.93
P2s A	0	2.34	1.34	190.51

Table 6.2 gives the atomic percentage derived from fits to the XPS data for graphene, QD, and QD-G. It can be deduced from the percentages that the value for C1s A at 285.03 eV increases in the QD-G sample compared to that of the QD sample; similarly the values for O1s at 531.28 and 533.13 eV also increase in the QD-G sample, consistent with the increased oxygen content attributable to the TOP/TOPO capping agents of the QDs.

To determine whether the shift in both absorbance and PL spectra is not due to an increase in the size of the QDs as a result of ripening processes due to the longer reaction times (generally the case with QDs) [42, 43], control reactions in which aliquots were removed from the reaction across a time series, both with and without the presence of graphene, were performed. UV-Vis and PL data indicate that the shift is not size or time dependent but is solely due to the interaction of the QDs with graphene. Figure 6.15 (left) is a composite of the UV-Vis data of the aliquots of QDs on graphene at the reaction time intervals of 4, 8, 12, 16, 20, and 30 min and the reference spectrum of QDs. It can be clearly seen that the absorption edge for all the aliquots at different time intervals remains unchanged at 590 nm, while that of the free QD is at 563 nm. Figure 6.15 (right) shows the corresponding PL spectra and

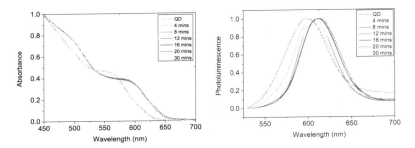

Figure 6.15 UV-Vis absorption spectrum (left) and PL spectrum (right) of QD, aliquots of QDs on graphene at different time intervals 4, 8, 12, 16, 20, and 30 min; the spectra are normalized to the absorption at 450 nm. Reprinted from Ref. [40]. Copyright (2014), with permission from Elsevier.

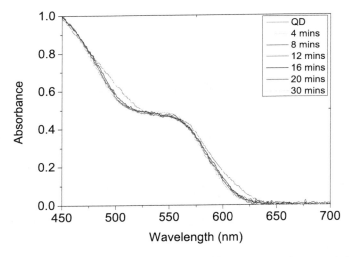

Figure 6.16 UV-Vis absorption spectrum of QD, aliquots of QDs with ODE at different time intervals 4, 8, 12, 16, 20, and 30 min; the spectra are normalized to the absorption at 450 nm. Reprinted from Ref. [40]. Copyright (2014), with permission from Elsevier.

the reference spectrum of QDs. The PL spectrum of the graphene-adsorbed QDs remains primarily at 612 nm irrespective of reaction time, compared to that of the nonadsorbed QDs at 597 nm.

Similarly, UV-Vis spectra of the samples obtained in the absence of graphene highlight the fact that the shift in the optical bands of the QDs is related to the interaction with graphene and not simply to an increase in the size of QDs as a result of unforeseen growth mechanisms during prolonged reaction times at elevated temperatures. Indeed, no evidence for any such growth was observed in the ODE medium. Figure 6.16 is the UV-Vis spectra of the aliquots of QDs with ODE at different time intervals at 4, 8, 12, 16, 20, and 30 min and the reference spectra of QD. It can be clearly seen that the absorption for all the aliquots at different time intervals remains unchanged at 563 nm, that is the absorption of the QD.

6.4 Conclusion and Outlook

In the present chapter the successful synthesis of high-quality CdSe QDs in a bench-top colloidal synthesis has been demonstrated. We observed a change in the phase of the CdSe QDs from cubic ZB to hexagonal WZ and back to the cubic ZB structure as an effect of reaction time and temperature—a unique phase shift, not reported previously despite the wide usage of similar colloidal methods. It provides new insights into the growth mechanisms of CdSe QDs.

Preformed, well-characterized CdSe QDs were successfully deposited onto graphene sheets, resulting in a regular patterning of QDs on the graphene surface, taking on near-ideal hexagonal packing within clusters. This indicates that the CdSe QDs display some particle–particle interactions, which are subsequently minimized by attaining the close-packed arrangement. However, these interactions have been shown not to be the driving mechanism for the 30 nm red shift observed in the CdSe absorption edge and the corresponding shift of 18 nm in the emission band. This can only be electronic in nature and represents a true coupling of the two systems—in effect the QDs display optical properties consistent with quantum confinement in a larger particle, even though the true core size of the QD particles is unchanged. This may indicate some degree of electronic quantum tunnelling between the two components. It is interesting that no optical bleaching due to fluorescence quenching was observed, despite this coupling of electronic systems, implying some coherence in the interaction. Finally, it has been demonstrated that the red shift cannot be attributed to particle growth as a result of enhanced reaction times but that it is purely due to the direct coupling of the QDs to graphene. This work has demonstrated that the optical properties of QDs may be enhanced by the conceptual ability to tune the absorption and emission bands via the extent of electronic coupling between the QDs and the graphene, further advancing the achievement of the use of QDs in various potential applications in fields of optics, biological imaging and sensing.

Whilst significant progress in the synthesis and characterization of CdSe QDs has been made in this chapter, there remain many avenues of research in the field of QD research; the authors recognize that the present work is one small step in that general direction and hope that it encourages others to continue along that path.

Acknowledgments

The authors would like to thank Fan Wang and Dr. Peter Reece from the School of Physics, the University of New South Wales, for the PL measurements; Dr. Katharine L. Page and Dr. Thomas Proffen (NPDF instrument scientist at the Los Alamos National Laboratory, New Mexico) for the PDF analysis; and Dr. Mohammad Choucair for providing the graphene samples. I would also like to thank Adam Micolich, Deborah Kane, and Peter Roger for their valuable inputs in the chapter.

References

1. Dabbousi, B. O., et al. (CdSe)ZnS Core–shell quantum dots: synthesis and characterization of a size series of highly luminescent nanocrystallites, *J. Phys. Chem. B*, **101**(46), 1997, 9463–9475.
2. Murray, C. B., Norris, D. J., and Bawendi, M. G. Synthesis and characterization of nearly monodisperse Cde (E = S, Se, Te) semiconductor nanocrystallites, *J. Am. Chem. Soc.*, **115**(19), 1993, 8706–8715.
3. Peng, X., and Thessing, J. Controlled synthesis of high quality semiconductor nanocrystals, *Struct. Bonding*, **118**, 2005, 79–119.

4. Peng, Z. A., and Peng, X. Formation of high-quality CdTe, CdSe, and CdS nanocrystals using CdO as precursor, *J. Am. Chem. Soc.*, **123**(1), 2001, 183–184.
5. Qu, L. H., Peng, Z. A., and Peng, X. G. Alternative routes toward high quality CdSe nanocrystals, *Nano Lett.*, **1**(6), 2001, 333–337.
6. Hickey, S. G., et al. Size and shape control of colloidally synthesized IV-VI nanoparticulate Tin(II) sulfide, *J. Am. Chem. Soc.*, **130**(45), 2008, 14978–14980.
7. Zhang, K., et al. Preparation, characterization, and fluorescence properties of well-dispersed core–shell CdS/carbon nanoparticles, *J. Mater. Sci.*, **46**(21), 2011, 6975–6980.
8. Miao, S. D., et al. Synthesis and characterization of cadmium phosphide quantum dots emitting in the visible red to near-infrared, *J. Am. Chem. Soc.*, **132**(16), 2010, 5613–5615.
9. Kim, Y.-T., et al. Electrochemical synthesis of CdSe quantum-dot arrays on a graphene basal plane using mesoporous silica thin-film templates, *Adv. Mater.*, **22**(4), 2010, 515–518.
10. Wang, L., et al. Rapid determination of the toxicity of quantum dots with luminous bacteria, *J. Hazard. Mater.*, **177**(1-3), 2010, 1134–1137.
11. Heersche, H. B., et al. Bipolar supercurrent in graphene, *Nature*, **446**(7131), 2007, 56–59.
12. Geim, A. K., and Novoselov, K. S. The rise of graphene, *Nat. Mater.*, **6**(3), 2007, 183–191.
13. Phillips, P. Mottness, *Ann. Phys.*, **321**(7), 2006, 1634–1650.
14. Zhang, Y., et al. Experimental observation of the quantum Hall effect and Berry's phase in graphene, *Nature*, **438**(7065), 2005, 201–204.
15. Lee, C., et al. Measurement of the elastic properties and intrinsic strength of monolayer graphene, *Science*, **321**(5887), 2008, 385–388.
16. Katsnelson, M. I., Graphene: carbon in two dimensions, *Mater. Today*, **10**(1-2), 2007, 20–27.
17. Kim, K. S., et al. Large-scale pattern growth of graphene films for stretchable transparent electrodes, *Nature*, **457**(7230), 2009, 706–710.
18. Paek, S.-M., Yoo, E., and Honma, I. Enhanced cyclic performance and lithium storage capacity of SnO_2/graphene nanoporous electrodes with three-dimensionally delaminated flexible structure, *Nano Lett.*, **9**(1), 2009, 72–75.
19. Stankovich, S., et al. Graphene-based composite materials, *Nature*, **442**(7100), 2006, 282–286.

20. Calandra, M., and Mauri, F. Electronic structure of heavily doped graphene: the role of foreign atom states, *Phys. Rev. B*, **76**(19), 2007, 161406-(1)–161406-(4).
21. Leenaerts, O., Partoens, B., and Peeters, F. Adsorption of H_2O, NH_3, CO, NO_2, and NO on graphene: a first-principles study, *Phys. Rev. B*, **77**(12), 2008, 125416-(1)–125416-(6).
22. Nethravathi, C., et al. Graphite oxide-intercalated anionic clay and its decomposition to graphene-inorganic material nanocomposites, *Langmuir*, **24**(15), 2008, 8240–8244.
23. Si, Y. C., and Samulski, E. T. Exfoliated graphene separated by platinum nanoparticles, *Chem. Mater.*, **20**(21), 2008, 6792–6797.
24. Cong, H. P., et al. Water-soluble magnetic-functionalized reduced graphene oxide sheets: in situ synthesis and magnetic resonance imaging applications, *Small*, **6**(2), 2010, 169–173.
25. Lim, S. J., et al. Synthesis and characterization of zinc-blende CdSe-based core/shell nanocrystals and their luminescence in water, *J. Phys. Chem. C*, **112**(6), 2008, 1744–1747.
26. Yang, Y. A., et al. Synthesis of CdSe and CdTe nanocrystals without precursor injection, *Angew. Chem., Int. Ed. Engl.*, **44**(41), 2005, 6712–6715.
27. Yu, K., et al. Effect of reaction media on the growth and photoluminescence of colloidal CdSe nanocrystals, *Langmuir*, **20**(25), 2004, 11161–11168.
28. Radulaski, M., Numerical Simulations of Electron-Phonon Interactions in Quantum Dots, Diploma thesis, 2011.
29. Xia, X., et al. Wurtzite and zinc-blende CdSe based core/shell semiconductor nanocrystals: structure, morphology and photoluminescence, *J. Lumin.*, **130**(7), 2010, 1285–1291.
30. Kanodarwala, F. K., et al., Phase transformations in CdSe quantum dots induced by reaction time, *Mater. Lett.*, **141**, 2015, 67–69.
31. Yeh, C. Y., et al. Zinc-blende–wurtzite polytypism in semiconductors, *Phys. Rev. B*, **46**, 1992, 10086–10097.
32. Talapin, D. V., et al. Seeded growth of highly luminescent CdSe/CdS nanoheterostructures with rod and tetrapod morphologies, *Nano Lett.*, **7**, 2007, 2951–2959.
33. Fiore, A., et al. Tetrapod-shaped colloidal nanocrystals of II–VI semiconductors prepared by seeded growth, *J. Am. Chem. Soc.*, **131**(6), 2009, 2274–2282.

34. Proffen, T., et al. Structural analysis of complex materials using the atomic pair distribution function: a practical guide, *Z. Kristallogr.*, **218**, 2003, 132–143.
35. Vesely, C. J., and Langer, D. W. Electronic core levels of the IIB-VIA compounds, *Phys. Rev. B*, **4**, 1971, 451–462.
36. Wagner, C. D., et al. Handbook of X-Ray Photoelectron Spectroscopy, Physical Electronics, MN, 1978.
37. Katari, J. E. B., Colvin, V. L., and Alivisatos, A. P. X-ray photoelectron spectroscopy of CdSe nanocrystals with applications to studies of the nanocrystal surface, *J. Phys. Chem.*, **98**, 1994, 4109–4117.
38. Wang, Y., et al. One-pot facile decoration of CdSe quantum dots on graphene nanosheets: novel graphene-CdSe nanocomposites with tunable fluorescent properties, *J. Mater. Chem.*, **21**(2), 2011, 562–566.
39. Choucair, M., Thordarson, P., and Stride, J. A. Gram-scale production of graphene based on solvothermal synthesis and sonication, *Nat. Nanotechnol.*, **4**(1), 2008, 30–33.
40. Kanodarwala, F. K., et al., Deposition of CdSe quantum dots on graphene sheets, *J. Lumin.*, **146**, 2014, 46–52.
41. Xia, Y. N., et al. Monodispersed colloidal spheres: old materials with new applications, *Adv. Mater.*, **12**(10), 2000, 693–713.
42. Neeleshwar, S., et al. Size-dependent properties of CdSe quantum dots, *Phys. Rev. B*, **71**(20), 2005, 201307-(1)–201307-(4).
43. Moreels, I., et al. Size-dependent optical properties of colloidal PbS quantum dots, *ACS Nano*, **3**(10), 2009, 3023–3030.

Biography

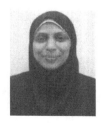

Fehmida K. Kanodarwala was born in Mumbai, India. She received her PhD degree in chemistry in 2012 from the University of New South Wales. Her PhD research dealt with the synthesis, characterization and functionalization of CdSe quantum dots. Dr. Kanodarwala is currently working as a postdoctoral fellow at the University of New South Wales, Australia, researching metal-organic framework nanocomposite membranes for gas separation. Her current interest is in nanoparticle synthesis and application for fuel gases.

Dr. Kanodarwala is a member of the Australian Research Council Nanotechnology Network and the Australian Microscopy & Microanalysis Society. She has attended a number of local and international conferences and has established several international collaborations.

Chapter 7

Design of Novel Nanostructured Photoanode Materials for Low-Cost and Efficient Dye-Sensitized Solar Cell Applications

Yang Bai,[a] Zhen Li,[b] Rose Amal,[c] and Lianzhou Wang[a]

[a]*Nanomaterials Centre, School of Chemical Engineering and Australian Institute for Bioengineering and Nanotechnology, University of Queensland, St. Lucia, Brisbane, QLD 4072, Australia*
[b]*Institute of Superconducting and Electronic Materials, Australian Institute of Innovative Materials, University of Wollongong, Squires Way, North Wollongong, NSW 2500, Australia*
[c]*School of Chemical Engineering, University of New South Wales, Sydney, NSW 2052, Australia*
ybai@unl.edu, l.wang@uq.edu.au

Dye-sensitized solar cells (DSSCs), known as the third generation of solar cells, are being considered as a promising alternative to expensive conventional silicon-based photovoltaic devices. This interest relates to low material cost, easy and inexpensive methods of fabrication, and relatively high power conversion efficiency for DSSCs. Inspired by the breakthrough work of Grätzel, much effort has been made to further improve the performance in the past decades. As one of the key components, the photoanode not only

---

Nanomaterials: Science and Applications
Edited by Deborah Kane, Adam Micolich, and Peter Roger
Copyright © 2016 Pan Stanford Publishing Pte. Ltd.
ISBN 978-981-4669-72-6 (Hardcover), 978-981-4669-73-3 (eBook)
www.panstanford.com

acts as the backbone for dye adsorption but also assumes the task of charge transport, which determines DSSC performance. The conventional TiO_2 nanoparticle (NP)-based photoanode suffers from inefficient charge transfer and light harvesting. To optimize the photoanode architecture, we show the design of novel nanostructured photoanode materials featuring large dye uptake ability, efficient charge transfer, and improved light harvesting. In this chapter, the first part provides a brief introduction to various aspects of DSSCs, including device structure, working principles, and characterization techniques. The second part reviews recent advances in the engineering of photoanode architectures, followed by a brief discussion regarding the stability and commercialization of DSSC technology. Our recent work will then be presented in the next section, focusing on the design of new photoanode materials for enhanced DSSC application. In the end, a relevant conclusion and outlook will be addressed for the future development of low-cost and efficient solar cells.

7.1 Introduction

The global consumption of energy is expected to double within the next 40 years [1]. This huge energy demand cannot be satisfied by accelerated consumption of conventional fossil fuels, which would aggravate environmental pollution and global warming. The development of renewable and clean energy technologies is vital to meeting the future energy needs of society. Various technologies have been developed to produce energy from natural renewable resources, including hydropower, wind power, and solar power (photovoltaic and solar thermal). A significant increase in renewable energy production is expected in the coming decades. Among these energy sources, solar power is the most abundant, providing 6000 times the world's current energy demand. Thus it is commonly considered as the ultimate solution toward clean and sustainable energy production in the future.

Photovoltaic cells convert solar energy directly into electricity. There has been exponential growth in fundamental research on photovoltaics and their transfer to the industrial market over the past decades. Conventional photovoltaic devices (first-generation solar cells) are based on single-/polycrystalline silicon (Si). The silicon solar cell is configured as a large-area p–n junction formed by placing a layer of p-type silicon into direct contact with a layer of n-type silicon. The electrons and holes are generated by photoexcitation at the interface region of a p–n junction, called the depletion region. The electrons and holes are separated by the electrical field across the junction and collected through an external load. A certified record efficiency of 27.6% was obtained by Amonix [2] using single-crystalline silicon. The purification of crystalline Si is an energy-intensive process, resulting in a high production cost for crystalline Si solar cells. Thin-film solar cells incorporating amorphous Si, CdTe, $CuInSe_2$ (CIS), and $CuInGaSe_2$ (CIGS) have been developed to reduce the material cost. These are called second-generation solar cells and have confirmed conversion efficiencies ranging from 13.5% to 19.9%. Higher efficiencies have been obtained using GaAs, InP, and InGaP III–V semiconductor multijunction solar cells, which take advantage of a greater portion of the solar spectrum. Multijunction solar cells bring the certified highest efficiency of 44.4% [2] and have thus replaced traditional Si cells in applications where cost is not a major issue. While second-generation photovoltaics has significantly reduced the dependence on high purity crystalline Si, the total production cost is only slightly lower due to the extremely expensive manufacturing technologies involved. Major breakthroughs are still required to meet the goal of low-cost clean energy production for widespread use.

The integration of nanostructured materials into photovoltaic devices provides an opportunity to develop lower-cost solar cells with relatively high efficiency. Dye-sensitized solar cells (DSSCs), also known as third-generation solar cells, have attracted considerable scientific and industrial interest over the past two decades [1, 3–6]. DSSCs first captured international attention in 1991 with the report of DSSCs with 7% efficiency by O'Regan and Grätzel [3]. Subsequent work quickly boosted the efficiency to 10% [7]. Development slowed briefly thereafter, until 2014, when a new record efficiency of 13% for liquid-junction DSSCs was achieved by using a new porphyrin dye SM315 [8]. DSSCs are traditionally fabricated using inexpensive oxide nanoparticles (NPs) and coordination complexes or organic dyes. The cell fabrication can avoid vacuum processing or high temperatures so that the technology can be easier to scale up to the terawatt level. DSSCs can also be fabricated using plastic substrates, enabling the possibility of flexible photovoltaic elements and novel concepts such as power windows. In addition, DSSCs show good performance under diffuse light conditions.

It is worth noting that the key to the breakthrough for DSSCs in 1991 was the introduction of a mesoporous TiO_2 NP-based photoanode with a high surface area. The photoanode film supports the sensitizer, collects the photogenerated electrons from the dye molecules, and provides the path for electron diffusion. Thus it is one of the crucial elements determining the DSSC performance. As a result, engineering of the photoanode has attracted tremendous attention during the last 20 years. We provide a focused review of recent research on the design of novel nanostructured photoanodes. Three key aspects are to be addressed: dye uptake ability, electron mobility, and light-harvesting efficiency. Prior to this, we will give an overview of the DSSC structure and working principles. To fully understand the working mechanism and complex interaction of its components, several frequently used analysis techniques will be presented, including the photovoltaic characteristic measurements and electrochemical methods. A discussion regarding the stability and commercialization of DSSC technology is also provided. We close with a survey of our recent work and a brief outlook for the development of low-cost efficient DSSCs.

7.2 How Does a Dye-Sensitized Solar Cell Work?

7.2.1 Operating Principles

A typical DSSC comprises four major parts: (1) a molecular sensitizer dye attached to a (2) porous TiO_2 film on a conducting glass substrate (fluorine-doped tin oxide [FTO]), which forms as a photoanode immersed in a (3) redox mediator electrolyte sandwiched with a (4) platinum-coated counterelectrode (CE). Figure 7.1 shows the typical operating principle of a DSSC cell and

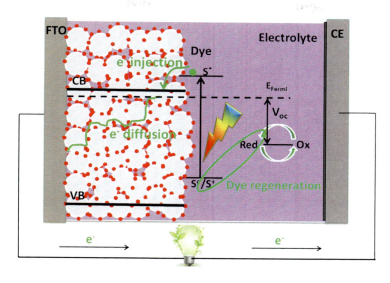

Figure 7.1 Operating principle and energy level scheme of a DSSC.

the operating cycle of DSSCs can be summarized as below:

$$\text{Photoanode}: S + h\upsilon \rightarrow S^* \quad \text{Photon absorption} \quad (7.1)$$

$$S^* \rightarrow S^+ + e^-_{TiO_2} \quad \text{Electron injection} \quad (7.2)$$

$$2S^+ + 3I^- \rightarrow 2S + I_3^- \quad \text{Dye regeneration} \quad (7.3)$$

$$\left.\begin{array}{l} S^+ + e^-_{TiO_2} \rightarrow S \\ I_3^- + 2e^-_{TiO_2} \rightarrow 3I^- \\ I_3^- + 2e^-_{FTO} \rightarrow 3I^- \end{array}\right\} \text{Recombination} \quad (7.4)$$

$$\text{Counterelectrode}: I_3^- + 2e^-_{Pt} \rightarrow 3I^- \quad \text{Iodide regeneration} \quad (7.5)$$

Light absorption is performed by the sensitizer (S), which is attached to the surface of a wide-bandgap semiconductor, usually a film consisting of TiO_2 NPs. After being photoexcited by the photons of sunlight (Eq. 7.1), electrons are injected into the conduction band (CB) of the oxide semiconductor from the dye (Eq. 7.2). Injected electrons in the CB of the TiO_2 film are transferred through the surface or the bulk of the interconnected TiO_2 NPs with diffusion toward the back contact (FTO). These electrons consequently reach the CE (cathode) through the external load. The photoexcited dye is regenerated by electron donation from the electrolyte penetrated into the porous film (Eq. 7.3). DSSCs are the only photovoltaic devices where light absorption and charge transfer are physically separated processes. Thus a DSSC essentially mimics the photosynthesis process used by plants. This separation offers the opportunity to individually tailor light absorption and charge transport and thereby bring gains in efficiency.

Most frequently, the electrolyte contains the iodide/triiodide couple as a redox shuttle. Other mediators such as copper (I/II) complexes [9] or the TEMPO/TEMPO+ redox couple [10] have also been investigated recently as an alternative to the iodide/triiodide system. The reduction of S^+ by iodide prevents any significant buildup of S^+ and thus intercepts the recapture of the CB electrons by S^+ at the surface. Furthermore it results in the production of triiodide ions in the electrolyte. The iodide is regenerated, in turn, by the reduction of the triiodide ions at the CE (Eq. 7.7), where the electrons are contributed via migration through the external load. Therefore, electricity is generated from sunlight by the device without any permanent chemical transformation; it is regenerative and stable. The theoretical maximum voltage of the device generated under illumination is known as the open-circuit voltage (V_{oc}). It corresponds to the energy difference between the redox potential of the mediator in the electrolyte and the Fermi level of the nanocrystalline film indicated with a dashed line in Fig. 7.1.

Nevertheless, there are certain undesirable reactions that can occur, which include the injected electrons recombining (i) with the oxidized dye (Eq. 7.4) or (ii) with the oxidized redox couple in the electrolyte at the TiO_2 surface (Eq. 7.5) or (iii) on the FTO surface as the incomplete cover of the FTO substrate by nanocrystalline TiO_2 (Eq. 7.6), resulting in loss in cell efficiency.

7.2.2 Key Components

It is crucial to understand the properties of the four components when striving for high power conversion efficiency.

7.2.2.1 Metal oxide photoanode

In DSSCs, the photoanode (working electrode) is usually a thin film of semiconductor, most commonly TiO_2. A semiconductor has two bands, one nominally fully occupied and one nominally empty. These are known as the valence band (VB) and the CB. The VB is the highest range of electron energies in which electrons are normally present at absolute zero temperature, whilst the CB is the level of electron energies higher than that of the VB, sufficient to allow electrons to move freely within the atomic lattice of the material. They are separated in energy by a gap where electrons cannot reside. For conduction to occur, electrons need to be excited from the VB to the CB, where there are sufficient unoccupied states to enable the electron to move through the material. The conductivity is tied to the magnitude of the energy gap, normally called the bandgap. Materials where the bandgap exceeds 4 eV are generally considered to be insulators [11]. The electrical conductivity of a semiconductor is intermediate between that of a conductor and that of an insulator. Another important energy level associated with semiconductors is the Fermi level. It is defined as the energy at which the probability of a quantum state being occupied by an electron is exactly half. For pure, undoped semiconductors, the Fermi level is located halfway between the VB and the CB.

TiO_2 is the most commonly used semiconductor in DSSCs, owing to its stability and relatively inexpensive cost. There are three crystalline polymorphs for TiO_2 in nature: rutile phase (tetragonal, space group P42/mnm, $E_g \approx 3.05$ eV), anatase phase (tetragonal, I41/amd, $E_g \approx 3.23$ eV), and brookite phase (orthorhombic, Pcab, $E_g \approx 3.26$ eV). The rutile phase TiO_2 is not widely used in DSSCs despite being thermodynamically stable and having a smaller bandgap, which makes it more suitable in absorbing the solar spectrum. The metastable anatase phase, which can be irreversibly transformed into the rutile phase by high-temperature processing, is preferable for three reasons: (a) An anatase TiO_2 NP film offers a high internal surface area for dye adsorption [12], (b) the anatase phase also has higher electric conductivity [12], and (c) the CB edge of the anatase phase is 0.1 eV higher, which should increase the cell's maximum open circuit voltage (V_{oc}).

The TiO_2 photoanode also mediates charge transport. The exact mechanics of this process is still under keen debate today [13–15]. Several competing interpretations have been advanced, including some based on diffusion [15] or the Montrol–Scher model for random displacement of charge carriers in disordered solids [14]. The effective electron diffusion coefficient is expected to depend on a number of factors, such as trap filling and space charge compensation by ionic motion in the electrolyte. Theoretical efforts will continue, as there is a need for further in-depth analysis of this intriguing charge percolation process in the photoanodes. The mesoporous structure of TiO_2 photoanodes assured efficient dye adsorption; however, it also has some drawbacks [16]: (1) The inherent conductivity of the film is very low, (2) the small size of the nanocrystalline particles does not support a built-in electric field, and (3) the electrolyte penetrates the porous film all the way to the back contact, making the semiconductor/electrolyte interface essentially 3D. The drawbacks of the mesoporous structure need to be overcome for further performance development of DSSCs with TiO_2 films.

Parallel to the study on DSSCs using TiO_2 photoanodes, extensive efforts have also been devoted to ZnO [17], In_2O_3 [18], Nb_2O_5 [19], SnO_2 [20], and Zn_2SnO_4 [21] as photoanodes. Among all these semiconductors, ZnO seems to have the greatest potential as an alternative to TiO_2 for enhanced DSSCs. ZnO possesses a similar energy band structure and physical properties to TiO_2 but has a much higher electronic mobility that would be favorable for electron transport. However, much work still needs to be done, since the efficiency achieved for DSSCs with ZnO is still much lower than that of DSSCs fabricated with typical TiO_2, let alone other materials.

7.2.2.2 Sensitizer for light absorption

The sensitizers in DSSCs play a critical role in absorbing light and generating electron–hole pairs. To achieve a high light-to-energy conversion efficiency, the sensitizer needs to satisfy several requirements, as follows [16]:

- The sensitizer should absorb light broadly across the UV and near-IR region with high molar absorptivity. The optimum absorption peak position is around 920 nm corresponding to an ideal bandgap of 1.35 eV.
- The energy levels of the sensitizer should match well with those of the semiconducting oxides and electrolyte. To minimize energy losses and to maximize the photovoltage, the excited state of the sensitizer should be only slightly above the CB edge of the semiconductor but sufficiently above the CB edge to provide an energetic driving force for the electron injection process. For the same reason, the ground state of the sensitizer needs to be aligned with the redox potential of the electrolyte for the regeneration of the sensitizer.
- Electron injection from the excited state to the CB of the semiconductor should be fast enough to outrun competing unwanted charge recombination.
- To decrease the interface resistance and to secure long-term stable bonding, sensitizers need to be strongly anchored onto the surface of the semiconductor film.
- The sensitizing materials should be stable enough in the working environment to sustain up to 20 years of operation under sunlight, that is, at least 10^8 redox turnovers.

To date, various sensitizing materials including metal complex dyes, metal-free organic dyes, natural dyes, and quantum dots (QDs) have been investigated and employed in DSSCs. In terms of conversion yield and long-term stability, the most popular sensitizers are metal complex dyes such as polypyridyl complexes of ruthenium (Ru) developed by the Grätzel group: N3, N719, and N749 (black dyes). The metal complex dyes are particularly promising and have the general structure $ML_2(X)_2$, where L stands for 2,2'-bipyridyl-4,4'-dicarboxylic acid, M is Ru, and X represents a halide, cyanide, thiocyanate, [7, 16], or water substituent. Chemical structures of N3, N749, and some other dyes are shown in Fig. 7.2. Since its discovery in 1993, the ruthenium complex cis-$RuL_2(NCS)_2$, known as N3 dye, has become the paradigm for heterogeneous charge transfer sensitizers for mesoporous solar cells [7]. In a subsequently

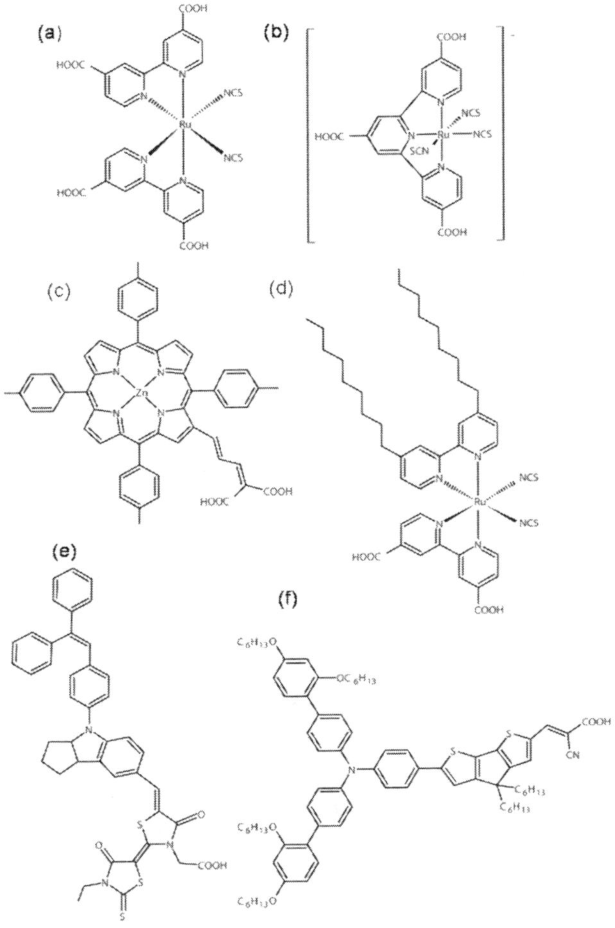

Figure 7.2 Chemical structures of some important dye molecules for DSSCs. (a) N3, (b) black dye N749, (c) porphyrin, (d) Z907, (e) indoline, and (f) donor-Q-acceptor organic dye Y123. Reprinted with permission from Ref. [5]. Copyright 2012, AIP Publishing LLC.

developed the N719 dye, two protons of N3 were replaced by a tetrabutylammonium (TBA) cation group. The deprotonation of N3 changes the polarity at the interface, positively shifting the CB edge of TiO_2 and increasing the photovoltage in DSSCs employing the

N719 dye. Though the photovoltaic performance of N3 and N719 is outstanding, there's significant room for further improvement if spectra coverage can be extended. The synthesis of a class of a black dye [22], which displays the panchromatic sensitization character over the whole visible range extending from the near-IR region up to 920 nm, offers an opportunity to increase the maximum current density of DSSCs over 20 mA/cm^2. Chiba et al. have recently achieved a record cell efficiency of 11.1% using a black dye called N749 [23].

Ru-based dyes have several drawbacks, some quite significant, that weigh against the relatively high efficiency they provide. These include the high cost of noble metals and complicated synthesis and purification processes. In terms of widespread commercialization, various types of metal-free organic dyes have been developed as low-cost sensitizers in DSSCs. These organic dyes generally consist of an electron donor, an electron acceptor, a conjugated spacer between donor and acceptor, and a surface-anchoring group. Apart from the cost-effectiveness, organic dyes have several other advantages over the Ru complex dyes, which have a larger molar extinction coefficient, more facile synthesis, and more flexibility in tuning the absorbing light spectrum. Thus, remarkable progress in organic dyes has been gained in recent years. DSSCs fabricated with donor-Q-acceptor dyes have shown efficiencies of ca. 10% [24–26]. The Grätzel group has recently reported DSSCs with a record efficiency of 13% using a new porphyrin dye SM315 with a high open-circuit voltage, V_{oc}, of 0.91 V, a short-circuit current density, J_{sc}, of 18.1 mA cm^{-2}, and a fill factor of 0.78 [8].

Inorganic semiconductor QDs have also been extensively studied as new sensitizers to replace conventional organic dyes in DSSCs because of their excellent properties: size-dependent and tunable energy bandgaps, broad excitation spectra, high extinction coefficient, multiple-exciton generation (MEG), and photostability [27–35]. QDs can be easily grown on or attached directly to the mesoporous oxide film by chemical bath deposition (CBD), or they can be anchored through a linker molecule. Figure 7.3 shows the energy levels of various semiconductor QDs [36]. Among all these QDs, cadmium chalcogenide (CdX, X = S, Se, or Te) have attracted more attention in quantum dot–sensitized solar cells (QDSSCs) over

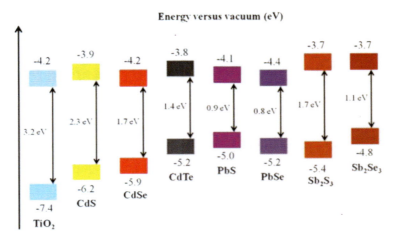

Figure 7.3 Energy levels vs vacuum of various semiconductor quantum dots (QDs). Reproduced with permission from Ref. [36], Copyright © 2013 Nature Publishing Group.

the last few years. Note that CdX absorbs light efficiently since it has a bulk material bandgap above 1.3 eV (bandgaps for CdS, CdSe, and CdTe are 2.25 eV, 1.73 eV, and 1.49 eV, respectively). By employing Mn^{2+} doping of CdS, Kamat et al. have obtained an efficiency of 5.4% for CdS/CdSe co-sensitized QDSSCs fabricated by a simple CBD method [37]. Recently, a record efficiency of 6.76% for QDSSCs was achieved by Wang et al. with the presynthesized CdTe/CdSe type II core/shell QDs as the sensitizer that was attached to the mesoporous TiO_2 layer via a linker molecule [35].

7.2.2.3 Electrolyte for electron transportation

As one of the key components of DSSCs, the electrolyte collects electrons at the cathode and transports the electrons back to the dye molecule. In terms of cell efficiency, the most widely used electrolyte is the iodide/triiodide (I^-/I_3^-) redox mediator in acetonitrile, containing 0.5 M LiI and 0.5 M I_2. Here iodide is the electron donor that reduces the oxidized sensitizer, and triiodide is the electron acceptor at the platinum electrode. The electron injection into the

TiO$_2$ CB occurs in the femtosecond time range, which is much faster than the electron recombination with I$_3^-$. The oxidized dye preferably reacts with I$^-$ than combining with the injected electrons. The I$_3^-$ then diffuses to the CE to capture electrons and, in turn, produce I$^-$. The iodide/triiodide electrolyte not only satisfies the energetic and kinetic requirements for efficient DSSCs but also has many other merits such as excellent stability and reversibility, low visible light absorption, and high diffusion constants. However, its redox potential is not well adapted to that of the presently employed sensitizers. The voltage loss resulting from the mismatch is 0.4 eV and 0.2 eV for the N3 dye and the black dye, respectively [38]. By avoiding this loss, the conversion efficiency of the N3 dye–based cell would be raised from 10% to 17%. The challenge for the chemist is to identify new redox couples that are well matched to the sensitizer, while maintaining all the advantages of the iodide/triiodide system.

New redox couples as alternatives to the I$^-$/I$_3^-$ pair have been investigated and tested in DSSCs. These include copper complexes [39], pseudohalogen redox couples (SeCN$^-$/(SeCN)$_3^-$, SCN$^-$/(SCN)$_3^-$) [40], Br/Br$_3^-$ [41], and the Co(II)/Co(III) complex [42–44]. The SeCN$^-$/(SeCN)$_3^-$ redox couple has shown an excellent efficiency of 7.5%, but the long-term stability is problematic [45]. An enhanced open-circuit voltage of DSSCs has been achieved by employing Br/Br$_3^-$ as the redox couple, which would enlarge the difference between the Fermi level of the working electrode and the redox energy level of the electrolyte [41]. Recently, a record efficiency of 13% was obtained by Grätzel's group by incorporating a Co(II)/Co(III) redox electrolyte in conjunction with a porphyrin dye [8].

Despite the good performance of the liquid electrolyte, the long-term durability of photovoltaic devices still needs to be improved. To overcome disadvantages such as the leakage of organic solvent, research has been conducted to develop new-generation electrolytes, for example, room-temperature ionic liquids [46], quasi-solid-state electrolytes [47], and solid-state electrolytes [48]. Another possible way to improve the stability of DSSCs is to develop encapsulation techniques [49].

7.2.2.4 Counterelectrodes

As a critical component in DSSCs, the CE collects electrons from external circuit and catalyzes the reduction of I_3^- to I^- [50–52], thereby realizing the regeneration of the sensitizer. Traditionally, platinum (Pt) is used as the CE catalyst, owing to its excellent catalytic activity for the reduction of triiodide to iodide as well as high electrical conductivity. However, the low abundance and high cost of Pt severely restricts its application for the large-scale fabrication of DSSCs. Therefore, it is highly desirable to exploit substitutes for Pt in order to further reduce the overall cost and make DSSCs more competitive among various photovoltaic devices for future commercialization.

In previous studies, several noble metal–free materials such as conductive organic polymers and carbon materials (graphite, graphene, and carbon nanotubes) have been explored as CEs in DSSCs [53–58]. More recent research has been devoted to the development of novel inorganic compounds as catalytic CE materials in DSSCs, such as sulfides [59–66], nitrides [67, 68], carbides [50, 68], selenides [69], oxides [70–72], etc.

Electrochemical impedance spectroscopy (EIS) [50, 73, 74] is always employed by using dummy cells to characterize the catalytic activity of these alternative CE catalysts. Figure 7.4a shows the scheme of a dummy cell that is assembled with two identical electrodes (CE/electrolyte/CE). As indicated in the equivalent circuit diagram shown in Fig. 7.4b, R_s represents the series resistance that is composed of the bulk resistance of CE materials, FTO substrate resistance, and contact resistance. The charge transfer resistance (R_{ct}) corresponds to the charge transfer process at the CE/electrolyte interfaces and changes inversely with the catalytic activity of different CEs. Z_w is the Warburg diffusion impedance, which arises from mass transport limitations due to the diffusion of the triiodide/iodide couple within the electrolyte. All these parameters can be determined by fitting the impedance spectra using the Z-view software and directly reflect the catalytic property of the examined catalyst. To further clarify the electrochemical characteristics of the electrode, Tafel polarization, together with cyclic voltammetry (CV) measurements, is carried out [50, 68, 71].

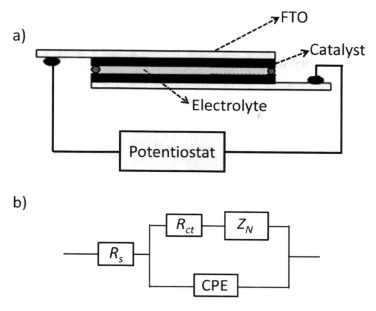

Figure 7.4 (a) Scheme of a dummy cell; (b) equivalent circuit diagram of a dummy cell with two identical electrodes.

7.3 Characterization Techniques

Besides investigations of the separate components, it is also essential to study the complete solar cell in order to fully understand the complex interaction of its components. Thus, a number of characterization techniques, including basic efficiency measurements and electrochemical methods, have been developed for DSSCs. With the assistance of these techniques, we were able to analyze the internal processes on complete cells under normal solar light conditions, which would assist the modeling of different electron transfer processes and the optimization of material components.

7.3.1 Photovoltaic Characteristic Measurements

The current density–voltage (J–V) characteristics of a DSSC cell under illumination are used to determine the overall power conversion efficiency (η). To compare solar cells tested in different laboratories all over the world, the efficiency is measured under a set of standard conditions. Specifically, the solar radiation incident on the cell should have a total power density of 100 mW/cm² with a spectral power distribution characterized as AM 1.5.[a]

The solar energy to electricity power conversion efficiency (η) of DSSC is calculated by the equation

$$\eta = \frac{J_{sc} V_{oc} FF}{P_{in}} \times 100\% \quad (7.6)$$

where J_{sc} is the short-circuit photocurrent density, V_{oc} is the open-circuit photovoltage, P_{in} is the incident light power per unit area, and FF is the fill factor, which is calculated by the equation

$$FF = \frac{P_{max}}{J_{sc} V_{oc}} = \frac{J_{max} V_{max}}{J_{sc} V_{oc}} \quad (7.7)$$

where J_{max} and V_{max} are the photocurrent density and photovoltage at the maximum obtainable power point, respectively, in $J-V$ curves of the solar cells.

The spectral response of DSSCs is determined by measuring the monochromatic incident photon-to-current conversion efficiency (IPCE), which is defined as

$$IPCE = \frac{\text{Quantity of collected electrons}}{\text{Quantity of incident photons}} = \frac{hc J_{sc}}{e\lambda P_{in}} \quad (7.8)$$

where λ, e, h, and c are the wavelength of incident light, elementary charge, Planck's constant, and speed of light, respectively.

7.3.2 Electrochemical Methods

Powerful electrochemical methods can be used to characterize all the components of DSSCs separately. This provides important information on the energy levels of the components, on the reversibility of electrochemical reactions, and on the kinetics of electrochemical processes. The standard equipment in electrochemistry is a potentiostat connected to a three-electrode cell, with a working electrode, a CE, and a reference electrode.

---

[a] The solar spectrum after traveling through the atmosphere to sea level with the sun directly overhead is referred to as AM1. AM 1.5 means 1.5 atmosphere thicknesses and corresponds to a solar zenith angle of 78°.

As one of the most commonly used electrochemical methods in DSSCs, the open-circuit voltage decay (OCVD) technique can be employed to examine the charge transfer kinetics of DSSCs. Before the measurement, DSSCs are illuminated under the simulated solar light to obtain a steady-state voltage, indicating the equilibrium between the electron photogeneration and the recombination of the photogenerated electrons by the I_3^- ions in the electrolyte is attained in the cells [75–77]. The V_{oc} as a function of time is recorded after the illumination is interrupted, while the cell is kept at open circuit. The decay of the V_{oc} is a sign of electron loss as a result of the charge recombination.

EIS is another major technique for understanding the kinetic processes of DSSCs [30, 50, 73, 77–80]. Under appropriate conditions, electron transport in the mesoporous TiO_2 film, electron recombination at the TiO_2–electrolyte interface, charge transfer at the CE, and diffusion of the redox species in the electrolyte can be distinguished on the basis of the spectral shapes of the impedance response with frequency. Figure 7.5 shows a typical impedance spectrum of a DSSC, together with its electrical equivalent model [81]. As shown in the model, r_{ct} is the charge transfer resistance of the charge recombination process between electrons in the mesoporous metal oxide film and ions in the electrolyte; C_m is the chemical capacitance of the mesoporous metal oxide film; r_t is the transport resistance of the electrons in the mesoporous metal oxide film; Z_d is the Warburg element showing the Nernst diffusion of ions in the electrolyte; R_{Pt} and C_{Pt} are the charge transfer resistance and double-layer capacitance at the CE (platinized transparent conducting oxide [TCO] plate), respectively; R_{TCO} and C_{TCO} are the charge transfer resistance and the corresponding double-layer capacitance at the exposed TCO–electrolyte interface, respectively; R_{CO} and C_{CO} are the resistance and capacitance at the TCO–TiO_2 contact, respectively; and R_S is the series resistance, including the sheet resistance of the TCO glass and the contact resistance of the cell. The steady-state transport resistance through the mesoporous network, transient diffusion coefficient, chemical capacitance at the metal oxide–electrolyte interface, and recombination resistance can be evaluated by fitting the impedance spectra using the Z-view software.

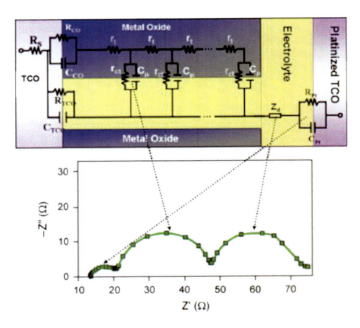

Figure 7.5 Electrical equivalent (top panel) and impedance spectrum (Nyquist plot) (bottom panel) of a typical DSSC. Reprinted from Ref. [81] with permission of the American Ceramic Society, www.ceramics.org All rights reserved.

In addition, photoelectrochemical techniques such as intensity-modulated photocurrent spectroscopy (IMPS), intensity-modulated photovoltage spectroscopy (IMVS) [82–84], and transient photocurrent/photovoltage [85, 86] have also been developed to study DSSCs under actual operating conditions.

7.4 Development of Nanostructured Photoanodes

The photovoltaic performance of DSSCs is closely related to the properties of a nanostructured photoanode film consisting of wide-bandgap semiconductors. Advanced nanotechnology has opened the door to developing new nanostructured materials for use in DSSCs. During the last two decades, intense efforts have been made to design and optimize photoanode nanostructures on the basis of

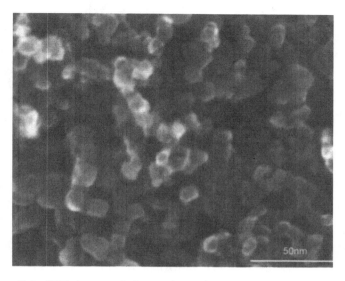

Figure 7.6 SEM image of the surface of a mesoporous anatase film. Reprinted by permission from Macmillan Publishers Ltd: *Nature* (Ref. [4]), copyright (2001).

three requisites: large surface area, high light-harvesting efficiency, and efficient charge transfer. The chemical and mechanical stability should also be taken into account in terms of achieving long lifetimes.

7.4.1 Mesoporous Nanoparticle Films

The impressive breakthrough of DSSCs in 1991 was achieved by using a mesoporous TiO_2 NP film, as shown in Fig. 7.6. Mesoporous NP films usually have pores between 2 and 50 nm in diameter and a continuous network that can be either ordered or disordered. So far, a wide range of TiO_2 NPs with desirable shape, phase, and crystallinity has been investigated for use as photoanodes in DSSCs. This is mainly because the films comprised of NPs provide a high surface area, which is beneficial for generating a large photocurrent and therefore high power conversion efficiency. Another advantage comes from the simple synthesis of NPs and the ease of film fabrication.

The internal network geometry within mesoporous films has a great influence on the electron transport dynamics of DSSCs. Discovered by Zukalova et al. in 2005, ordered mesoporous TiO_2 nanocrystalline films showed enhanced solar conversion efficiency by about 50% compared to conventional films consisted of randomly oriented anatase nanocrystals with the same thickness [87]. The ordered TiO_2 nanocrystalline films were prepared by layer-by-layer deposition using Pluronic P123 as a template. The 0.95 μm thick randomly oriented anatase film showed a conversion efficiency of only 2.21% under standard global AM 1.5 solar conditions, while the cell with ordered mesoporous TiO_2 nanocrystalline film yielded an enhanced efficiency of 4.04% finally [87].

Besides, a comparison of photovoltaic performance for DSSCs using anatase- and rutile-phase TiO_2 NPs was demonstrated by Park et al. [12]. For the same film thickness, the V_{oc} of the dye-sensitized rutile and anatase films is essentially the same, whereas the short-circuit photocurrent of the rutile-based cell is about 30% lower than that of the anatase-based cell because of lesser dye adsorption due to a smaller surface area compared with that of the anatase film. However, a hybrid TiO_2 photoanode composed of a mixture of anatase and rutile TiO_2 exhibited higher conversion efficiency than that of pure anatase. The anatase–rutile (71% anatase and 29% rutile) based DSSC showed superior performance with an efficiency of 6.8% than the pure anatase (efficiency, $\eta = 5.3\%$) for the same crystalline size and surface area (26 nm, Brunauer–Emmett–Teller (BET) 57 m^2/g) [88].

Great attention has been invested in constructing photoanodes using anatase TiO_2 nanocrystals with more reactive (001) facets for high-performance DSSCs [76, 89–91], since the work by Lu et al. showing that uniform anatase TiO_2 single crystals with a high percentage (47%) of (001) facets were successfully synthesized [92]. Nanosized anatase TiO_2 single crystals with different percentages of exposed (001) facets (see Fig. 7.7) have been employed as photoanodes in DSSCs. Figure 7.7a–c demonstrates the evolution of the morphology of the nanocrystals as a function of the HF concentration. The geometry of the NSCT-a (Fig. 7.7a,e,g) can be considered as a decahedron with dominant (001) facets at the bottom and top, and the calculated percentage of exposed (001)

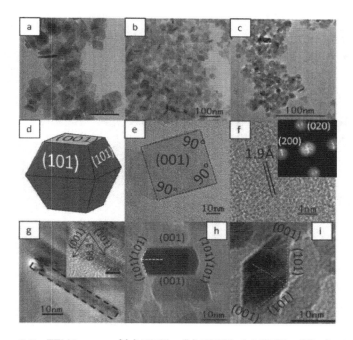

Figure 7.7 TEM images of (a) NSCT-a, (b) NSCT-b, (c) NSCT-c, (d) schematic crystallographic structure of TiO_2 single crystal, (e) top view and (g) side view of a nanosized single crystal of NSCT-a, (f) the inset of (g) high-resolution TEM images recorded from (e) and (g), respectively, and the inset of (f) fast-Fourier transform (FFT) pattern recorded from (f) indexed to the (001) zone. (h, i) Side views of the nanosized single crystals of NSCT-b and NSCT-c. Reprinted with permission from Ref. [76]. Copyright © 2011 WILEY-VCH.

facets was ca. 80%. By diluting the HF concentration, a decrease in the lateral size and an increase in the thickness can be observed in NSCT-b (Fig. 7.7b,h). The percentage of exposed (001) facets was estimated to be ca. 38%. Furthermore, the size of NSCT-c (Fig. 7.7c,i) shrank to ca. 9 nm with a percentage of exposed (001) facets less than 10%. When applied in DSSCs, over 40% enhancement of conversion efficiency was achieved for the cell based on anatase single crystals with ca. 80% of (001) facets compared to that based on Degussa P25 [76].

To further enhance the conversion efficiency of DSSCs, the posttreatment of TiO$_2$ NP films by TiCl$_4$ is generally required. TiCl$_4$ treatments provide several benefits [93–96]: (1) interparticular necking, (2) increased binding sites, (3) suppressed interfacial charge recombination, and (4) a positive shift in the TiO$_2$ CB edge. As a result, increased dye loading, improved electron injection, and more efficient charge transfer are obtained in the posttreated TiO$_2$ NP films.

7.4.2 Light-Scattering and LSPR Effects

One major drawback of conventional TiO$_2$ NP photoanodes is the negligible light scattering of the films due to their small particle size ranging typically from ca. 20–30 nm. This results in a low light-harvesting efficiency. An optical scattering layer on top has been proposed as it could enhance the light harvesting by localizing the incident light within the photoanode. So far, an array of light-scattering materials has been investigated, including TiO$_2$ mesoporous microspheres [97, 98], hollow spheres [99–101], and mirror-like NPs [90, 102].

Bifunctional nano-embossed hollow spherical TiO$_2$ (NeHS TiO$_2$) particles [100] have been utilized as efficient light scatterers. The cross section of the bilayer structure is shown in Fig. 7.8. NeHS particles show excellent property in scattering the incoming light, as confirmed by reflectance spectroscopy. Substantial improvement has been achieved when the NeHS-containing layer is used as a secondary layer in DSSCs. Despite the improved light harvesting due to such microsized hollow spherical TiO$_2$, the accessible surface for dye loading is usually sacrificed. To address this issue, another approach was proposed using submicrometer-sized TiO$_2$ beads [103] with abundant mesopores, as shown in Fig. 7.9. These crystalline, mesoporous TiO$_2$ beads have a surface area up to 108.0 m^2 g^{-1} and tunable pore size varying from 14.0 to 22.6 nm through a facile combination of sol–gel and solvothermal processes. Such mesoporous TiO$_2$ beads have an average diameter of ca. 830 nm and are composed of anatase TiO$_2$ nanocrystals. Compared to the benchmark P25 electrode, the 12.3 µm thick TiO$_2$ electrode made from the mesoporous TiO$_2$ beads achieved a 27% increase

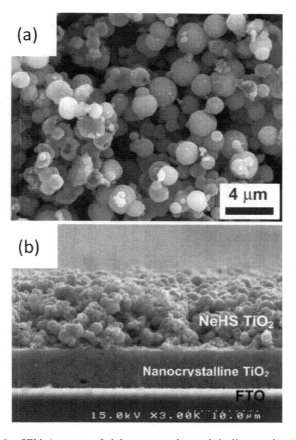

Figure 7.8 SEM images of (a) nano-embossed hollow spherical TiO$_2$ (NeHS TiO$_2$) and (b) the cross section of a bilayer structure showing the nanocrystalline TiO$_2$ underlayer and NeHS TiO$_2$ overlayer. Reprinted with permission from Ref. [100]. Copyright © 2008 WILEY-VCH.

in conversion efficiency. In addition, the mesoporous TiO$_2$ beads possessed higher IPCE values shown in Fig. 7.9h over a wide range (from 370 to 750 nm) than P25 films with similar thickness. Polydisperse ZnO aggregates with similar structure as TiO$_2$ beads was also demonstrated by Cao et al. for use as photoanode materials in DSSCs and a much higher efficiency has been obtained compared to that of conventional ZnO NP-based photoanode films [104–106].

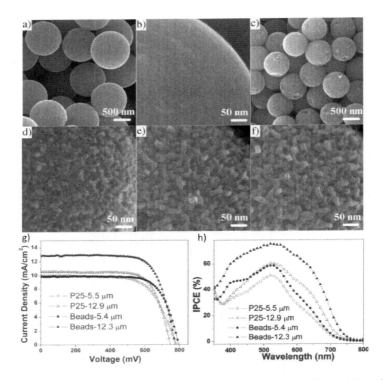

Figure 7.9 SEM images of the precursor material, sample S1 (a, b), and the calcined mesoporous TiO_2 beads obtained after a solvothermal process with different amounts of ammonia; sample S2 contained no ammonia (c, d), sample S3 contained 0.5 mL ammonia (e), and sample S4 contained 1.0 mL ammonia (f); I–V curves (g) and IPCE (h) of the TiO_2 electrodes prepared from either P25 nanoparticles or mesoporous TiO_2 beads (sample S4) at two film thicknesses. Reprinted with permission from Ref. [103]. Copyright © 2009 WILEY-VCH.

Besides the scattering effect by prolonging the light pathway, another emerging approach toward panchromatic light harvesting in DSSCs utilizes the localized surface plasmon resonance (LSPR) of noble metal nanostructures [107–113]. Surface plasmons are oscillations of charge density that can exist at the interface between two media with electric permittivity of opposite signs. When both the energy and the momentum of the incident light match the energy and momentum of the plasmons, the incident light can

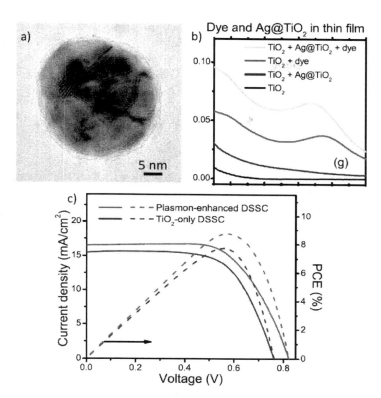

Figure 7.10 (a) TEM image of Ag@TiO$_2$ nanoparticle, (b) optical absorption spectra of Ag@TiO$_2$ NPs, ruthenium dye molecules, and their mixtures in the matrix of a TiO$_2$ thin film, and (c) current density and PCE of the most efficient plasmon-enhanced DSSC. Reprinted with permission from Ref. [109], Copyright 2011 American Chemical Society.

be strongly coupled to the plasmons [114]. In principle, noble metal nanostructures could amplify the light harvesting in DSSCs by either scattering light enabling a longer optical path length, by a dipole–dipole interaction and resonant energy transfer or by near-field coupling between the surface plasmon polariton and the dye-excited state [108]. Recently Belcher et al. successfully synthesized a core/shell Ag@TiO$_2$ nanostructure, as shown in Fig. 7.10b. The extremely thin shell is utilized to prevent recombination and back reaction as well as preventing metal NPs from corrosion by the electrolyte in DSSCs. By incorporating a small amount of Ag@TiO$_2$ NPs (0.1 wt%) into the TiO$_2$ photoanode, the overall conversion efficiency was significantly increased from 7.8% to 9.0%. In addition, the thickness of photoanode could be decreased by 25% with improved electron collection [109].

7.4.3 Higher-Order Nanostructures

Another major drawback of the conventional TiO$_2$ NP photoanodes is the low transport efficiency of electrons, which imposes an upper limit on the film thickness. In a film composed of TiO$_2$ NPs, electrons diffuse to the surface of the collector electrode (e.g., FTO substrate) through a zigzag pathway [80] and may easily recombine with the oxidizing species, predominately triiodide ions in the electrolyte, thus reducing the efficiency. Therefore, 1D TiO$_2$ [115–120] and ZnO nanostructures [80, 121, 122] and 2D [76, 123] and 3D [124–126] TiO$_2$ and ZnO nanostructures have attracted recent attention in facilitating electron transport in DSSCs.

Sung et al. reported the synthesis of nanorods from the necking of truncated TiO$_2$ NPs [127]. A comparison of electron transport and charge recombination characteristics between NP- and nanorod-based photoanodes in DSSCs was examined by stepped light-induced transient measurements of photocurrent and voltage (SLIM-PCV) under front-side illumination. The average electron diffusion length of the nanorod film was much longer than that of the NP film due to the decreased intercrystalline contacts between grain boundaries. Enhanced conversion efficiency by 40% was finally achieved for nanorod-based DSSCs, owing to their excellent carrier transport behavior.

Recent studies show that randomly packed nanorods (nanowires [NWs]) may not be the best structure to promote carrier mobility in photoanodes as the number of grain boundaries for the electrons to pass through cannot be significantly reduced via such a simple strategy. Thus, considerable attention has been given to vertically aligned 1D nanostructures such as ordered NW and nanotube (NT) arrays. Almost all the solution-phase prepared TiO$_2$ NW arrays on FTO substrates were rutile TiO$_2$ because of a very small lattice mismatch between FTO and rutile TiO$_2$ [118, 128–130]. However,

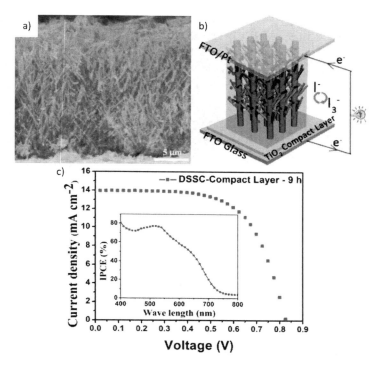

Figure 7.11 (a) SEM image of a hierarchical anatase TiO2 nanowire array, (b) schematic diagram, and (c) photovoltaic characteristics of DSSC based on an anatase TiO2 nanowire photoanode. Reproduced with permission from Ref. [131]; copyright © 2013 Nature Publishing Group.

compared to rutile structures, superior photovoltaic performance was normally obtained for anatase TiO_2 resulting from higher dye loading and a faster electron transport rate [12]. Wu et al. recently reported a facile one-step hydrothermal fabrication of hierarchical anatase TiO_2 NW arrays consisting of long TiO_2 NW trunks and short nanorod branches on FTO glass [131]. Figure 7.11a is a cross-sectional field emission scanning electron microscopy (SEM) image showing oriented TiO_2 NW arrays grown vertically on an FTO substrate with an average length of 18 µm. The photovoltaic characteristics of TiO_2 nanostructured films prepared at different hydrothermal reaction times (1, 2, 3, 6, 9, 12, hours) have been studied. By introducing a TiO_2 compact layer (Fig. 7.11b) ahead of the hydrothermal process, a high efficiency of 7.34% was achieved with the optimized hierarchical anatase TiO_2 nano-architecture array film.

Vertical arrays of ZnO NWs were also explored as photoanode candidates in DSSCs. ZnO with 1D features can be easily synthesized by facile chemical methods because of a highly anisotropic crystal structure. Therefore, various types of 1D ZnO nanostructures have been reported [122, 123, 132, 133]. The positive aspects of the ZnO NW are its low resistivity of 0.3–2.0 $\Omega \cdot cm$, high electron concentration of $1-5 \times 10^{18}$ cm^{-3}, high mobility of 1–5 $cm^2/V\ s$, and high electron diffusivity of 0.05–0.5 cm^2/s. ZnO NW array–based DSSCs were firstly introduced by Law et al. in 2005 [121]. Despite the suppressed electron trapping and improved charge collection, DSSCs fabricated with ZnO NW arrays exhibited much lower energy conversion efficiency than those with TiO_2 NPs, mainly due to the low accessible surface area for dye adsorption.

To address the challenge in synthesis of vertically ordered nanostructures with a high internal surface area, Xu et al. demonstrated a convenient approach that involves alternate cycles of NW growth and a self-assembled monolayer coating process for synthesizing multilayer assemblies of ZnO NW arrays for high-efficiency DSSCs [134]. The assembled multilayer ZnO NW arrays possess an internal surface area more than five times larger than what one can possibly obtain with single-layer NW arrays. An SEM image of a four-layer assembly of ZnO NW arrays, in which each layer has a thickness of ca. 10 μm, is shown in Fig. 7.12a. Figure 7.12b,c compares the photovoltaic characteristics of DSSCs comprised of ZnO NW arrays with different layers. An efficiency of 7.0% was finally obtained for the four-layer assembly, which is comparable to that of TiO_2 NP–based DSSCs.

The development of well-aligned TiO_2 NT arrays with a hollow cavity structure is proposed as another strategy to increase the internal surface area for vertically ordered nanostructures. Traditionally, TiO_2 NTs are produced via the anodization of a Ti substrate. Though the electron diffusion length is expected to be significantly increased, a serious problem is that NT arrays grown on opaque Ti metal are detrimental to efficient light harvesting, as such NT-based DSSCs need to be illuminated from the backside. During

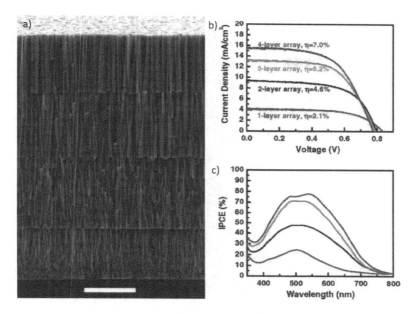

Figure 7.12 (a) SEM image of a four-layer assembly of ZnO nanowire arrays (scale bar: 10 μm), (b) $J-V$ characteristics, and (c) IPCE of DSSCs fabricated using TiO_2-coated multilayer assemblies of ZnO nanowire arrays. Reprinted with permission from Ref. [134], Copyright 2013 American Chemical Society.

backside illumination, much of the incident light will be blocked by the CE as well as the electrolyte, resulting in at least 20% decrease in conversion efficiency. Therefore, recent efforts have been focused on direct growth [135, 136] and/or detachment and transfer [120, 137] of ordered TiO_2 NT arrays for front-illuminated DSSCs. By using a nanoporous alumina templating method, highly ordered TiO_2 NTs were successfully fabricated by Kang et al. on FTO substrates [119]. A modified sol–gel route was employed to infiltrate the alumina pores with $Ti(OC_3H_7)_4$, which was subsequently converted into TiO_2 NTs, as shown in Fig. 7.13. The average external diameter, tube length, and wall thickness achieved were 295 nm, 6–15 μm, and 21–42 nm, respectively.

Recently, Li and coworkers reported the use of detachment and transfer to fabricate strongly adhering, transparent NT arrays on

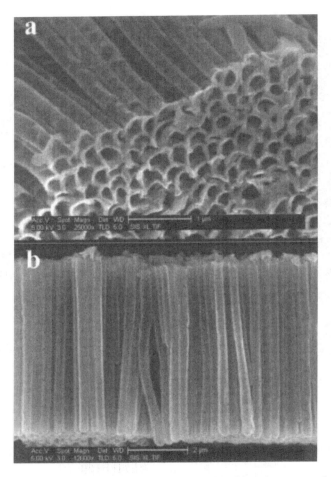

Figure 7.13 SEM images of (a) top-down and (b) side views of TiO2 nanotube arrays after removal of the anodized alumina template. The average TiO2 nanotube outer diameter and length are 295 nm and 6.1 μm, respectively. Reprinted with permission from Ref. [119]; copyright © 2013 American Chemical Society.

FTO glass for front-illuminated NT DSSCs [120]. The ordered NT arrays were detached from the NT Ti substrate, annealed, by means of a second anodization, at 20 V for 4 hours, and then transferred, inverted, onto a FTO substrate. A DSSC cell fabricated with the transparent and inverted NT photoanode shows a significantly

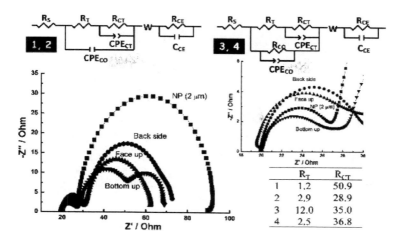

Figure 7.14 Nyquist plots obtained from electrochemical impedance spectra (EIS) measured for corresponding DSSC devices under AM 1.5 illumination at open-circuit condition. Top models show the equivalent circuits used to fit the EIS results. Reproduced from Ref. [120] with permission of the Royal Society of Chemistry.

improved efficiency of 6.24% compared to that of a conventional back-illuminated device ($\eta = 4.61\%$). The charge transfer kinetics of NT arrays was finally examined by impedance spectra. The impedance results were fitted according to the equivalent circuits shown in Fig. 7.14. The smaller charge transport resistance for the DSSC device based on inverted NT structure provides solid evidence to confirm its superior charge transfer property.

Lately, a novel bottom-up 3D host–passivation–guest (H–P–G) electrode concept was demonstrated. It differs from conventional hierarchical structures and enables structural control on the electron extraction, CB, and recombination dynamics, as well as the optical scattering in photovoltaic devices [126]. This new type of electrode is exemplified herein by incorporating it into a DSSC photoanode, as shown in Fig. 7.15b, to significantly improve the photocurrent, fill factor, and, most importantly, photovoltage. The cross-sectional SEM image (Fig. 7.15a) clearly shows the high pore connectivity throughout the 3D open structure as well as the significant disorder inherited from the polystyrene template. It is

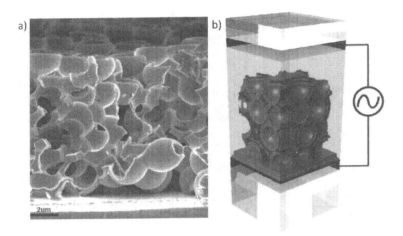

Figure 7.15 (a) Cross-sectional view of a disordered TiO$_2$ passivated 3D Al/ZnO backbone and (b) schematic representation of a 3D DSSC. Reprinted with permission from Ref. [126], Copyright 2011 American Chemical Society.

an additional advantage of the 3D macroporous structure that the backbone only uses a small volume fraction of the 3D film, and in this case the high degree of necking between the templating spheres and the very thin film of metal oxide host deposited leave the vast majority of the volume for filling with the guest materials. By using this novel 3D H–P–G morphology partially filled with anatase NPs, an increase in photovoltage of up to 110 mV was achieved. It is believed that the straightforward and simple bottom-up fabrication technique produces a highly optically scattering 3D photoanode material that could enhance light harvesting and charge extraction and reduce interfacial recombination to significantly increase the cell photovoltage, photocurrent, and fill factor in various low-cost photovoltaic technologies.

Despite the various fancy nanostructured materials and concepts proposed above, there is still much room for further optimizing photoanode nanostructures. To sum up, to substantially improve the power conversion efficiency of DSSCs, much more effort should be devoted to the design of novel nanostructured photoanode materials with both higher light harvesting and promoted charge transfer

Table 7.1 Recent state-of-the-art DSSCs based on liquid junctions

Published date	Device description	η (%)	Ref. no.
June 23, 2006	Black dye/I^-/I_3^-	11.1	[23]
Nov. 4, 2011	YD2-o-C8 dye/Co (II/III)	12.3	[138]
Jan. 3, 2012	Black dye + Y1 co-adsorbent/I^-/I_3^-	11.4	[139]
Feb. 2, 2014	SM315 dye/Co (II/III)	13	[8]

efficiency without sacrificing the large surface area for sufficient dye adsorption.

7.5 Stability and Commercial Development of DSSCs

In terms of large-scale practical use, the working lifetime is just as important as efficiency for DSSCs. However, considering the balance of systems and module manufacturing costs, it is impractical to commercialize solar cells with lab-scale efficiencies of less than 10%. Therefore, the majority of past research efforts have been devoted to improving efficiencies beyond this threshold. To date, the efficiency of DSSCs has been enhanced to 13%. Table 7.1 shows some of the recent efficiency values for state-of-the-art DSSCs based on liquid junctions. Nonetheless, increasing attention has recently been paid to stability as well.

Over the last two decades, a vast amount of tests have been carried out to scrutinize the stability of DSSCs by both academic and industrial institutions [6, 140]. In the early development stage of DSSCs, the quality of device sealing was sometimes not good enough during cell testing, causing leakage of the volatile solvents. This problem has been solved by improving the sealing method in most research groups, including industrial enterprises. Long-term light-soaking experiments performed over thousands of hours [141, 142] under full or even concentrated sunlight have confirmed the intrinsic stability of current DSSC embodiments. Molecular engineering for new sensitizers, together with the use of robust and nonvolatile electrolytes such as ionic liquids, enables the stable operation of DSSC devices under high temperature at around 85°C

[143]. These extensive studies provide the possibility that DSSCs are able to match the stability requirements needed to sustain outdoor operation for at least 20 years [144].

A combination of high efficiency, long-term stability, and low cost is always required for the successful commercialization of any photovoltaic technology. Certified DSSC module efficiencies have recently reached 9.9% [2]. Apart from the material abundance and ease of manufacture, DSSCs also perform relatively better under diffuse light conditions and at higher temperatures. DSSCs also offer opportunities to design devices with a large flexibility in shape, color, and transparency. Thus new commercial opportunities would be opened up with integration into different products. So far, a number of companies such as BASF, Bosch, and Corus in Europe and Toyota, Sharp, Panasonic, Sony, Fujikura, and Samsung in Asia have shown their interest in DSSCs [6]. A large-volume production line has been set up by the company G24i, in Wales. Many research companies such as Dyesol (Australia), Solaronix (Switzerland), and Peccell (Japan) have been focusing on selling material components and equipment [6]. DSSCs are now just on the verge of commercialization as the pilot plants and small manufacturing facilities have become feasible.

7.6 Our Recent Work on Design of Novel Nanostructured Photoanodes

Over the past two decades, apart from the search for more efficient and stable dyes, the design of novel photoanode materials has also seen much effort since the breakthrough work by Grätzel. Initially our work was mainly focused on tailoring of photoanode architecture to improve the electron transfer efficiency. Therefore ZnO NW networks featuring excellent charge transport were selected and in situ grown within conventional TiO_2 NP films by a simple hydrothermal method. The optimized hybrid photoanode consisting of a ZnO NW network as the direct pathway for electron transport exhibited an increased efficiency of 8.44%. This is a remarkable 26.9% improvement compared with that of the benchmark TiO_2 photoanode under the same testing conditions.

However, the insufficient dye adsorption with increasing of ZnO NWs limited further enhancement of the efficiency. To further improve efficiency, porous titania nanohybrids (NHs) were successfully prepared by hybridizing the exfoliated titania nanosheets (NSs) with anatase TiO_2 NPs. Various characterizations revealed that NHs as photoanodes play a trifunctional role (light harvesting, dye adsorption, and electron transfer) in improving the efficiency of DSSCs. The optimized photoanode consisting of layered NHs demonstrated a higher efficiency of 10.1%.

7.6.1 ZnO NW/TiO_2 NP Hybrid Photoanode

Conventional DSSCs are fabricated using mesoporous TiO_2 NP films [4], which have a high surface area accessible to the dye. This results in sufficient dye adsorption and thus high conversion efficiency. However, a major drawback of the conventional TiO_2 NP photoanode in DSSCs is inefficient electron transport, which imposes an upper limit on the film thickness. In a film composed of anatase TiO_2 NPs, the electron diffusion coefficient is more than 2 orders of magnitude lower than that in single-crystal TiO_2 [145]. As shown in Fig. 7.16, electrons in the TiO_2 NP film diffuse to the surface of the collector electrode (e.g., FTO substrate) through a zigzag pathway. In the electron transfer process, electrons may recombine with oxidizing species, predominately triiodide ions in the electrolyte, thus reducing the DSSC efficiency. Therefore, how to efficiently transfer electrons and reduce their recombination with redox species is believed to be the key step in achieving high-efficiency DSSCs.

Fabrication of films from 1D nanostructures that can provide a direct rather than zigzag pathway for electron transfer compared to 0D NP analogues has proven to be an effective way to facilitate electron transport [117, 121, 146–150]. For instance, Law et al. found the electron diffusion coefficient of ZnO NWs is several hundred times higher than that of ZnO or TiO_2 NP films [121]. Using NWs or NTs, the electron lifetime in electrode films can be improved by three times that in NP films [115]. In addition to the efficient electron transport, NWs with tunable lengths in the range of hundreds of nanometers to micrometers can serve as light-scattering centers to increase the optical length in the film, thus enhancing the light-harvesting efficiency. This effect is similar to that of large particles [99, 101], which has been demonstrated both experimentally and theoretically [151, 152]. In contrast, TiO_2 NPs used in most conventional DSSCs are in the size range of ca. 20–30 nm, which is much smaller than the wavelength of visible light, resulting in less light scattering. However, the overall conversion efficiency of DSSCs using 1D nanostructures is still much lower than that of the particulate systems [153], which is mainly due to the insufficient internal surface area of 1D structures for dye adsorption, thus leading to lower photocurrent as a result of less photogenerated electrons.

As mentioned above, both large surface area and high charge transfer efficiency are essential to constitute an excellent photoanode [154]. The combination of ZnO NPs/ZnO NWs in photoanodes for DSSCs has been investigated by Prof. Cao's group [155] and significant enhancement in power conversion efficiency was demonstrated. However, the overall power conversion efficiency is lower than 5%. In this work, we report an innovative experimental design for in situ growth of a ZnO NW network within a conventional mesoporous TiO_2 NP film for use as a photoanode. Our idea is to intentionally introduce a small amount of a ZnO NW network in the TiO_2 NP film by a seed-mediated wet-chemical method to facilitate the interfacial contact of two components. In this way, the presence of a 1D ZnO NW network will play two vital roles, increasing light scattering and promoting electron transfer. Figure 7.16 illustrates two electron diffusion processes in conventional TiO_2 NPs and our TiO_2 NP/ZnO NW hybrid photoanode, respectively. In the conventional TiO_2 photoelectrode, electrons transport via a zigzag pathway through the NPs and are readily trapped by surface states. This results in an increase in electron–hole recombination. Whereas in the hybrid TiO_2–ZnO photoelectrode, we hypothesize that the presence of ZnO NWs embedded in a TiO_2 film would increase the light scattering and more importantly form a heterojunction free of band discontinuities with a built-in potential [156, 157], leading to much facilitated electron diffusion from TiO_2 NPs to ZnO NWs. An enhanced overall conversion efficiency of 8.44% for a TiO_2 NP/ZnO NW hybrid photoanode was achieved—a noticeable

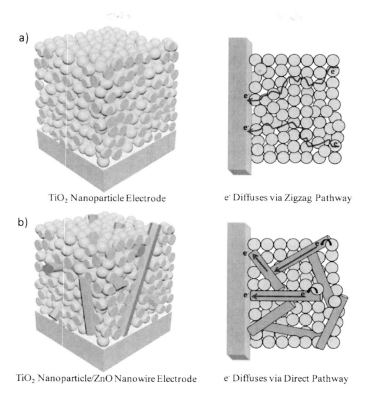

Figure 7.16 Schematic illustration of electron (e$^-$) diffuse transport in (a) a conventional nanoparticle electrode and (b) a nanoparticle/nanowire network electrode. Reproduced with permission from Ref. [80]. Copyright © 2012 WILEY-VCH.

26.9% improvement compared to the photoelectrode made of the benchmark TiO_2 paste under the same testing conditions. Various characterizations confirmed our hypothesis and the feasibility of using new hybrid photoanodes for efficiency improvement of DSSCs. Reflectance spectra demonstrate that the light-harvesting efficiency of the TiO_2/ZnO hybrid films was higher than that of bare TiO_2 films due to the effective light-scattering of ZnO NWs. The EIS study indicates the excellent electron transport property of hybrid films. Thus, the use of an in situ grown ZnO NW network in TiO_2 films may shed new insights into the fine-tuning of photoanode structures for further efficiency improvement in DSSCs.

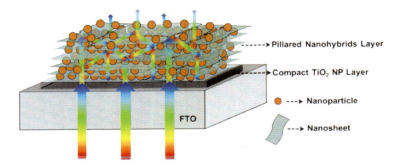

Figure 7.17 Idealized schematic diagram of photoanodes based on layered NHs for light scattering. Reproduced with permission from Ref. [77], Copyright 2012 American Chemical Society.

7.6.2 Porous Titania NS/NP Hybrid Photoanode

Even though the light-harvesting and charge transfer efficiency can be enhanced by introducing an optical light-scattering layer and fabrication of films from 1D and 2D nanostructures, respectively, the surface area that is accessible to the dye is usually sacrificed, resulting in insufficient dye adsorption and thus limited conversion efficiency. Thereby how to efficiently transfer electrons and harvest light without compromising the dye adsorption is believed to be one of the key challenges in achieving high-efficiency DSSCs.

Layered NHs obtained by pillaring semiconducting NPs such as CdS, α-Fe_2O_3, and TiO_2 [158–161] into layered inorganic compounds [162–167] have recently drawn growing attention in photocatalysis, due to their large surface area, as well as suppressed electron–hole recombination because of electron transfer between guest and host [159, 160, 168]. Titania NSs ($Ti_{0.91}O_2$) derived from delamination of layered compounds have unique structural feature of ultimate 2D anisotropy, with extremely small thickness in the subnano- to nanometer scales. These characteristics usually lead to new physical and chemical properties for the NSs [169]. In addition, the exfoliation of layered metal oxides into 2D NSs [170, 171] ($Ti_{0.91}O_2$ NSs) makes it possible to pillar large-sized (TiO_2) NPs into the interlayer space of host materials through an exfoliation-restacking process of NSs and guest particles [160, 172, 173].

The obtained pillared NHs possess highly controllable physical and chemical properties [159, 174–176]. In particular, due to the enlarged interlayer distance, the total surface area is significantly increased, facilitating chemical adsorption or reaction. Moreover, the energy band difference between guest and host will enhance the charge transfer between them [168, 177]. Apart from the high surface area and enhanced electron transfer efficiency, the large-sized 2D NSs that constitute the layered NHs can also act as an ideal optical scatter [178]. In this regard, the layered titania NHs are expected to be promising photoanode candidates, playing a trifunctional role (light harvesting, dye adsorption, and electron transfer) for high-efficiency DSSCs.

In this work, we report layered NHs prepared by hybridizing exfoliated titanate NSs ($Ti_{0.91}O_2$) with anatase TiO_2 NPs for use as photoanodes in DSSCs. Our key strategy was to use the exfoliation-reassembly strategy to introduce TiO_2 NPs ranging from 7 to 9 nm into the interlayers of 2D exfoliated $Ti_{0.91}O_2$ NSs without deterioration of their fundamental crystal structures. In this way, the porosity and surface area of the NHs are expected to be significantly enlarged, which is beneficial for sufficient dye adsorption. Additionally submicrometer-sized NSs will play a vital role in increasing the light scattering, as shown in Fig. 7.17. In addition, we hypothesize that electron–hole recombination would be effectively suppressed due to the charge transfer between guest and host in the layered NH system [159, 160, 168]. An enhanced overall conversion efficiency of 10.1% for layered titania NS/NP hybrid photoanodes was achieved, a 29.5% improvement compared to the photoelectrode made of the benchmark Degussa TiO_2 P25 under the same testing conditions. Various characterizations confirmed our hypothesis and the feasibility of using new layered NH photoanodes for efficiency improvement of DSSCs. Reflectance spectra demonstrate that the light-harvesting efficiency of the NH films was significantly higher than that of the P25 film due to the effective light scattering of $Ti_{0.91}O_2$ NSs. The larger surface area of the layered NH films leading to increased dye loading is verified by Brunauer–Emmett–Teller (BET) specific surface area measurements. In addition, not only the dark current potential scan but also the open-circuit voltage decay (OCVD) and impedance spectra indicate a lower charge recombination for photoelectrodes fabricated with NHs. Therefore, layered NHs may lead to a new way to fine-tuning photoanode structures for high-efficiency DSSCs as well as boosting the efficiency of QDSSCs.

7.7 Conclusions and Outlook

During the past two decades, tremendous attention has been paid to DSSCs from both academic and industry communities, owing to their relatively high efficiency and especially low cost and ease of production, which can avoid the expensive and energy-intensive high vacuum and materials purification steps. As a critical component that directly determines the power conversion efficiency of DSSCs, the engineering of photoanode architectures has seen intense efforts in further increasing light harvesting and facilitating electron transport. In this chapter, we primarily presented a brief introduction of the device structure, working principle, and characterization techniques to give a general knowledge of DSSCs. A focused review was then provided as a key part of the recent advances that center on the development of nanostructured photoanodes from three key aspects: dye uptake ability, electron mobility, and light-harvesting efficiency. Subsequently the stability and commercial development of DSSCs were summarized. We finally showed some of our recent work in this area.

Apart from the merits of DSSC technology mentioned above, better performance under diffuse light conditions and large flexibility in shape, color, and transparency also help open up new commercial opportunities. In terms of successful and fully commercialization in the near future, a combination of high efficiency, long-term stability, and low cost is required for DSSCs. Increasing efficiency will still be the primary driver that enables DSSCs to compete with other thin-film technologies. The trifunctional concept, which aims at improving charge transfer and light-harvesting efficiency without sacrificing dye uptake ability, should be always taken into account in the future design of novel nanostructured photoanodes. Additionally, optimizing energetic alignment of cell components (redox couple and sensitizer), while maintaining appropriate kinetics, could boost the efficiency above 15% or even close to 17%. The next breakthrough will likely require changing multiple cell components simultaneously. Therefore, a comprehensive understanding of the chemistry and physics of DSSCs needs to be addressed so that rational approaches can identify such material combinations without excessively long-term trial-and-error–based development processes.

Though relatively good stability has been demonstrated through accelerated aging tests, it should be noted that no standard protocol exists to define the procedures for relevant testing. Much research effort should be devoted not only to the development of encapsulation technology or novel device structures such as solid-state thin films but also to the establishment of standard procedures for accelerated testing of DSSC stability.

From the perspective of large-scale application of DSSCs, the low cost of both materials and manufacturing processes should always be considered as a critical factor in commercial development. The exploration of noble metal-free sensitizers and electrocatalysts would drive the DSSC community toward a new generation of cost-effective DSSCs. On the other hand, the design of modules and integration of processing steps should lead toward high throughput at low cost without sacrificing performance.

With the intense efforts of academic researchers, and growing interest from the industrial community, continued advancement of DSSC technology in addressing all these challenges should be expected.

Acknowledgments

We are grateful for the financial support of the Australian Research Council (ARC). YB gratefully acknowledges the scholarship provided by the University of Queensland and the China Scholarship Council. YB also acknowledges the ARC Centre of Excellence for Functional Nanomaterials, in which some of the experimental work was carried out.

References

1. Grätzel, M. Mesoscopic solar cells mesoscopic solar cells, in *Solar Energy*, Richter, C., Lincot, D., and Gueymard, C., eds., Springer, New York, 2013, 79–96.
2. Green, M. A., Emery, K., Hishikawa, Y., Warta, W., and Dunlop, E. D. Solar cell efficiency tables (version 42), *Prog. Photovoltaics*, **21**(5), 2013, 827–837.
3. O'Regan, B., and Gratzel, M. A low-cost, high-efficiency solar cell based on dye-sensitized colloidal TiO_2 films, *Nature*, **353**(6346), 1991, 737–740.
4. Grätzel, M. Photoelectrochemical cells, *Nature*, **414**(6861), 2001, 338–344.
5. Baxter, J. B. Commercialization of dye sensitized solar cells: present status and future research needs to improve efficiency, stability, and manufacturing, *J. Vac. Sci. Technol., A*, **30**(2), 2012, 020801-020801-19.
6. Hagfeldt, A., Boschloo, G., Sun, L. C., Kloo, L., and Pettersson, H., Dye-sensitized solar cells, *Chem. Rev.*, **110**(11), 2010, 6595–6663.
7. Nazeeruddin, M. K., Kay, A., Rodicio, I., R. Humphry-Baker, Mueller, E., Liska, P., Vlachopoulos, N., and Graetzel, M. Conversion of light to electricity by cis-X2bis(2,2'-bipyridyl-4,4'-dicarboxylate)ruthenium (II) charge-transfer sensitizers (X = Cl^-, Br^-, I^-, CN^-, and SCN^-) on nanocrystalline titanium dioxide electrodes, *J. Am. Chem. Soc.*, **115**(14), 1993, 6382–6390.
8. Mathew, S., Yella, A., Gao, P., Humphry-Baker, R., CurchodBasile, F. E., Ashari-Astani, N., Tavernelli, I., Rothlisberger, U., NazeeruddinMd, K., and Grätzel, M. Dye-sensitized solar cells with 13% efficiency achieved through the molecular engineering of porphyrin sensitizers, *Nat. Chem.*, **6**(3), 2014, 242–247.
9. Brugnati, M., Caramori, S., Cazzanti, S., Marchini, L., and Bignozzi, C. A. Electron transfer mediators for photoelectrochemical cells based on Cu (I) metal complexes, *Int. Photoenergy, J.*, **2007**, 2008, Article ID 80756.
10. Zhang, Z., Chen, P., Murakami, T. N., Zakeeruddin, S. M., and Gratzel, M. The 2,2,6,6-tetramethyl-1-piperidinyloxy radical: an efficient, iodine-free redox mediator for dye-sensitized solar cells, *Adv. Funct. Mater.*, **18**(2), 2008, 341–346.
11. Singh, R., Green, M. A., and Rajkanan, K. Review of conductor-insulator-semiconductor (CIS) solar cells, *Sol. Cells*, **3**(2), 1981, 95–148.

12. Park, N.-G., Van de Lagemaat, J., and Frank, A. Comparison of dye-sensitized rutile-and anatase-based TiO_2 solar cells, *J. Phys. Chem. B*, **104**(38), 2000, 8989–8994.
13. Ennaoui, A., Fiechter, S., Pettenkofer, C., Alonso-Vante, N., Büker, K., Bronold, M., Höpfner, C., and Tributsch, H. Iron disulfide for solar energy conversion, *Sol. Energy Mater. Sol. Cells*, **29**(4), 1993, 289–370.
14. Soedergren, S., Hagfeldt, A., Olsson, J., and Lindquist, S.-E. Theoretical models for the action spectrum and the current-voltage characteristics of microporous semiconductor films in photoelectrochemical cells, *J. Phys. Chem.*, **98**(21), 1994, 5552–5556.
15. de Jongh, P.E., and Vanmaekelbergh, D. Trap-limited electronic transport in assemblies of nanometer-size TiO_2 particles, *Phys. Rev. Lett.*, **77**(16), 1996, 3427–3430.
16. Grätzel, M. Perspectives for dye-sensitized nanocrystalline solar cells, *Prog. Photovoltaics*, **8**(1), 2000, 171–185.
17. Martinson, A. B. F., Elam, J. W., Hupp, J. T., and Pellin, M. J. ZnO nanotube based dye-sensitized solar cells ZnO nanotube based dye-sensitized solar cells, *Nano Lett.*, **7**(8), 2007, 2183–2187.
18. Furube, A., Murai, M., Watanabe, S., Hara, K., Katoh, R., and Tachiya, M. Near-IR transient absorption study on ultrafast electron-injection dynamics from a Ru-complex dye into nanocrystalline In2O3 thin films: comparison with SnO_2, ZnO, and TiO_2 films. *J. Photochem. Photobiol., A*, **182**(3), 2006, 273–279.
19. Ai, X., Guo, J. C., Anderson, N. A., and Lian, T. Q. Ultrafast electron transfer from Ru polypyridyl complexes to Nb_2O_5 nanoporous thin films, *J. Phys. Chem. B*, **108**(34), 2004, 12795–12803.
20. Ai, X., Anderson, N. A., Guo, J. C., and Lian, T. Q. Electron injection dynamics of Ru polypyridyl complexes on SnO_2 nanocrystalline thin films, *J. Phys. Chem. B*, **109**(15), 2005, 7088–7094.
21. Tan, B., Toman, E., Li, Y., and Wu, Y. Zinc stannate (Zn_2SnO_4) dye-sensitized solar cells, *J. Am. Chem. Soc.*, **129**(14), 2007, 4162–4163.
22. Nazeeruddin, K., M., Pechy, P., and Grätzel, M. Efficient panchromatic sensitization of nanocrystalline TiO_2 films by a black dye based on a trithiocyanato-ruthenium complex, *Chem. Commun.*, **1997**(18), 1997, 1705–1706.
23. Chiba, Y., Islam, A., Watanabe, Y., Komiya, R., Koide, N., and Han, L. Dye-sensitized solar cells with conversion efficiency of 11.1%, *Jpn. J. Appl. Phys., Part 2*, **45**(24/28), 2006, L638–L640.

24. Hagberg, D. P., Edvinsson, T., Marinado, T., Boschloo, G., Hagfeldt, A., and Sun, L. A novel organic chromophore for dye-sensitized nanostructured solar cells, *Chem. Commun.*, **2006**(21), 2006, 2245–2247.
25. Ito, S., Zakeeruddin, S. M., Humphry-Baker, R., Liska, P., Charvet, R., Comte, P., Nazeeruddin, M. K., P. Péchy, Takata, M., Miura, H., Uchida, S., and Grätzel, M. High-efficiency organic-dye-sensitized solar cells controlled by nanocrystalline-TiO_2 electrode thickness, *Adv. Mater.*, **18**(9), 2006, 1202–1205.
26. Hara, K., Sato, T., Katoh, R., Furube, A., Ohga, Y., Shinpo, A., Suga, S., Sayama, K., Sugihara, H., and Arakawa, H. Molecular design of coumarin dyes for efficient dye-sensitized solar cells, *J. Phys. Chem. B*, **107**(2), 2002, 597–606.
27. Nozik, A. J. Exciton multiplication and relaxation dynamics in quantum dots: applications to ultrahigh-efficiency solar photon conversion, *Inorg. Chem.*, **44**(20), 2005, 6893–6899.
28. Nozik, A. J. Multiple exciton generation in semiconductor quantum dots, *Chem. Phys. Lett.*, **457**(1–3), 2008, 3–11.
29. Kamat, P. V. Quantum dot solar cells. Semiconductor nanocrystals as light harvesters, *J. Phys. Chem. C*, **112**(48), 2008, 18737–18753.
30. Lee, H., Wang, M., Chen, P., Gamelin, D. R., Zakeeruddin, S. M., M. Grätzel, and Nazeeruddin, M. K. Efficient CdSe quantum dot-sensitized solar cells prepared by an improved successive ionic layer adsorption and reaction process, *Nano Lett.*, **9**(12), 2009, 4221–4227.
31. Ruhle, S., Shalom, M., and Zaban, A., Quantum-dot-sensitized solar cells, *ChemPhysChem*, **11**(11), 2010, 2290–2304.
32. Lee, Y.-L., and Lo, Y.-S. Highly efficient quantum-dot-sensitized solar cell based on co-sensitization of CdS/CdSe, *Adv. Funct. Mater.*, **19**(4), 2009, 604–609.
33. Mora-Sero, I., and Bisquert, J. Breakthroughs in the development of semiconductor-sensitized solar cells, *J. Phys. Chem. Lett.*, **1**(20), 2010, 3046–3052.
34. Lee, J.-W., Son, D.-Y., Ahn, T. K., Shin, H.-W., Kim, I. Y., Hwang, S.-J., Ko, M. J., Sul, S., Han, H., and Park, N.-G. Quantum-dot-sensitized solar cell with unprecedentedly high photocurrent, *Sci. Rep.*, **3**, 2013, Article ID 1050.
35. Wang, J., Mora-Seró, I., Pan, Z., Zhao, K., Zhang, H., Feng, Y., Yang, G., Zhong, X., and Bisquert, J. Core/shell colloidal quantum dot exciplex states for the development of highly efficient quantum-dot-sensitized solar cells, *J. Am. Chem. Soc.*, **135**(42), 2013, 15913–15922.

36. Rhee, J. H., Chung, C.-C., and Diau, E. W.-G. A perspective of mesoscopic solar cells based on metal chalcogenide quantum dots and organometal-halide perovskites, *NPG Asia Mater.*, **5**(10), 2013, e68–e85.
37. Santra, P.K., and Kamat, P. V. Mn-doped quantum dot sensitized solar cells: a strategy to boost efficiency over 5%, *J. Am. Chem. Soc.*, **134**(5), 2012, 2508–2511.
38. Michael, G. Dye-sensitized solar cells, *J. Photochem. Photobiol., C*, **4**(2), 2003, 145–153.
39. Hattori, S., Wada, Y., Yanagida, S., and Fukuzumi, S. Blue copper model complexes with distorted tetragonal geometry acting as effective electron-transfer mediators in dye-sensitized solar cells, *J. Am. Chem. Soc.*, **127**(26), 2005, 9648–9654.
40. Oskam, G., Bergeron, B. V., Meyer, G. J., and Searson, P. C. Pseudohalogens for dye-sensitized TiO_2 photoelectrochemical cells, *J. Phys. Chem. B*, **105**(29), 2001, 6867–6873.
41. Wang, Z.-S., Sayama, K., and Sugihara, H. Efficient eosin Y dye-sensitized solar cell containing Br^-/Br^{3-} electrolyte, *J. Phys. Chem. B*, **109**(47), 2005, 22449–22455.
42. Sapp, S. A., Elliott, C. M., Contado, C., Caramori, S., and Bignozzi, C. A. Substituted polypyridine complexes of Cobalt(II/III) as efficient electron-transfer mediators in dye-sensitized solar cells, *J. Am. Chem. Soc.*, **124**(37), 2002, 11215–11222.
43. Cameron, P. J., Peter, L. M., Zakeeruddin, S. M., and Grätzel, M. Electrochemical studies of the Co(III)/Co(II)(dbbip)2 redox couple as a mediator for dye-sensitized nanocrystalline solar cells, *Coord. Chem. Rev.*, **248**(13–14), 2004, 1447–1453.
44. Nusbaumer, H., Zakeeruddin, S. M., Moser, J.-E., and Grätzel, M. An alternative efficient redox couple for the dye-sensitized solar cell system, *Chem. Eur. J.*, **9**(16), 2003, 3756–3763.
45. Cao, Y., Zhang, J., Bai, Y., Li, R., Zakeeruddin, S. M., M. Grätzel, and Wang, P. Dye-sensitized solar cells with solvent-free ionic liquid electrolytes, *J. Phys. Chem. C*, **112**(35), 2008, 13775–13781.
46. Wang, P., Zakeeruddin, S. M., Comte, P., Exnar, I., and Grätzel, M. Gelation of ionic liquid-based electrolytes with silica nanoparticles for quasi-solid-state dye-sensitized solar cells, *J. Am. Chem. Soc.*, **125**(5), 2003, 1166–1167.
47. Wang, P., Zakeeruddin, S. M., Moser, J. E., Nazeeruddin, M. K., Sekiguchi, T., and Gratzel, M. A stable quasi-solid-state dye-sensitized solar cell

with an amphiphilic ruthenium sensitizer and polymer gel electrolyte, *Nat. Mater.*, **2**(6), 2003, 402–407.

48. Bach, U., Lupo, D., Comte, P., Moser, J. E., Weissortel, F., Salbeck, J., Spreitzer, H., and Gratzel, M. Solid-state dye-sensitized mesoporous TiO_2 solar cells with high photon-to-electron conversion efficiencies, *Nature*, **395**(6702), 1998, 583–585.

49. Choi, H., Kang, S. O., Ko, J., Gao, G., Kang, H. S., Kang, M. S., Nazeeruddin, M. K., and Grätzel, M. An efficient dye-sensitized solar cell with an organic sensitizer encapsulated in a cyclodextrin cavity, *Angew. Chem.*, **121**(32), 2009, 6052–6055.

50. Wu, M., Lin, X., Hagfeldt, A., and Ma, T. Low-cost molybdenum carbide and tungsten carbide counter electrodes for dye-sensitized solar cells, *Angew. Chem., Int. Ed.*, **50**(15), 2011, 3520–3524.

51. Boschloo, G., and Hagfeldt, A. Characteristics of the iodide/triiodide redox mediator in dye-sensitized solar cells, *Acc. Chem. Res.*, **42**(11), 2009, 1819–1826.

52. Papageorgiou, N. Counter-electrode function in nanocrystalline photoelectrochemical cell configurations, *Coord. Chem. Rev.*, **248**(13–14), 2004, 1421–1446.

53. Roy Mayhew, J. D., Bozym, D. J., Punckt, C., and Aksay, I. A. Functionalized graphene as a catalytic counter electrode in dye-sensitized solar cells, *ACS Nano*, **4**(10), 2010, 6203–6211.

54. Xia, J. B., Chen, L., and Yanagida, S. Application of polypyrrole as a counter electrode for a dye-sensitized solar cell, *J. Mater. Chem.*, **21**(12), 2011, 4644–4649.

55. Xue, Y., Liu, J., Chen, H., Wang, R., Li, D., Qu, J., and Dai, L., Nitrogen-doped graphene foams as metal-free counter electrodes in high-performance dye-sensitized solar cells, *Angew. Chem.*, **124**(48), 2012, 12290–12293.

56. Das, S., Sudhagar, P., Verma, V., Song, D., Ito, E., Lee, S. Y., Kang, Y. S., and Choi, W. Amplifying charge-transfer characteristics of graphene for triiodide reduction in dye-sensitized solar cells, *Adv. Funct. Mater.*, **21**(19), 2011, 3729–3736.

57. Brennan, L. J., Byrne, M. T., Bari, M., and Gun'ko, Y. K. Carbon nanomaterials for dye-sensitized solar cell applications: a bright future, *Adv. Energy Mater.*, **1**(4), 2011, 472–485.

58. Wu, J. H., Li, Q. H., Fan, L. Q., Lan, Z., Li, P. J., Lin, J. M., and Hao, S. C. High-performance polypyrrole nanoparticles counter electrode for dye-sensitized solar cells, *J. Power Sources*, **181**(1), 2008, 172–176.

59. Lin, J. Y., Chan, C. Y., and Chou, S. W. Electrophoretic deposition of transparent MoS2-graphene nanosheet composite films as counter electrodes in dye-sensitized solar cells, *Chem. Commun.*, **49**(14), 2013, 1440–1442.
60. Wu, M. X., Wang, Y. D., Lin, X., Yu, N. S., Wang, L., Wang, L. L., Hagfeldt, A., and Ma, T. L. Economical and effective sulfide catalysts for dye-sensitized solar cells as counter electrodes, *Phys. Chem. Chem. Phys.*, **13**(43), 2011, 19298–19301.
61. Wang, M. K., Anghel, A. M., Marsan, B., Cevey Ha, N.-L., Pootrakulchote, N., Zakeeruddin, S. M., and Grätzel, M. CoS supersedes Pt as efficient electrocatalyst for triiodide reduction in dye-sensitized solar cells, *J. Am. Chem. Soc.*, **131**(44), 2009, 15976–15977.
62. Kung, C.-W., Chen, H.-W., Lin, C.-Y., Huang, K.-C., Vittal, R., and Ho, K.-C. CoS acicular nanorod arrays for the counter electrode of an efficient dye-sensitized solar cell, *ACS Nano*, **6**(8), 2012, 7016–7025.
63. Sun, H. C., Qin, D., Huang, S. Q., Guo, X. Z., Li, D. M., Luo, Y. H., and Meng, Q. B. Dye-sensitized solar cells with NiS counter electrodes electrodeposited by a potential reversal technique, *Energy Environ. Sci.*, **4**(8), 2011, 2630–2637.
64. Chen, X., Hou, Y., Zhang, B., Yang, X. H., and Yang, H. G. Low-cost SnSx counter electrodes for dye-sensitized solar cells, *Chem. Commun.*, **49**(51), 2013, 5793–5795.
65. Xin, X. K., He, M., Han, W., Jung, J., and Lin, Z. Q. Low-cost copper zinc tin sulfide counter electrodes for high-efficiency dye-sensitized solar cells, *Angew. Chem.*, **123**(49), 2011, 11943–11946.
66. Yi, L. X., Liu, Y. Y., Yang, N. L., Tang, Z. Y., Zhao, H. J., Ma, G. H., Su, Z. G., and Wang, D. One dimensional CuInS2-ZnS heterostructured nanomaterials as low-cost and high-performance counter electrodes of dye-sensitized solar cells, *Energy Environ. Sci.*, **6**(3), 2013, 835–840.
67. Li, G. R., Wang, F., Jiang, Q. W., Gao, X. P., and Shen, P. W. Carbon nanotubes with titanium nitride as a low-cost counter-electrode material for dye-sensitized solar cells, *Angew. Chem. Int. Ed.*, **122**(21), 2010, 3735–3738.
68. Wu, M. X., Lin, X., Wang, Y. D., Wang, L., Guo, W., Qi, D. D., Peng, X. J., Hagfeldt, A., Grätzel, M., and Ma, T. L. Economical Pt-free catalysts for counter electrodes of dye-sensitized solar cells, *J. Am. Chem. Soc.*, **134**(7), 2012, 3419–3428.
69. Gong, F., Wang, H., Xu, X., Zhou, G., and Wang, Z.-S. In situ growth of Co0.85Se and Ni0.85Se on conductive substrates as high-performance

counter electrodes for dye-sensitized solar cells, *J. Am. Chem. Soc.*, **134**(26), 2012, 10953–10958.

70. Cheng, L., Hou, Y., Zhang, B., Yang, S., Guo, J. W., Wu, L., and Yang, H. G. Hydrogen-treated commercial WO3 as an efficient electrocatalyst for triiodide reduction in dye-sensitized solar cells, *Chem. Commun.*, **49**(53), 2013, 5945–5947.

71. Hou, Y., Wang, D., Yang, X. H., Fang, W. Q., Zhang, B., Wang, H. F., Lu, G. Z., Hu, P., Zhao, H. J., and Yang, H. G. Rational screening low-cost counter electrodes for dye-sensitized solar cells, *Nat. Commun.*, **4**, 2013, 1583.

72. Hou, Y., Chen, Z. P., Wang, D., Zhang, B., Yang, S., Wang, H. F., Hu, P., Zhao, H. J., and Yang, H. G. Highly electrocatalytic activity of RuO_2 nanocrystals for triiodide reduction in dye-sensitized solar cells, *Small*, **10**(3), 2013, 484–492.

73. Wang, Q., Moser, J.-E., and Grätzel, M. Electrochemical impedance spectroscopic analysis of dye-sensitized solar cells, *J. Phys. Chem. B*, **109**(31), 2005, 14945–14953.

74. Kern, R., Sastrawan, R., Ferber, J., Stangl, R., and Luther, J. Modeling and interpretation of electrical impedance spectra of dye solar cells operated under open-circuit conditions, *Electrochim. Acta*, **47**(26), 2002, 4213–4225.

75. Zaban, A., Greenshtein, M., and Bisquert, J. Determination of the electron lifetime in nanocrystalline dye solar cells by open-circuit voltage decay measurements, *ChemPhysChem*, **4**(8), 2003, 859–864.

76. Wu, X., Chen, Z. G., Lu, G. Q., and Wang, L. Z. Nanosized anatase TiO_2 single crystals with tunable exposed (001) facets for enhanced energy conversion efficiency of dye-sensitized solar cells, *Adv. Funct. Mater.*, **21**(21), 2011, 4167–4172.

77. Bai, Y., Xing, Z., Yu, H., Li, Z., Amal, R., and Wang, L. Porous titania nanosheet/nanoparticle hybrids as photoanodes for dye-sensitized solar cells, *ACS Appl. Mater. Interfaces*, **5**(22), 2013, 12058–12065.

78. Wang, Q., Ito, S., Grätzel, M., Fabregat-Santiago, F., Mora-Seró, I., Bisquert, J., Bessho, T., and Imai, H. Characteristics of high efficiency dye-sensitized solar cells, *J. Phys. Chem. B*, **110**(50), 2006, 25210–25221.

79. Kuang, D., Uchida, S., Humphry-Baker, R., Zakeeruddin, S. M., and Grätzel, M. Organic dye-sensitized ionic liquid based solar cells: remarkable enhancement in performance through molecular design of indoline sensitizers, *Angew. Chem., Int. Ed.*, **47**(10), 2008, 1923–1927.

80. Bai, Y., Yu, H., Li, Z., Amal, R., Lu, G. Q., and Wang, L. Z. In situ growth of a ZnO nanowire network within a TiO$_2$ nanoparticle film for enhanced dye-sensitized solar cell performance, *Adv. Mater.*, **24**(43), 2012, 5850–5856.
81. Jose, R., Thavasi, V., and Ramakrishna, S. Metal oxides for dye-sensitized solar cells, *J. Am. Ceram. Soc.*, **92**(2), 2009, 289–301.
82. Zhang, D., Yoshida, T., Oekermann, T., Furuta, K., and Minoura, H. Room temperature synthesis of porous nanoparticulate TiO$_2$ films for flexible dye-sensitized solar cells, *Adv. Funct. Mater.*, **16**(9), 2006, 1228–1234.
83. Liao, J.-Y., Lei, B.-X., Chen, H.-Y., Kuang, D.-B., and Su, C.-Y. Oriented hierarchical single crystalline anatase TiO$_2$ nanowire arrays on Ti-foil substrate for efficient flexible dye-sensitized solar cells, *Energy Environ. Sci.*, **5**(2), 2012, 5750–5757.
84. Wang, H., Nicholson, P. G., Peter, L., Zakeeruddin, S. M., and Grätzel, M. Transport and interfacial transfer of electrons in dye-sensitized solar cells utilizing a Co (dbbip) 2 redox shuttle, *J. Phys. Chem. C*, **114**(33), 2010, 14300–14306.
85. Ahn, K.-S., Kang, M.-S., Lee, J.-W., and Kang, Y. S. Effects of a surfactant-templated nanoporous TiO interlayer on dye-sensitized solar cells, *J. Appl. Phys.*, **101**, 2007, 084312.
86. Kang, S. H., Choi, S.-H., Kang, M.-S., Kim, J.-Y., Kim, H.-S., Hyeon, T., and Sung, Y.-E. Nanorod based dye sensitized solar cells with improved charge collection efficiency, *Adv. Mater.*, **20**(1), 2008, 54–58.
87. Zukalova, M., Zukal, A., Kavan, L., Nazeeruddin, M. K., Liska, P., and Gratzel, M. Organized mesoporous TiO$_2$ films exhibiting greatly enhanced performance in dye-sensitized solar cells, *Nano Lett.*, **5**(9), 2005, 1789–1792.
88. Han, H. W., Zan, L., Zhong, J. S., and Zhao, X. Z. A novel hybrid nanocrystalline TiO$_2$ electrode for the dye-sensitized nanocrystalline solar cells, *J. Mater. Sci.*, **40**(18), 2005, 4921–4923.
89. Yu, J., Fan, J., and Lv, K. Anatase TiO$_2$ nanosheets with exposed (001) facets: improved photoelectric conversion efficiency in dye-sensitized solar cells, *Nanoscale*, **2**(10), 2010, 2144–2149.
90. Zhang, H. M., Han, Y. H., Liu, X. L., Liu, P., Yu, H., Zhang, S. Q., Yao, X. D., and Zhao, H. J. Anatase TiO$_2$ microspheres with exposed mirror-like plane (001) facets for high performance dye-sensitized solar cells (DSSCs), *Chem. Commun.*, **46**(44), 2010, 8395–8397.
91. Jung, M.-H., Chu, M.-J., and Kang, M. G. TiO$_2$ nanotube fabrication with highly exposed (001) facets for enhanced conversion efficiency of solar cells, *Chem. Commun.*, **48**(41), 2012, 5016–5018.

92. Yang, H. G., Sun, C. H., Qiao, S. Z., Zou, J., Liu, G., Smith, S. C., Cheng, H. M., and Lu, G. Q., Anatase TiO_2 single crystals with a large percentage of reactive facets, *Nature*, **453**(7195), 2008, 638–641.
93. Sommeling, P. M., O'Regan, B. C., Haswell, R. R., Smit, H. J. P., Bakker, N. J., Smits, J. J. T., Kroon, J. M., and van Roosmalen, J. A. M. Influence of a $TiCl_4$ post-treatment on nanocrystalline TiO_2 films in dye-sensitized solar cells, *J. Phys. Chem. B*, **110**(39), 2006, 19191–19197.
94. Ito, S., Murakami, T. N., Comte, P., Liska, P., C. Grätzel, Nazeeruddin, M. K., and Grätzel, M. Fabrication of thin film dye sensitized solar cells with solar to electric power conversion efficiency over 10%, *Thin Solid Films*, **516**(14), 2008, 4613–4619.
95. Wang, J., and Lin, Z. Q. Dye-sensitized TiO_2 nanotube solar cells with markedly enhanced performance via rational surface engineering, *Chem. Mater.*, **22**(2), 2010, 579–584.
96. Brennan, T. P., Bakke, J. R., Ding, I. K., Hardin, B. E., Nguyen, W. H., Mondal, R., Bailie, C. D., Margulis, G. Y., Hoke, E. T., Sellinger, A., McGehee, M. D., and Bent, S. F. The importance of dye chemistry and $TiCl_4$ surface treatment in the behavior of Al_2O_3 recombination barrier layers deposited by atomic layer deposition in solid-state dye-sensitized solar cells, *Phys. Chem. Chem. Phys.*, **14**(35), 2012, 12130–12140.
97. Huang, F. Z., Chen, D. H., Zhang, X. L., Caruso, R. A., and Cheng, Y. B. Dual-function scattering layer of submicrometer-sized mesoporous TiO_2 beads for high-efficiency dye-sensitized solar cells, *Adv. Funct. Mater.*, **20**(8), 2010, 1301–1305.
98. Yan, K. Y., Qiu, Y. C., Chen, W., Zhang, M., and Yang, S. H. A double layered photoanode made of highly crystalline TiO_2 nanooctahedra and agglutinated mesoporous TiO_2 microspheres for high efficiency dye sensitized solar cells, *Energy Environ. Sci.*, **4**(6), 2011, 2168–2176.
99. Wu, X., Lu, G. Q., and Wang, L. Shell-in-shell TiO_2 hollow spheres synthesized by one-pot hydrothermal method for dye-sensitized solar cell application, *Energy Environ. Sci.*, **4**(9), 2011, 3565–3572.
100. Koo, H. J., Kim, Y. J., Lee, Y. H., Lee, W. I., Kim, K., and Park, N. G. Nano-embossed hollow spherical TiO_2 as bifunctional material for high-efficiency dye-sensitized solar cells, *Adv. Mater.*, **20**(1), 2008, 195–199.
101. Qian, J. F., Liu, P., Xiao, Y., Jiang, Y., Cao, Y. L., Ai, X. P., and Yang, H. X. TiO_2-coated multilayered SnO_2 hollow microspheres for dye-sensitized solar cells, *Adv. Mater.*, **21**(36), 2009, 3663–3667.

102. Yu, H., Bai, Y., Zong, X., Tang, F. Q., Lu, G. Q. M., and Wang, L. Z. Cubic CeO2 nanoparticles as mirror-like scattering layers for efficient light harvesting in dye-sensitized solar cells, *Chem. Commun.*, **48**(59), 2012, 7386–7388.
103. Chen, D., Huang, F., Cheng, Y.-B., and Caruso, R. A. Mesoporous anatase TiO_2 beads with high surface areas and controllable pore sizes: a superior candidate for high-performance dye-sensitized solar cells, *Adv. Mater.*, **21**(21), 2009, 2206–2210.
104. Zhang, Q. F., and Cao, G. Z. Nanostructured photoelectrodes for dye-sensitized solar cells, *Nano Today*, **6**(1), 2011, 91–109.
105. Zhang, Q., Chou, T. P., Russo, B., Jenekhe, S. A., and Cao, G., Aggregation of ZnO nanocrystallites for high conversion efficiency in dye-sensitized solar cells, *Angew. Chem.*, **120**(13), 2008, 2436–2440.
106. Zhang, Q., Chou, T. P., Russo, B., Jenekhe, S. A., and Cao, G. Polydisperse aggregates of ZnO nanocrystallites: a method for energy-conversion-efficiency enhancement in dye-sensitized solar cells, *Adv. Funct. Mater.*, **18**(11), 2008, 1654–1660.
107. Standridge, S. D., Schatz, G. C., and Hupp, J. T. Distance dependence of plasmon-enhanced photocurrent in dye-sensitized solar cells, *J. Am. Chem. Soc.*, **131**(24), 2009, 8407–8409.
108. Brown, M. D., Suteewong, T., Kumar, R. S. S., D'Innocenzo, V., Petrozza, A., Lee, M. M., Wiesner, U., and Snaith, H. J. Plasmonic dye-sensitized solar cells using core-shell metal- insulator nanoparticles, *Nano Lett.*, **11**(2), 2010, 438–445.
109. Qi, J., Dang, X., Hammond, P. T., and Belcher, A. M. Highly efficient plasmon-enhanced dye-sensitized solar cells through metal@ oxide core–shell nanostructure, *ACS Nano*, **5**(9), 2011, 7108–7116.
110. Hou, W., Pavaskar, P., Liu, Z., Theiss, J., Aykol, M., and Cronin, S. B. Plasmon resonant enhancement of dye sensitized solar cells, *Energy Environ. Sci.*, **4**(11), 2011, 4650–4655.
111. Choi, H., Chen, W. T., and Kamat, P. V. Know thy nano neighbor. Plasmonic versus electron charging effects of metal nanoparticles in dye-sensitized solar cells, *ACS Nano*, **6**(5), 2012, 4418–4427.
112. Gangishetty, M. K., Lee, K. E., Scott, R. W. J., and Kelly, T. L. Plasmonic enhancement of dye sensitized solar cells in the Red-to-NIR region using triangular core-shell Ag@ SiO_2 nanoparticles, *ACS Appl. Mater. Interfaces*, **5**(21), 2013, 11044–11051.
113. Dang, X., Qi, J., Klug, M. T., Chen, P.-Y., Yun, D. S., Fang, N. X., Hammond, P. T., and Belcher, A. M. Tunable localized surface plasmon-

enabled broadband light-harvesting enhancement for high-efficiency panchromatic dye-sensitized solar cells, *Nano Lett.*, **13**(2), 2013, 637–642.

114. Ding, B., Lee, B. J., Yang, M., Jung, H. S., and Lee, J.-K., Surface-plasmon assisted energy conversion in dye-sensitized solar cells, *Adv. Energy Mater.*, **1**(3), 2011, 415–421.

115. Ohsaki, Y., Masaki, N., Kitamura, T., Wada, Y., Okamoto, T., Sekino, T., Niihara, K., and Yanagida, S. Dye-sensitized TiO_2 nanotube solar cells: fabrication and electronic characterization, *Phys. Chem. Chem. Phys.*, **7**(24), 2005, 4157–4163.

116. Zhu, K., Vinzant, T. B., Neale, N. R., and Frank, A. J. Removing structural disorder from oriented TiO_2 nanotube arrays: reducing the dimensionality of transport and recombination in dye-sensitized solar cells, *Nano Lett.*, **7**(12), 2007, 3739–3746.

117. Adachi, M., Murata, Y., Takao, J., Jiu, J. T., Sakamoto, M., and Wang, F. M. Highly efficient dye-sensitized solar cells with a titania thin-film electrode composed of a network structure of single-crystal-like TiO_2 nanowires made by the "oriented attachment" mechanism, *J. Am. Chem. Soc.*, **126**(45), 2004, 14943–14949.

118. Liu, B., and Aydil, E. S. Growth of oriented single-crystalline rutile TiO_2 nanorods on transparent conducting substrates for dye-sensitized solar cells, *J. Am. Chem. Soc.*, **131**(11), 2009, 3985–3990.

119. Kang, T.-S., Smith, A. P., Taylor, B. E., and Durstock, M. F. Fabrication of highly-ordered TiO_2 nanotube arrays and their use in dye-sensitized solar cells, *Nano Lett.*, **9**(2), 2009, 601–606.

120. Li, L.-L., Chen, Y.-J., Wu, H.-P., Wang, N. S., and Diau, E. W.-G. Detachment and transfer of ordered TiO_2 nanotube arrays for front-illuminated dye-sensitized solar cells, *Energy Environ. Sci.*, **4**(9), 2011, 3420–3425.

121. Law, M., Greene, L. E., Johnson, J. C., Saykally, R., and Yang, P. Nanowire dye-sensitized solar cells, *Nat. Mater.*, **4**(6), 2005, 455–459.

122. Xu, F., and Sun, L., Solution-derived ZnO nanostructures for photoanodes of dye-sensitized solar cells, *Energy Environ. Sci.*, **4**(3), 2011, 818–841.

123. Lin, C. Y., Lai, Y. H., Chen, H. W., Chen, J. G., Kung, C. W., Vittal, R., and Ho, K. C. Highly efficient dye-sensitized solar cell with a ZnO nanosheet-based photoanode, *Energy Environ. Sci.*, **4**(9), 2011, 3448–3455.

124. Wei, Y., Xu, C., Xu, S., Li, C., Wu, W., and Wang, Z. L. Planar waveguide–nanowire integrated three-dimensional dye-sensitized solar cells, *Nano Lett.*, **10**(6), 2010, 2092–2096.

125. Tétreault, N., E. Horváth, Moehl, T., Brillet, J., Smajda, R., Bungener, S., Cai, N., Wang, P., Zakeeruddin, S. M., and Forró, L. High-efficiency solid-state dye-sensitized solar cells: fast charge extraction through self-assembled 3D fibrous network of crystalline TiO_2 nanowires, *ACS Nano*, **4**(12), 2010, 7644–7650.

126. Tétreault, N., Arsenault, É., Heiniger, L.-P., Soheilnia, N., Brillet, J., Moehl, T., Zakeeruddin, S., Ozin, G. A., and Grätzel, M. High-efficiency dye-sensitized solar cell with three-dimensional photoanode, *Nano Lett.*, **11**(11), 2011, 4579–4584.

127. Kang, S. H., Choi, S. H., Kang, M. S., Kim, J. Y., Kim, H. S., Hyeon, T., and Sung, Y. E. Nanorod-based dye-sensitized solar cells with improved charge collection efficiency, *Adv. Mater.*, **20**(1), 2008, 54–58.

128. Feng, X., Shankar, K., Varghese, O. K., Paulose, M., Latempa, T. J., and Grimes, C. A. Vertically aligned single crystal TiO_2 nanowire arrays grown directly on transparent conducting oxide coated glass: synthesis details and applications, *Nano Lett.*, **8**(11), 2008, 3781–3786.

129. Wang, H. E., Chen, Z. H., Leung, Y. H., Luan, C. Y., Liu, C. P., Tang, Y. B., Yan, C., Zhang, W. J., Zapien, J. A., Bello, I., and Lee, S. T. Hydrothermal synthesis of ordered single-crystalline rutile TiO_2 nanorod arrays on different substrates, *Appl. Phys. Lett.*, **96**(26), 2010, 263104–263104.

130. Yu, H., Pan, J., Bai, Y., Zong, X., Li, X., and Wang, L. Hydrothermal synthesis of a crystalline rutile TiO_2 nanorod based network for efficient dye-sensitized solar cells, *Chem. Eur. J.*, **19**(40), 2013, 13569–13574.

131. Wu, W.-Q., Lei, B.-X., Rao, H.-S., Xu, Y.-F., Wang, Y.-F., Su, C.-Y., and Kuang, D.-B. Hydrothermal fabrication of hierarchically anatase TiO_2 nanowire arrays on FTO glass for dye-sensitized solar cells, *Sci. Rep.*, **3**, 2013, Article ID 1352.

132. Wang, M. L., Huang, C. G., Cao, Y. G., Yu, Q. J., Guo, W., Huang, Q. F., Liu, Y., Huang, Z., Huang, J. Q., Wang, H., and Deng, Z. H. The effects of shell characteristics on the current-voltage behaviors of dye-sensitized solar cells based on ZnO/TiO_2 core/shell arrays, *Appl. Phys. Lett.*, **94**(26), 2009, 263506–263509.

133. Zhang, Q., Dandeneau, C. S., Zhou, X., and Cao, G. ZnO Nanostructures for dye-sensitized solar cells, *Adv. Mater.*, **21**, 2009, 4087–4108.

134. Xu, C., Wu, J., Desai, U. V., and Gao, D. Multilayer assembly of nanowire arrays for dye-sensitized solar cells, *J. Am. Chem. Soc.*, **133**(21), 2011, 8122–8125.

135. Ito, S., Ha, N.-L. C., Rothenberger, G., Liska, P., Comte, P., Zakeeruddin, S. M., Pechy, P., Nazeeruddin, M. K., and Gratzel, M. High-efficiency (7.2%) flexible dye-sensitized solar cells with Ti-metal substrate for nanocrystalline-TiO_2 photoanode, *Chem. Commun.*, **2006**(38), 2006, 4004–4006.

136. Lee, S., Noh, J. H., Han, H. S., Yim, D. K., Kim, D. H., Lee, J.-K., Kim, J. Y., Jung, H. S., and Hong, K. S. Nb-Doped TiO_2: a new compact layer material for TiO_2 dye-sensitized solar cells, *J. Phys. Chem. C*, **113**(16), 2009, 6878–6882.

137. Park, J. H., Lee, T. W., and Kang, M. G. Growth, detachment and transfer of highly-ordered TiO_2 nanotube arrays: use in dye-sensitized solar cells, *Chem. Commun.*, **2008**(25), 2008, 2867–2869.

138. Yella, A., Lee, H.-W., Tsao, H. N., Yi, C., Chandiran, A. K., Nazeeruddin, M. K., Diau, E. W.-G., Yeh, C.-Y., Zakeeruddin, S. M., and Grätzel, M. Porphyrin-sensitized solar cells with cobalt (II/III)–based redox electrolyte exceed 12 percent efficiency, *Science*, **334**(6056), 2011, 629–634.

139. Han, L., Islam, A., Chen, H., Malapaka, C., Chiranjeevi, B., Zhang, S., Yang, X., and Yanagida, M. High-efficiency dye-sensitized solar cell with a novel co-adsorbent, *Energy Environ. Sci.*, **5**(3), 2012, 6057–6060.

140. Lenzmann, F., and Kroon, J., Recent advances in dye-sensitized solar cells, *Adv. OptoElectron.*, **2007**, 2007, Article ID 65073.

141. Pettersson, H., and Gruszecki, T. Long-term stability of low-power dye-sensitised solar cells prepared by industrial methods, *Sol. Energy Mater. Sol. Cells*, **70**(2), 2001, 203–212.

142. Wang, Z.-S., Cui, Y., Dan-oh, Y., Kasada, C., Shinpo, A., and Hara, K. Molecular design of coumarin dyes for stable and efficient organic dye-sensitized solar cells, *J. Phys. Chem. C*, **112**(43), 2008, 17011–17017.

143. Kubo, W., Kitamura, T., Hanabusa, K., Wada, Y., and Yanagida, S. Quasi-solid-state dye-sensitized solar cells using room temperature molten salts and a low molecular weight gelator, *Chem. Commun.*, **2002**(4), 2002, 374–375.

144. Grätzel, M. Recent advances in sensitized mesoscopic solar cells, *Acc. Chem. Res.*, **42**(11), 2009, 1788–1798.

145. Forro, L., Chauvet, O., Emin, D., Zuppiroli, L., Berger, H., and Levy, F. High mobility n-type charge carriers in large single crystals of anatase (TiO_2), *J. Appl. Phys.*, **75**(1), 1994, 633–635.

146. Law, M., Goldberger, J., and Yang, P. D. Semiconductor nanowire and nanotube, *Annu. Rev. Mater. Res.*, **34**(1), 2004, 83–122.

147. Yu, K.H., and Chen, J. H. Enhancing solar cell efficiencies through 1-D nanostructures, *Nanoscale Res. Lett.*, **4**(1), 2009, 1–10.
148. Wong, D. K. P., Ku, C. H., Chen, Y. R., Chen, G. R., and Wu, J. J. Enhancing electron collection efficiency and effective diffusion length in dye-sensitized solar cells, *ChemPhysChem*, **10**(15), 2009, 2698–2702.
149. Leschkies, K. S., Divakar, R., Basu, J., Enache-Pommer, E., Boercker, J. E., Carter, C. B., Kortshagen, U. R., Norris, D. J., and Aydil, E. S. Photosensitization of ZnO nanowires with CdSe quantum dots for photovoltaic devices, *Nano Lett.*, **7**(6), 2007, 1793–1798.
150. Seol, M., Kim, H., Tak, Y., and Yong, K. Novel nanowire array based highly efficient quantum dot sensitized solar cell, *Chem. Commun.*, **46**(30), 2010, 5521–5523.
151. Yoon, J. H., Jang, S. R., Vittal, R., Lee, J., and Kim, K. J. TiO_2 nanorods as additive to TiO_2 film for improvement in the performance of dye-sensitized solar cells, *J. Photochem. Photobiol., A*, **180**(1–2), 2006, 184–188.
152. Nazeeruddin, M. K., Splivallo, R., Liska, P., Comte, P., and Gratzel, M. A swift dye uptake procedure for dye sensitized solar cells, *Chem. Commun.*, 2003(12), 1456–1457.
153. Grätzel, M. Conversion of sunlight to electric power by nanocrystalline dye-sensitized solar cells, *J. Photochem. Photobiol., A*, **164**(1), 2004, 3–14.
154. Luo, Y. H., Li, D. M., and Meng, Q. B. Towards optimization of materials for dye-sensitized solar cells, *Adv. Mater.*, **21**(45), 2009, 4647–4651.
155. Yodyingyong, S., Zhang, Q., Park, K., Dandeneau, C. S., Zhou, X., Triampo, D., and Cao, G. ZnO nanoparticles and nanowire array hybrid photoanodes for dye-sensitized solar cells, *Appl. Phys. Lett.*, **96**(7), 2010, 073115/1–073115/3.
156. Law, M., Greene, L. E., Radenovic, A., Kuykendall, T., Liphardt, J., and Yang, P. $ZnO–Al_2O_3$ and $ZnO–TiO_2$ core-shell nanowire dye-sensitized solar cells, *J. Phys. Chem. B*, **110**(45), 2006, 22652–22663.
157. Pang, S., Xie, T. F., Zhang, Y., Wei, X., Yang, M., Wang, D. J., and Du, Z. L. Research on the effect of different sizes of ZnO nanorods on the efficiency of TiO_2-based dye-sensitized solar cells, *J. Phys. Chem. C*, **111**(49), 2007, 18417–18422.
158. Fujishiro, Y., Uchida, S., and Sato, T. Synthesis and photochemical properties of semiconductor pillared layered compounds, *Int. J. Inorg. Mater.*, **1**(1), 1999, 67–72.

159. Kim, T. W., Hur, S. G., Hwang, S. J., Park, H., Choi, W., and Choy, J. H. Heterostructured Visible-light-active photocatalyst of chromia-nanoparticle-layered titanate, *Adv. Funct. Mater.*, **17**(2), 2007, 307–314.
160. Choy, J. H., Lee, H. C., Jung, H., Kim, H., and Boo, H. Exfoliation and restacking route to anatase-layered titanate nanohybrid with enhanced photocatalytic activity, *Chem. Mater.*, **14**(6), 2002, 2486–2491.
161. Geng, F., Ma, R., Nakamura, A., Akatsuka, K., Ebina, Y., Yamauchi, Y., Miyamoto, N., Tateyama, Y., and Sasaki, T. Unusually stable ~100-fold reversible and instantaneous swelling of inorganic layered materials, *Nat. Commun.*, **4**, 2013, 1632–1639.
162. Paek, S.-M., Jung, H., Park, M., Lee, J.-K., and Choy, J.-H. An inorganic nanohybrid with high specific surface area: TiO_2-pillared MoS_2, *Chem. Mater.*, **17**(13), 2005, 3492–3498.
163. Shibata, T., Takanashi, G., Nakamura, T., Fukuda, K., Ebina, Y., and Sasaki, T. Titanoniobate and niobate nanosheet photocatalysts: superior photoinduced hydrophilicity and enhanced thermal stability of unilamellar Nb_3O_8 nanosheet, *Energy Environ. Sci.*, **4**(2), 2011, 535–542.
164. Ko, J., Kim, I., Hwang, S., and Jung, H. Study on the structural and photocatalytic properties for pore size tailored SnO_2-pillared layered titanate nanohybrids, *J. Nanosci. Nanotechnol.*, **11**(2), 2011, 1726–1729.
165. Xu, B.-H., Lin, B.-Z., Wang, Q.-Q., Pian, X.-T., Zhang, O., and Fu, L.-M. Anatase TiO_2-pillared hexaniobate mesoporous nanocomposite with enhanced photocatalytic activity, *Microporous Mesoporous Mater.*, **147**(1), 2012, 79–85.
166. Lin, B., He, L., Zhu, B., Chen, Y., and Gao, B., Visible-light photocatalytic activity of mesoporous nanohybrid assembled by tantalotungstate nanosheets and manganese ions, *Catal. Commun.*, **29**(0), 2012, 166–169.
167. Lin, B.-Z., Li, X.-L., Xu, B.-H., Chen, Y.-L., Gao, B.-F., and Fan, X.-R. Improved photocatalytic activity of anatase TiO_2-pillared $HTaWO6$ for degradation of methylene blue, *Microporous Mesoporous Mater.*, **155**(0), 2012, 16–23.
168. Yanagisawa, M., Uchida, S., Fujishiro, Y., and Sato, T. Synthesis and photocatalytic properties of titania pillared $H_4Nb_6O_{17}$ using titanyl acylate precursor, *J. Mater. Chem.*, **8**(12), 1998, 2835–2838.

169. Liu, G., Wang, L., Yang, H. G., Cheng, H.-M., and Lu, G. Q., Titania-based photocatalysts-crystal growth, doping and heterostructuring, *J. Mater. Chem.*, **20**(5), 2010, 831–843.
170. Akatsuka, K., Takanashi, G., Ebina, Y., Haga, M.-a., and Sasaki, T. Electronic band structure of exfoliated titanium- and/or niobium-based oxide nanosheets probed by electrochemical and photoelectrochemical measurements, *J. Phys. Chem. C*, **116**(23), 2012, 12426–12433.
171. Osada, M., and Sasaki, T., 2D Oxide nanosheets: controlled assembly and applications, *ECS Trans.*, **50**(6), 2013, 111–116.
172. Sasaki, T., Watanabe, M., Hashizume, H., Yamada, H., and Nakazawa, H. Macromolecule-like aspects for a colloidal suspension of an exfoliated titanate. Pairwise association of nanosheets and dynamic reassembling process initiated from it, *J. Am. Chem. Soc.*, **118**(35), 1996, 8329–8335.
173. Sasaki, T., and Watanabe, M. Osmotic swelling to exfoliation. exceptionally high degrees of hydration of a layered titanate, *J. Am. Chem. Soc.*, **120**(19), 1998, 4682–4689.
174. Paek, S. M., Jung, H., Lee, Y. J., Park, M., Hwang, S. J., and Choy, J. H. Exfoliation and reassembling route to mesoporous titania nanohybrids, *Chem. Mater.*, **18**(5), 2006, 1134–1140.
175. Kim, T. W., Ha, H. W., Paek, M. J., Hyun, S. H., Baek, I. H., Choy, J. H., and Hwang, S. J. Mesoporous iron oxide-layered titanate nanohybrids: soft-chemical synthesis, characterization, and photocatalyst application, *J. Phys. Chem. C*, **112**(38), 2008, 14853–14862.
176. Kim, T. W., Hwang, S. J., Jhung, S. H., Chang, J. S., Park, H., Choi, W., and Choy, J. H. Bifunctional heterogeneous catalysts for selective epoxidation and visible light driven photolysis: nickel oxide-containing porous nanocomposite, *Adv. Mater.*, **20**(3), 2008, 539–542.
177. Choy, J. H., Lee, H. C., Jung, H., Kim, H., and Boo, H. Exfoliation and restacking route to anatase-layered titanate nanohybrid with enhanced photocatalytic activity, *Chem. Mater.*, **14**(6), 2002, 2486–2491.
178. Qiu, Y. C., Chen, W., and Yang, S. H. Facile hydrothermal preparation of hierarchically assembled, porous single-crystalline ZnO nanoplates and their application in dye-sensitized solar cells, *J. Mater. Chem.*, **20**(5), 2010, 1001–1006.

Biography

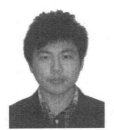

Yang Bai (born in 1988) received his BS in inorganic nonmetal material engineering (2010) from the Central South University (China). He is currently a PhD student in the School of Chemical Engineering and Nanomaterials Centre, University of Queensland. His research interests mainly focus on the design of novel nanostructured photoelectrode (including photoanode and counterelectrode) materials for low-cost and efficient dye-sensitized solar cells (DSSCs) and quantum dot–sensitized solar cells (QDSSCs).

Chapter 8

Gas Transport Properties and Transport-Based Applications of Electrospun Nanofibers

Dahua Shou,[a] Lin Ye,[a] and Jintu Fan[b]

[a] *School of Aerospace, Mechanical and Mechatronic Engineering, University of Sydney, NSW 2006, Australia*
[b] *Department of Fiber Science & Apparel Design, Cornell University, Ithaca, NY 14853-4401, USA*
dhshou@gmail.com

Electrospun nanofibers have found great applications in numerous areas, including filtration, protective clothing, tissue engineering, thermal insulation, and fuel cells. These fibers have several unique properties such as extremely small radius, high surface areas, high porosity, and relatively high mechanical performance. For gas transport–based applications, electrospun nanofibers significantly increase filtration efficiency at a given pressure drop of gas flow, and they are also known as good candidates of breathable protective clothing with high convective flow resistance but low moisture diffusive resistance. However, the related transport properties (i.e., gas flow and vapor diffusion) in the nanoscale fibrous media are difficult

---

Nanomaterials: Science and Applications
Edited by Deborah Kane, Adam Micolich, and Peter Roger
Copyright © 2016 Pan Stanford Publishing Pte. Ltd.
ISBN 978-981-4669-72-6 (Hardcover), 978-981-4669-73-3 (eBook)
www.panstanford.com

to explain using the continuum mechanics. This chapter presents mechanistic models for the main transport phenomena in order to advance the in-depth understanding of the relationship between the structure, transport, and functionality of electrospun nanofibers. A brief introduction of the recent progress in electrospinning is also provided.

8.1 Introduction to Electrospun Nanofibers

8.1.1 The Big World of Small Fibers

In comparison to commercial microfibers (Fig. 8.1a), nanofibers (Fig. 8.1b) have unique properties of high surface areas, extremely small diameter, high porosity, and good mechanical performance [1]. The novel features of nanofibers give rise to their wide applications in various fields, including filtration [2], protective clothing [3], tissue engineering [4], thermal insulation [5], and fuel cells [6]. Recently, electrospinning has gained increasing popularity as a powerful and versatile method to fabricate nanofibers (Fig. 8.1b), whereas an electrical charge is used to draw fine fibers from a liquid solution [7].

Specifically, some applications rely on the excellent transport properties (i.e., gas flow and vapor diffusion) of electrospun nanofibers [8]. For example, electrospun nanofibers are used as efficient filters for removing fine particles from a gas stream [9]. Unlike macroscopic transport problems in mass, momentum, or energy, as described on the basis of the traditional continuum assumption for microfibers, the movements and interactions of the nanoscale entities tend to be discrete random walkers in the microscopic world, and thus the continuum mechanics becomes somewhat unavailable to explain the transport behaviors [10]. As such, this chapter aims at systematically describing the connection between microstructures and nanoscale transport properties of electrospun nanofibers. Specifically, we will analyze the effect of structural parameters such as fiber radius and porosity on gas flow and vapor diffusion in the two significant transport-based applications, filtration and protective clothing.

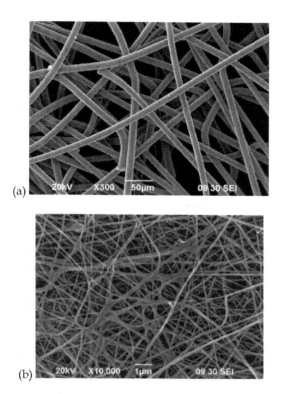

Figure 8.1 SEM images of (a) a conventional microfiber nonwoven and (b) a nylon 6 electrospun nanofiber mat.

8.1.2 What Is Electrospinning?

Electrospinning has a long history. The original concept was first observed in 1882 by Rayleigh [11] and investigated in detail on electrospraying by Zeleny [12]. The fundamental study on electrically driven jets laid the groundwork for electrospinning by Taylor in 1969 [13]. The term "electrospinning," derived from "electrostatic spinning," was introduced by Reneker in 1994 [14]. Since the 1990s and especially in the past decade, electrospinning has received more attention because of an increasing interest in nanotechnology. Superfine polymer fiber assemblies with diameters down to nanometers can be readily produced by this technique [1].

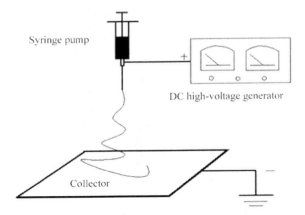

Figure 8.2 A typical electrospinning setup.

Electrospinning is typically conducted at standard ambient temperature and pressure (SATP). The typical setup of electrospinning apparatus is illustrated in Fig. 8.2. Basically, an electrospinning system consists of four major components: a high direct current (DC) voltage power supply, a controllable flow rate pump, a spinneret (e.g., a pipette needle), and a grounded collector (usually a metal screen, plate, or rotating mandrel). Before electrospinning, solid polymers are dissolved in certain solvents, and then the liquid polymer solutions are introduced into the pump for spinning nanofibers.

In the electrospinning process, very fine fibers (typically with fiber radius 25–500 nm) can be drawn from a polymer solution by an electrical charge with a high voltage of several tens of kilovolts [1]. The polymer solution is driven by the pump toward a tiny needle-like spinneret, which is subjected to an electric field. Then, the liquid surface is coated with charge and is elongated out of the spinneret to form a conical shape known as a Taylor cone. When the electric field reaches a critical value, the electrical force at the surface of the polymer solution or polymer melts can overcome the surface tension and thus a charged jet is ejected from the tip of the Taylor cone. The solvent evaporates, whilst travelling through the air, leaving behind a solid polymer fiber randomly deposited on the metal screen collector. If the molecular cohesion of the solvent is

Table 8.1 Effect of electrospinning parameters on fiber diameter and morphology

Parameter	Viscosity	Concentration	Molecular weight	Surface tension	Voltage	Flow rate
Parameter value	↗	↗	↗	↗	↗	↗
Fiber diameter	↗	↗	↗	↗	↗	↗
Bead number	↘	↘	↘	↗	↘	↗

sufficient, the charged liquid stream of polymer solution does not break up when accelerating toward the collector. As a whole, the elongating process of the fiber from solution to solid results in the formation of relatively uniform fibers with nanometer-scale radii.

8.1.3 What Affects Electrospun Nanofibers?

The electrospinning process is governed by many parameters, such as solution concentration, viscosity, conductivity, molecular weight, surface tension, applied voltage, tip-to-collector distance, flow rate, and the humidity and temperature of the surroundings. These parameters determine the fiber morphology and diameter as a result of electrospinning (see Table 8.1). Electrospun nanofibers of the desired morphology and radii can thus be generated on the basis of proper manipulation of these parameters [15].

Solution viscosity plays a critical role in determining the fiber radius and morphology during electrospinning [16]. Generally, an increase in solution viscosity gives rise to a larger and more uniform distribution of fiber radii [16]. No continuous fiber formation occurs at very low solution viscosity and the ejection of jets from the polymer solution via a needle is difficult at very high viscosity. Furthermore, only beads or bead-like fibers are formed as surface tension becomes the dominant factor at very low viscosity. As such, this leads to a probably optimal viscosity required for electrospinning.

Researchers have observed a power law relationship between polymer solution concentration and fiber radius—an increase in solution concentration increases fiber radius [17]. At a very low solution concentration, we get mostly beads with some fibers mixed in.

With increasing concentration there is an evolution from spherical beads to spindle-like and finally cylindrical fibers due to increasing viscosity resistance [17]. An optimal solution concentration for electrospinning exists. The formation of nanofibers is prohibited at very high solution concentrations by the inability of the solution flow at the needle spinneret [18].

The molecular weight of the polymer is correlated to the solution viscosity [1]. Generally in electrospinning, polymer solutions of high molecular weight have been adopted as they provide the adequate viscosity for generating fibers. If the molecular weight of the solution is too low, this leads to the generation of beads instead of fibers. Higher-molecular-weight solutions form fibers with larger radii.

A decrease in the surface tension of the nanofiber solution has benefits of producing fibers without beads at a lower voltage [19]. On the other hand, the higher surface tension imposes a higher probability of instability of the jets and the bloom of sprayed droplets [20].

A certain threshold voltage is required to form a fiber, but there is some dispute about the effect of applied voltage on both the electrospinning process and the resulting fiber radius. Some authors have reported that higher voltages result in larger radius fibers due to greater ejection of polymer solution [21]. Conversely, others have shown fiber narrowing with increased electrostatic repulsive force and applied voltage [21].

The flow rate of the polymer solution driven by the pump is important in determining the jet velocity and the material transfer rate. A relatively lower flow rate is generally preferable, leaving the solvent adequate time for evaporation [22]. In contrast, a high flow rate may lead to beads and bead-like fibers because of inadequate drying time before the liquid fiber reaches the collector. It has also shown that fiber radius increases with increasing flow rate of the polymer solution.

A conductive collector is used to collect the final product [23]. Aluminum foil is one of the most widely used collectors, in addition to conductive paper, conductive cloth, wire mesh, pin, parallel or gridded bars [24], rotating rods, rotating wheels [25], and a nonsolvent liquid, for example, a methanol coagulation bath. The nanofibers are generally randomly deposited on the collector due to the bending instability of the charged jet [26]. Nowadays, aligned fibers are of wide interest and have been fabricated by using a rotating drum or rotating wheel-like metal frame as the collector [23].

It is noted that these applications are somewhat limited by the problems of producing sufficient electrospun nanofibers to make adequate fabric areas in an acceptable time. For this reason, many high-output but cost-effective electrospinning techniques are presented, such as multineedle electrospinning [27], needle-less electrospinning, [28], and bubble electrospinning [29].

8.1.4 Transport-Based Applications: Filters and Protective Clothing

The diameter of an electrospun fiber is always in the nanoscale. Thus these solid fibers have a nanoscale surface texture that yields different mechanisms of interaction with other materials and phases compared to macroscale fibers [30]. Electrospun nanofibers also possess the features of a high specific surface area [1]. Their high surface area makes electrospun nanofibers potentially applicable in various activities desiring a higher degree of physical contact, for example, capturing fine particles by physical attachment or providing high resistance for fluid [1].

The use of electrospun nanofiber mats as efficient filters is well established [31]. van der Waals forces are the key capturing forces between the fibers and the targeted particles [32]. The filter is generally characterized by their collection efficiency and pressure drop for air filtration. For nanofibrous filters, they have much higher collection efficiency for microparticles and especially nanoparticles than commercial microfibrous filters, whereas the pressure drop is only slightly increased or even unchanged [33]. Since the thin nanowebs are suffering from relatively poor bulk mechanical properties during high-pressure-drop filtration, electrospun nanofiber webs are layered over a microfiber substrate.

Electrospun nanofiber mats are also considered as excellent candidates of protective clothing, since they have a high moisture vapor penetration rate, convective flow resistance, and toxic chemical resistance [31]. At the early stages, electrospun nanofibers were employed for textile and clothing applications, yet they are actually hard to produce in a woven pattern due to the difficulty in handling the numerous but barely visible nanofibers. However, they have the potential to produce seamless nonwoven-like garments with multiple functionalities (i.e., flame, chemical, environmental protection) by mixing nanofibers into layers or layering nanofibers onto microfiber substrates [34].

8.1.5 Limitations of Transport Modeling: Flow and Diffusion

Gas flow and vapor diffusion are two main mass transport mechanisms involved in applications of electrospun nanofibers in filtration and protective clothing. The stream topology of gas flow in a fibrous filter is critical to the transport properties of particles and to filtration performances. The quality of protecting clothing is mainly determined by gas flow resistance and vapor diffusivity simultaneously.

The slow flow through fibrous porous media is generally dominated by viscosity at a low Reynolds number, and the effects of gravity and inertia become negligible [35]. From a macroscopic view, permeability of fibrous media can be defined by Darcy's law [36]:

$$\langle \mathbf{u} \rangle = -\frac{K}{\mu} \nabla p \tag{8.1}$$

where K is Darcy's permeability, μ is the fluid viscosity, ∇p is the pressure gradient, and $\langle \mathbf{u} \rangle$ is the average fluid velocity. Darcy's equation, as an expression of conservation of momentum, originated from determining the permeability of porous media empirically in the 1850s [36].

The movement of vapor molecules caused by the concentration difference in a porous medium is known as diffusion [37]. It takes place when the concentration of the molecules is higher in one region than the other. Diffusivities are calculated by postulating the flux moving from regions of high to low concentration by using Fick's law [37]:

$$J = -D_b \nabla C \tag{8.2}$$

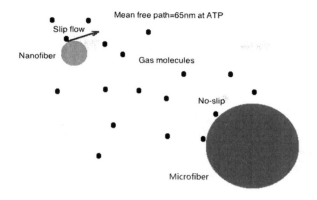

Figure 8.3 Gas molecules near a nanofiber and a microfiber.

where J is the diffusion flux and measures the amount of migrated diffusive molecules, D_b is the bulk diffusion coefficient in open space without any confinement, and C is the concentration of diffusive molecules.

Unlike macroscopic problems in mass, momentum, or energy transport, as described by the traditional continuum mechanics, the movements and interactions of the nanoscale entities tend to be random walkers in the microscopic world of electrospun nanofiber webs. For gas flow, the air molecule velocities are random near the surface of the fibers, as seen in Fig. 8.3. Continuum theory assumes that the average velocity of molecules fully in contact with the solid boundary of a microfiber is zero. This assumption is not strictly correct for nanofibers, as their radius is comparable to the mean free path of fluid molecules (average distance covered by a moving molecular between successive collisions with other molecules) and only a fraction of the air molecules actually contact the nanofibers [38]. The molecules that don't collide with the nanofibers contribute to slip flow [38].

For diffusion in porous media with large pores, movement of molecules is mainly blocked by their intermolecular collisions, and thus bulk diffusion occurs according to the continuum mechanics. However, when the pore radius is comparable with the mean free path of diffusion molecules, molecular wall collisions suffering from

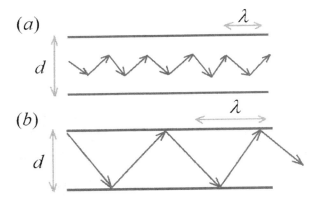

Figure 8.4 Schematic drawing of a molecule in a (a) microscale and a (b) nanoscale cylindrical tube with diameter d.

greater transport resistances will dominate [9]. A nanoscale mass transport known as Knudsen diffusion occurs, as seen in Fig. 8.4.

To sum up, gas flow and vapor diffusion in the nanoscale fibrous media are difficult to explain using the continuum mechanics. Mechanistic models accounting for these two transport behaviors are desirable, which will advance the in-depth understanding of the relationship between the structure, transport, and functionality of electrospun nanofibers.

8.2 Filters and Protective Clothing

8.2.1 Filters

8.2.1.1 Evaluation of filtration performance

Filtration efficiency E is defined as the fraction of particles collected by a fibrous filter [9]:

$$E = \frac{N_{in} - N_{out}}{N_{in}} \quad (8.3)$$

where N is the number of particles. Fibrous filters are different from a net or a sieve. A sieve will be 100% efficient in the capture of particles that are larger than its pores and this process is known as surface filtration. A net is based on depth filtration and thus thick

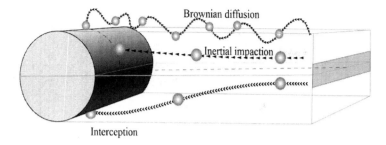

Figure 8.5 Illustration of mechanisms of particle collection by a fiber, including intercepion, Brownian diffusion, and interial impaction.

fibrous filters are more efficient than thin ones that are never 100% efficient.

The filtration efficiency of fibrous filters increases with increasing solid fiber volume fraction (FVF) or decreasing fiber radius. This, unfortunately, yields an increase in pressure drop Δ_p. Thus filter performance is judged, especially in industry, using a quality factor (QF) defined as [2]

$$QF = \frac{\ln(1-E)}{\Delta p} \qquad (8.4)$$

A good filter is often considered as one with a high filtration efficiency at a given pressure drop or simply a high QF.

8.2.1.2 Mechanisms of particle filtration

When particles within a gas stream approach a fiber, they may be trapped by the fiber due to the simultaneous action of several mechanisms, including interception, inertial impaction, and Brownian diffusion (Fig. 8.5) [2]. Gravitational settling is generally negligible for fine particles [2]. Interception indicates a particle is captured by a fiber when the distance from the center of the particle to the fiber is less than the particle radius. Inertial impaction occurs when heavier particles deviate from original gas streamlines and touch the fibers due to their inertia. Brownian filtration happens because of the random diffusive movement of particles suspended in a gas stream.

Modern filtration theory is based on the principle of single-fiber efficiency (SFE) [2]. The SFE is used to characterize the population of removed particles and is defined as the quotient of the number of particles captured by a unit length of fiber and the total number of particles in the undisturbed mainstream passing through the projected area [9]. An assumption of no particle rebound from the fiber is commonly made. In general, a single fiber has very low collection efficiency, but fiber bundles or filter layers can perform better. The SFE is built mainly on the cell approximation [39, 40], which portrays the fibrous medium as a collection of unit cells consisting of a solid fiber surrounded by flow streams. The size of the flow stream is given by the porosity or the FVF of the filter. However, this assumption is only strictly met if the fibers are parallel and distributed homogeneously.

The filtration efficiency E_f of a fibrous filter system is obtained as follows:

$$E_f = 1 - \exp(-4ch\delta/\pi d_f) \tag{8.5}$$

where c is the FVF, d_f is the fiber diameter, δ is the total SFE, and h is the filter thickness.

The total SFE is the sum of SFEs due to interception, inertial impaction, and Brownian diffusion:

$$E_f = E_{\text{inter}} + E_{\text{iner}} + E_{\text{Br}} \tag{8.6}$$

where E_{inter}, E_{Br}, and E_{iner} are SFEs due to interception, Brownian diffusion, and inertial impaction, respectively. They have the following expressions [2]:

$$E_{\text{inter}} = \frac{1 + \left(\frac{r_p}{r_f}\right)\left[2\ln\left(1 - \frac{r_p}{r_f}\right) - (1-c) + \left(1 + \frac{r_p}{r_f}\right)^{-2} - \frac{c}{2}\left(1 + \frac{r_p}{r_f}\right)^3\right]}{2f(c)} \tag{8.7}$$

$$E_{\text{iner}} = \frac{\left(\frac{d_p^2 \rho_p u}{18 d_f \mu}\right)\left[(29.6 - 28c^{0.62})\left(\frac{r_p}{r_f}\right)^2 - 27.5\left(\frac{r_p}{r_f}\right)^{2.8}\right]}{2f^2(c)} \tag{8.8}$$

$$E_{\text{Br}} = 2.9\left(\frac{1-c}{f(c)}\right)^{\frac{1}{3}}\left(\frac{d_f u}{D}\right)^{-2/3} \tag{8.9}$$

where D is the particle diffusion coefficient, r_p is the particle radius, ρ_p is the density of particles, and $f(c)$ is the hydrodynamic factor and is given by $f(c) = 0.25\ln c - 0.25 + 0.25c^2$ [41]. $f(c)$ characterizes the flow stream that is critical to the SFE of the above three filtration mechanisms. $f(c)$ is dependent on the geometrical arrangement, FVF, and fiber radius of the fibrous filter [41].

An electrospun nanofibrous filter commonly consists of a pad of loosely and randomly layered fibers. In addition, noncontinuum transport phenomena are observed in nanoscale regime. Thus, the above equations (Eqs. 8.7–8.9) based on ordered-packed fibers and continuum assumption do not agree with experimental results [42]. Therefore, empirical coefficients are often added to make the formulas valid by comparison to experiments and simulations [43, 44].

8.2.1.3 Measurement of particle filtration

Filtration efficiency of electrospun nanofiber mats is calculated by measuring the concentration of particles before and after passing through the mats [45]. Polydisperse NaCl particles have been widely used as testing particles and are created by a collision atomizer (Model 3079, TSI Inc.). Next, the generated particles go into an electrostatic classifier (Model 3080, TSI Inc.) and go out with a desired monodisperse size distribution. Fine particles of 50, 70, 100, 150, 200, 300, and 400 nm in diameter are chosen before the electrically neutralization using a Kr-85 aerosol neutralizer (Model 3077, TSI Inc.). Then, the concentration of NaCl particles is measured in the scanning mobility particle sizer (SMPS, Model 3936, TSI Inc.). In addition, the SMPS measures concentrations and sizes of the upstream and downstream NaCl particles, and finally the collection efficiency of electrospun nanofiber filters are calculated.

In Fig. 8.6, the pressure drop of nylon 6 electrospun nanofiber mats is measured at different values of concentration of the polymer solution, tip-to-collector distance, and solution flow rate [45]. A lower pressure drop is observed at a higher concentration of the polymer solution, a longer tip-to-collector distance, or a higher flow rate. In comparison to the melt-blown microfiber nonwovens, the pressure drop is much higher in electrospun nanofibrous media with a much smaller fiber size. In addition, the pressure drop of electrospun nanofibers is higher than high-efficiency particulate

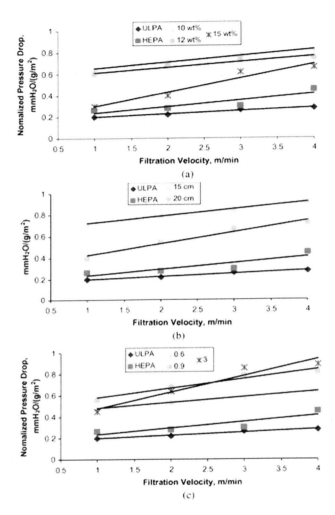

Figure 8.6 Pressure drop of nylon 6 electrospun nanofiber mats under different (a) concentration, (b) distance, and (c) feed rate. Reprinted from Ref. [45], Copyright (2013), with permission from Elsevier.

absorption (HEPA) and ultralow penetration air (ULPA)-grade filter media.

The filtration efficiency shown in Fig. 8.7 may also vary from different fiber sizes, in addition to the influence of different particle

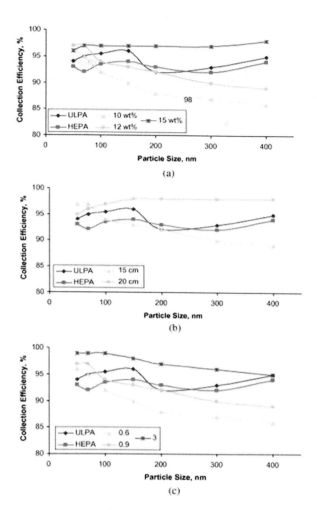

Figure 8.7 Collection efficiency of nylon 6 under different (a) concentration, (b) distance, and (c) feed rate. Reprinted from Ref. [45], Copyright (2013), with permission from Elsevier.

sizes. It is demonstrated that electrospun nanofiber filters have relatively higher filtration efficiency for very fine particles of 50 nm than that for coarse particles. In addition, the larger fibers (>100 nm in diameter) generally lead to a higher collection efficiency.

It is noted that electrospun nanofiber webs result in higher filtration efficiency and a higher pressure drop than conventional microfiber nonwovens. Thus, it would be of interest to revisit the filtration performance when electrospun nanofibers are layered on the microfiber substrate, considering the competition and interplay of the pressure drop or filtration efficiency between the dual layers.

8.2.2 Protective Clothing

8.2.2.1 Good candidates for protective systems

The convective flow resistance and vapor diffusive resistance of electrospun nanofibers are comparable to those of microporous polytetrafluoroethylene (PTFE) membranes, which have been used as a key component of protective systems [8]. However, electrospun nanofibers have a cost that is 30%–50% lower and better elongation than PTFE at a given protective performance [46]. Another advantage is that electrospun nanofiber mats may be sprayed onto a desired flexible, 3D scaffold [47]. Compared to microfibers, electrospun nanofibers of much finer radius have enhanced tensile strength due to the gradual ordering of the molecular chains and modest increase in the crystallinity of the fibers [48]. Additionally, the size effect results from the densely packed lamellae and fibrillar structures aligned with the fiber axis [48].

8.2.2.2 Measurement of diffusive and convective flow resistances

Water vapor diffusion resistance and convective gas flow resistance of electrospun fiber mats have been measured simultaneously by an automated dynamic moisture permeation cell (DMPC), as shown in Fig. 8.8 [49]. Gas flows at a given temperature and concentration of water vapor enter the test cell, and then the water vapor concentration and flow rates of the upstream and downstream of the gas are recorded. The transport of water vapor is considered as pure diffusion, solely driven by vapor concentration differences, when no pressure difference across the mat sample applies.

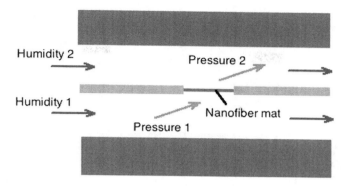

Figure 8.8 Convection/diffusion experiment in a dynamic moisture permeation cell.

The resistance of convective gas flow is given by Darcy's law:

$$R_D = \frac{A \Delta p}{\mu Q} \qquad (8.10)$$

where R_D is Darcy's flow resistance (m^{-1}), μ is the gas viscosity (17.85 × 10^{-6} kgm^{-1}s for N_2 at 20°C), Q is the total volumetric flow rate (m^{3}s^{-1}), A is the area of the test sample (m^2), and Δp is the pressure drop across the mat samples (Pa).

The total diffusion resistance as the sum of the diffusion resistances due to the sample (R_i) and the boundary air layers (R_b)

$$R_i + R_b = \frac{A \Delta C}{m} \qquad (8.11)$$

where R_i is the diffusion resistance of sample (sm^{-1}), R_b is the diffusion resistance of boundary air layers (sm^{-1}), m is the mass flux of water vapor across the sample (kgs^{-1}), A is the area of the test sample (m^2), and ΔC is the log mean water vapor concentration difference between top and bottom nitrogen streams (kgm^{-3}). The diffusion resistance of nanofiber layer can be calculated by subtracting the diffusion resistance of the boundary gas layer [8].

8.2.2.3 Breathable electrospun nanofibers

Figure 8.9 shows the comparison of the convective flow resistance between two electrospun nanofiber mats and several commercial microfiber webs [50]. In addition, the electrospun fiber mats are

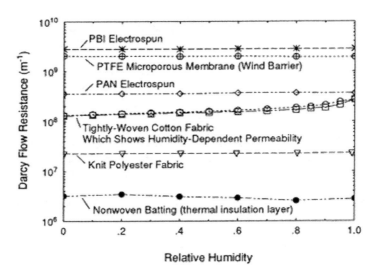

Figure 8.9 Convective gas flow resistances of commercial fabrics and electrospun nonwovens. Reprinted from Ref. [8], Copyright (2001), with permission from Elsevier.

found to have much higher convective flow resistance than those common microfiber-based clothing materials.

Gas slip occurs at the fiber surface when the mean free path of gas molecules becomes comparable to the fiber radius of electrospun nanofibers [16]. When this takes place, the pressure drop predicted by the continuum model is found to decrease by a factor of 1/3 for a fiber diameter of 65 nm by comparison to coarse fibers [8].

Figure 8.10 indicates the excellent water vapor diffusivity of electrospun nanofiber mats. The mats are very breathable with respect to allowing evaporative cooling for thin and lightweight protective clothing systems. The water vapor diffusion resistance of electrospun nanofiber mats is much smaller than the commercially used membrane-like laminates, which are widely used as highly breathable materials. Besides, the relative humidity has negligible influence on the diffusion transport behavior of these polymer membranes mats [51].

The strain effect on transport properties of electrospun nanofiber mats is investigated [49]. As expected, stretching the

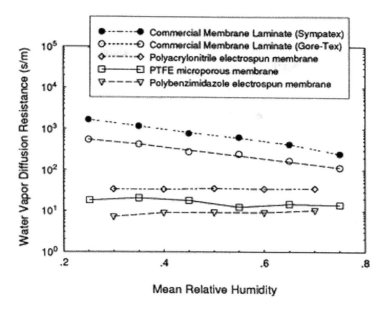

Figure 8.10 Water vapor transport properties of electrospun nonwovens. Reprinted from Ref. [8], Copyright (2001), with permission from Elsevier.

mats opens up the pores between fiber mats, decreasing the gas flow resistance. Fortunately, the decrease in flow resistance still remains within the "windproof" category of protective clothing. On the other hand, the diffusion resistance of water vapor negligibly varies against strains [49]. As such, electrospun nanofiber mats with simultaneously high rates of water vapor diffusivity and high gas flow resistances are promising breathable protective candidates under an applied strain.

8.2.3 A Call for Nanoscale Transport Models

From particle filtration in fibrous filters to the breathable property of protective clothing, gas flow past electrospun fibrous membranes is an essential phenomenon that has wide applications in scientific and industrial environments. One of the most important parameters for measuring the flow resistance or the species separation efficiency involved in those applications is permeability.

Permeability has been extensively explored over several decades [9, 39, 40, 52, 53]. The assumption that the fibrous media are homogeneous, with orderly fiber alignments, appears widely in these models. However, available electrospun fibers are always disorderedly and randomly distributed [54]. This variation can result in the predicted permeability differing from that in reality. More importantly, the permeability of electrospun nanofibers is underestimated by existing models that generally assume a no-slip flow condition at the fiber surface, which is inaccurate when the fiber size is comparable with the mean free path of air molecules, λ (i.e., $\lambda = 65$ nm for air in normal temperature and pressure) [55]. In fact, only the minority of the air molecules near nanofibers collide with the fiber surface, while the rest of the molecules without contacting the nanofibers continue their principal flow motion with a slip velocity.

Darcy's law is generally valid for flow in the continuum region with a pore size or fiber size much larger than λ. In addition, Darcy's law can be applied in the slip and transition regimes with Klinkenberg's or Knudsen's correction when the pore size is comparable with λ [56]. However, Darcy's law does not work with a pore size much smaller than λ. Gas molecules flow with minimal interaction with neighboring molecules and thus the continuum assumption breaks down [56]. As a general rule, Darcy's law can be used to characterize the flow behavior in electrospun nanofiber mats, since the minimum fiber radius is comparable to λ.

Gas diffusion as a concentration-driven transport across electrospun nanofibers also exists in filters and protective clothing. The application of Fick's law based on Eq. 8.2 requires the determination of the effective diffusivity. Various experimental techniques have therefore been developed to directly measure the diffusive flux against the directional concentration gradient or the effective diffusivity across fibrous materials [8, 57, 58] or to determine the evaporative resistance to moisture vapor diffusion (i.e., inverse to the effective diffusivity) [59, 60]. Recently, electrochemical diffusimetry, based on the analogy between Fick's and Ohm's laws, was also applied to measure the effective diffusivity of different carbon paper gas diffusion layers [61].

In general, gas diffusion slows down when diffusive molecules must follow tortuous pathways through the open pores of fibrous media. Moreover, the diffusion of molecules is hindered due to their frequent collisions with the solid wall in nanoscale pores [62]. For gas diffusion in the ordinary regime, where the pore size of the media is much greater than the mean free path of gas molecules, molecule–molecule collisions predominate and the diffusion coefficient is not sensitive to pore size. When the pore size is comparable with λ, however, molecule–wall collisions increase and the gas diffusivity decreases with the decrease in pore size [63]. In this transitional regime, the equivalent diffusivity, D_{Tr}, D_{Tr} is described by the Bosanquet equation [64]:

$$D_{Tr} = \left(\frac{1}{D_b} + \frac{1}{D_{Kn}} \right)^{-1} \tag{8.12}$$

where $K_n = \lambda/\langle d \rangle$ is the Knudsen number, $\langle d \rangle$ is the average pore diameter, D_b is bulk diffusivity, and D_{Kn} is the Knudsen diffusivity. The value of bulk diffusivity, D_b, is given by kinetic theory as $\lambda u/3$ with $K_n \ll 1$ in the ordinary regime [65], and D_{Kn} is expressed as $\langle d \rangle u_m/3$, with $K_n \gg 1$ in the Knudsen regime or free molecular regime [66], where u_m is the mean velocity of molecules.

Although nanoscale gas transport behaviors in simple geometry have been studied, there are few mechanistic models of transport properties for the complex electrospun nanofiber mats. Here, we will present our nanoscale transport models in the next section.

8.3 Gas Flow in Nanofibrous Media

8.3.1 Background of Gas Flow

In the context of permeability prediction, limited Stokes flow within a unit cell has been calculated to determine the flow behavior of circular fibers in a square array [39, 40, 53, 67–70]. On the basis of the widely used Kuwabara's expression of flow field around a fiber [39], Brown [9] developed a permeability model of ordered nanofibers, taking into account slip velocity in terms of dimensionless drag at the fiber surface. However, electrospun fibrous media are composed of fibers randomly located in horizontal planes (Fig. 8.1b) and the above models that are based on ordered arrangements of fibers cannot provide accurate predictions of through-plane permeability. Hosseini and Tafreshi [55] numerically mimicked the microstructures of randomly layered electrospun nanofibers by a μ-randomness algorithm. Slip flow was particularly considered to occur at the fiber surface of generated electrospun nanofibers and a higher permeability was found, as compared to that predicted by classical models of ordered fibers [55].

Here, we present a theoretical model that can accurately determine the through-plane permeability of an electrospun fiber layer as a function of randomness of fiber distribution and fiber size (or nanoscale effect). The cell of orthogonal fibers is chosen as the basic element to better characterize microstructures of the fibrous layer. The new cells with random size and distribution will be used to simulate the real architectures of electrospun fibrous mats in cubic space. Furthermore, the influences of the fiber radius or the nanoscale effect on the through-plane permeability will be extensively analyzed after validation of the model by numerical and experimental results.

8.3.2 Present Model of Gas Flow

A typical representative schematic for fibrous media is an ordered array of unidirectional fibers, as shown in Fig. 8.11. Under the condition of a low Reynolds number (Reynolds number <<1), steady flow through the representative cell is governed by the Stokes equation. As mentioned earlier, the nonslip assumption is not strictly correct when the fiber radius is comparable to the mean free path of air molecules. For the flow around a fiber, the tangential velocity is proportional to the tangential stress when partial slip occurs, and the first-order slip boundary condition is used [9]:

$$\mathbf{u}_s = \lambda \frac{\partial u}{\partial n} \tag{8.13}$$

where $\mathbf{u}_s$ is the slip velocity on the surface of fibers and n corresponds to the normal direction of the fiber surface. Generally, gas flow through coarse fibers is in a continuum regime ($10^{-3} > K_n$), while the flow field around nanofibers and microfibers is typically in a slip regime ($10^{-3} < K_n < 0.25$) or a transition regime

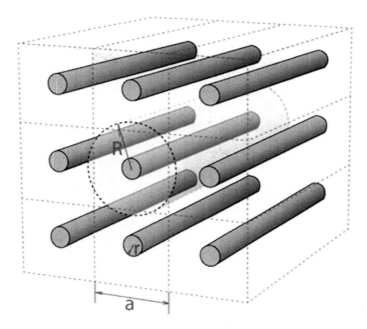

Figure 8.11 A unit cell of a single fiber in an ordered array of parallel fibers.

$(0.25 < K_n < 10)$ [55]. Here, the Knudsen number is defined as λ/r, where r is the fiber radius. Since λ is also defined as the slip coefficient in Eq. 8.13, the slip velocity can be alternatively expressed as

$$\mathbf{u}_s = K_n \frac{\partial u}{\partial n} r \qquad (8.14)$$

The basic element of fibers in square packing can be a square cross section with edge length a, as shown in Fig. 8.11. A circular cell is assumed to have an identical area and permeability as the square in Fig. 8.11 when the fiber fraction of the medium is low [39]. Thus, the radius of the effective circular cell is $R = r/\sqrt{c}$. For continuous flow on the surface of the circular cell, the internal flow velocity is equal to the mean velocity of the external effective medium. In addition, the flow vorticity vanishes due to the symmetry of flows between adjacent cells [39]. On the basis of the above boundary conditions, the permeability of the unit cell as a function of the FVF is given by [71]

$$K = \frac{-0.5\ln(c) - 0.75 + c - 0.25c^2 + 2K_n\left[-0.5\ln(c) - 0.25 + 0.25c^2\right]}{4c(1+2K_n)} r^2$$
(8.15)

Compared to the parallel-fiber-based assumption, the unit cell of orthogonal fibers is closer to the real electrospun fiber layers (Fig. 8.1b). The difficulty in determining the permeability of fiber layers composed of crossing fibers is that the flows of subpopulations are interdependent [72]. In 1986, Jackson and James [73] proposed the first permeability estimate for 3D fiber arrays, which is expressed in terms of unweighted local flow resistances in three principal directions in cubic space. Recently, Mattern and Deen [72] introduced more mixing rules for predicting the permeability of fiber assemblies. By comparing different mixing rules with multiple experimental results, Mattern and Deen [72] found volume-weighted resistivity to be the most reliable model or optimum blend, which was later validated by the work of Tamayol and Bahrami [74]. Here, the volume-averaged resistivity model is adopted to estimate the through-plane permeability of a unit cell of orthogonal fibers. The volume-averaged resistivity scheme is given by [72]

$$K(c) = \left[\frac{c_{\text{norm},x}}{c} K^{-1}_{\text{norm},x}(c) + \frac{c_{\text{norm},y}}{c} K^{-1}_{\text{norm},y}(c) + \frac{c_{\text{par},z}}{c} K^{-1}_{\text{par},z}(c)\right]^{-1}$$
(8.16)

where "norm" means normal to the flow direction and "par" means parallel to the flow direction.

The layered orthogonal fibers are normal to the flow direction and thus the local FVF $c_{\text{par},z}$ tends to zero. The local FVFs are assumed to be identical as the fibrous structure is isotropic between the two principal directions, that is, x direction and y direction. The permeability estimate based on Eq. 8.16 is found to be equal to Eq. 8.15, with $c_{\text{norm},x} = c_{\text{norm},y} = c/2$. Therefore, the orthogonal fibers have the same permeability as that of fiber alignments under given the FVF. In fact, the fiber crosses in a fibrous medium lead to a decrease in the permeability, whereas the enlarged pores between crossed fibers increase the permeability by comparison to parallel-fiber arrays. The competition between the two mechanisms superimposed with each other yields an approximately constant permeability.

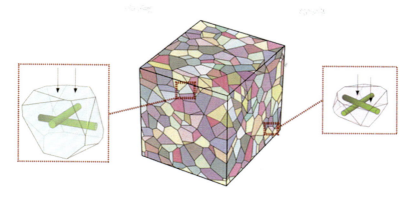

Figure 8.12 Cells of random size and distribution in cubic space.

This result shows that through-plane permeability is not sensitive to variation of in-plane fiber orientation, which has been verified by the finite-volume numerical simulation of Tahir and Tafreshi [75].

Then, more realistic fibrous media composed of randomly placed cells of orthogonal fibers are considered (Fig. 8.12). The Voronoi tessellation method [76] is used to quantify the size distribution of these cells. Cell center points are assumed to be randomly located, and each point is contained by a polygonal cell, whose boundary walls are defined by the midvertical planes of the lines joining the points. Such a polygonal cell is called a Voronoi cell. Kuwabara [39] has verified that the circular unit cell has the same permeability with the square cell under the same area or volume. Following Kuwabara's model, we assume each polygon cell of orthogonal fibers having aidentical permeability with the cuboidal cell under the same volume, and the volume distribution of polygonal cells with constant fiber volume V_f in each cell is used to characterize the randomness of fiber distribution. The through-plane permeability of fibrous layers of fully random arrangement is

$$K = \frac{-0.6\ln(c) - 0.74 + c - 0.25c^2 + 2K_n\left[-0.6\ln(c) - 0.14 + 0.25c^2\right]}{4c(1 + 2K_n)} r^2$$

(8.17)

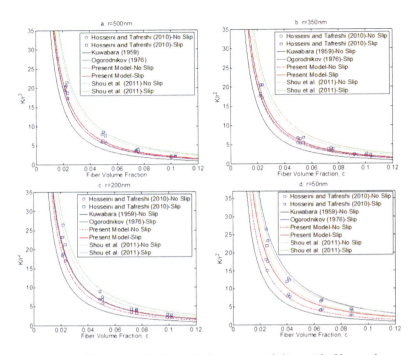

Figure 8.13 Variation of dimensionless permeability with fiber volume fraction for through-plane flow past the plane defined by randomly distributed nanofibers with a fiber radius of (a) 500 nm, (b) 350 nm, (c) 200 nm, and (d) 50 nm.

8.3.3 What Can Be Found from the Flow Model?

To examine the accuracy of our model for electrospun nanofiber layers, we compare the predicted permeabilites with the numerical results of Hosseini and Tafreshi [55], the empirical correlation of Ogorodnikov [77], and the analytical model [71] in Fig. 8.13. Kuwabara's model [39] for coarse fibers is also added for comparison. Ogorodnikov's model [77] is expressed as follows:

$$K/r^2 = \frac{-0.5 \ln(c) - 0.5 + 1.15 K_n (1-c)^4}{4c} \qquad (8.18)$$

We also compare our model with Kuwabara's model [39], which is widely used for determining the through-plane permeability of ordered fibers. The model of Ref. [39] is given by

$$K/r^2 = \frac{-0.5\ln(c) - 0.75 + c - 0.25c^2}{4c} \quad (8.19)$$

As seen from Fig. 8.13, our model agrees closely with the numerical data and empirical correlation of the through-plane permeability of nanofibers with different fiber radii: 500 nm (Fig. 8.13a), 350 nm (Fig. 8.13b), 200 nm (Fig. 8.13c), and 50 nm (Fig. 8.13d). With the decrease of fiber radius from 500 nm to 50 nm, the effect of slip flow is greatly enhanced and the dimensionless permeability is increased. When the fiber radius is 500 nm, the permeabilities with or without the slip effect are close to each other, indicating that slip flow might be negligible in this regime. Nevertheless, the through-plane permeability considering slip flow is increased by a factor of approximately 1/2 compared to that based on the continuum flow hypothesis when the fiber radius decreases to 50 nm. It is easy to understand that a wider pore size distribution leads to more large pores and therefore a higher permeability of the fibrous system at a given FVF and fiber radius, since permeability scales with the square of pore size. It is also shown that all the predicted permeabilities with the slip effect are much higher than Kuwabara's model [39] for an ordered-fiber array without the slip effect, as expected.

8.4 Vapor Diffusion in Nanofibrous Media

8.4.1 Background of Vapor Diffusion

The effective diffusion coefficient D_{eff} is widely expressed in terms of bulk diffusivity D_b, porosity ε, and tortuosity τ [78]:

$$D_{\text{eff}} = \frac{\varepsilon}{\tau} D_b \quad (8.20)$$

Realistic fibrous structures often contain fibers orientated in an uncontrolled manner. As such, it is difficult to determine the tortuosity through solving diffusion equations [79]. Monte Carlo numerical investigations were conducted to simulate the diffusion process, and semi-empirical correlations were obtained by curve-fitting the numerical results [80]. The semi-empirical formula is expressed as follows:

$$D_{\text{eff}} = \varepsilon \left(\frac{\varepsilon - \varepsilon_p}{1-\varepsilon_p} \right)^\alpha D_b \qquad (8.21)$$

Where ε_p and α are constants determined by geometrical arrangements of the fibrous medium.

Tomographic methods have also been applied to explore the diffusion in simulated porous media, such as soil, sandstone, and batteries [81, 82]. However, the task of extracting tomographic information is somewhat very complex, requiring extensive data for the reconstruction of the 3D fibrous structure [83].

Many porous media have a wide pore size distribution, and thus three types of diffusion mechanisms (i.e. bulk diffusion, transition diffusion, and Knudsen diffusion) co-exist simultaneously [84]. Recently, the effective diffusivity was simple expressed in a composite form [84]:

$$D_{\text{eff}} \varepsilon = D_b \varepsilon_1 + D_{\text{Tr}} \varepsilon_2 + D_{K_n} \varepsilon_3 \qquad (8.22)$$

where ε_1, ε_2, and ε_3 are the average porosities in the ordinary regime, transition regime, and Knudsen regime, respectively.

Although significant studies have been conducted on modeling vapor diffusion in fibrous materials, they are always limited to oversimplified structures. In addition, little research of Knudsen diffusion has been carried out in the nanofibrous medium because it is difficult to correlate the nanoscale transport to the microstructure.

Many natural objects, such as rivers, coastlines, and lakes, are found to have a self-similar feature at a wide range of scales. This property is called fractality [85]. Natural fractal objects do not always display exact self-similarity but possess statistical self-similarity, indicating that they are self-similar in some average sense. A fractal object is related to the length scale by a power law [85]:

$$M(l) \approx l^{D_0} \qquad (8.23)$$

where D_0 is the fractal dimension, $M(l)$ can be a quantity, or length, or volume, or area of the object, and l is the length scale. Fortunately, the pore size distribution and the pore length are found to be fractal in fibrous media [86–88]. As such, we apply fractal theory to quantify the correlation of effective diffusivity to fiber radius and porosity.

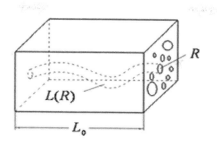

Figure 8.14 Fibrous porous media composed bundles of tortuous tubes. With kind permission from Springer Science+Business Media: From Ref. [54].

8.4.2 Present Model of Vapor Diffusion

The following assumptions are made: (1) The interconnected pores in fibrous media form a bundle of tortuous tubes (Fig. 8.14), (2) the distribution of tube sizes and tube lengths is statistically fractal-like, (3) fibers have a uniform radius, (4) fibers are impermeable, and (5) gas diffusion is in a steady state.

For a fractal porous medium, the pore number is correlated with the pore radius via a power law [89]:

$$N(l \geq R) = (R_{max}/R)^{D_f} \quad (8.24)$$

where D_f is the pore area fractal dimension, $1 < D_f < 2$ in two dimensions, and R and R_{max} are the pore radius and the maximum pore radius, respectively. In fact, the pores are not always uniform and have irregular shapes, so we use the area-equivalent radius R to characterize the pore size. The total pore number N_t, from the minimum pore radius R_{min} to the maximum pore radius R_{max}, is obtained by $(R_{max}/R_{min})^{D_f}$. In addition, the difference of the pore number with the radius lying between R and $R+dR$ is calculated by differentiating Eq. 8.24:

$$dN = -D_f R_{max}^{D_f} R^{-D_f-1} dR \quad (8.25)$$

The total diffusive fluxes, Q, is obtained by integrating the diffusion flux of individual tubes $q(R)$ on the basis of Eq. 8.25:

$$Q = \int_{R_{min}}^{R_{max}} q(R) dN \quad (8.26)$$

where, $q(R) = j(R)A(R)$, $j(R)$ is the diffusion rate, and $A(R) = \pi R^2$ is the cross-sectional area of a single tube. The total cross-sectional area of tubes, A_p is obtained by the following integration:

$$A_p = \int_{R_{min}}^{R_{max}} A(R) dN \qquad (8.27)$$

And the total cross-sectional area of the fibrous medium, A_t, is [90]

$$A_t = A_p/\varepsilon \qquad (8.28)$$

Gas diffusion flux $q(R)$ through a single tortuous tube is given by [91]

$$q(R) = -A(R)D_{equ}(R)\frac{\Delta C}{L(R)} \qquad (8.29)$$

where $D_{equ}(R)$ is the equivalent diffusivity of a tube, which has the same form with D_{Tr} in Eq. 8.12. Thus, $D_{equ}(R)$ can be expressed in terms of kn and D_b:

$$D_{equ}(R) = \frac{u}{3}\left(\frac{1}{2R} + \frac{1}{\lambda}\right)^{-1} = \frac{1}{1+K_n} D_b \qquad (8.30)$$

On the basis of Eq. 8.30, $D_{equ}(R)$ becomes D_b and D_{K_n} for upper and lower values of K_n, respectively. Therefore, the equivalent diffusivity covers the diffusive mechanisms throughout the range of length scales.

$L(R)$ is the tortuous length of a tube, as seen in Fig. 8.14, which is fractally related to the pore radius [92, 93]:

$$L(R) = L_0 \tau(R) = L_0^{D_\tau} R^{1-D_\tau} \qquad (8.31)$$

where D_τ is the tortuosity fractal dimension and L_0 is the straight length of a tube, equal to the root of the total crossing area [92, 93]. As the tortuosity is determined solely by the geometrical structures of porous media, it should be independent of diffusion mechanisms. However, it was found experimentally [94], numerically, and theoretically [65] that tortuosity in the Knudsen regime (τ_{K_n}) is greater than tortuosity in the ordinary regime (τ). It was found that $\tau_{K_n} = 3\tau$ in a single cylindrical tube [65, 78], and the increase of Knudsen tortuosity is due to the different path distributions resulting from the wall reflections of gas molecules [65]. Tomadakis and Sotirchos [78] numerically determined the modified tortuosity

(τ_M) in a semi-empirical fashion: $\tau_M = (\tau + \tau_{K_n} K_n)/(1 + K_n)$. Applying this to Eq. 8.31, we have the modified length of a tortuous tube:

$$L(R) = \frac{L_0 (\tau + \tau_{K_n} K_n)}{1 + K_n} = \frac{(\tau + 3K_n)}{1 + K_n} L_0^{D_\tau} R^{1-D_\tau} \quad (8.32)$$

Substituting Eqs. 8.27–8.32 into Eq. 8.26, we obtain a compact model of dimensionless effective diffusivity for porous media [54]:

$$\frac{D_{\text{eff}}}{D_b} = \frac{\varepsilon L_0^{D_\tau} (2 - D_f) \int_{R_{\min}}^{R_{\max}} \frac{2R^{D_\tau + 1 - D_f}}{2R + 3\lambda} dN}{\left[1 - \left(\frac{R_{\min}}{R_{\max}}\right)^{2-D_f}\right] R_{\max}^{2-D_f}} \quad (8.33)$$

The mean pore radius of fibrous media can be obtained on the basis of the following relationship [95, 96]:

$$\langle R \rangle = \frac{\varepsilon}{1 - \varepsilon} r \quad (8.34)$$

where $\langle R \rangle$ is the mean pore radius and r is the fiber radius. The mean pore radius can also be given by [86]

$$\langle R \rangle = \int_{R_{\min}}^{R_{\max}} R_f(R) \, dR = \frac{D_f}{D_f - 1} R_{\min} \quad (8.35)$$

On the basis of Eq. 8.34 and Eq. 8.35, $R_{\min}$ in Eq. 8.33 can be expressed as a function of fiber radius. Then, we can derive the dimensionless effective diffusivity expressed in terms of the fiber radius [54]:

$$\frac{D_{\text{eff}}}{D_b} = \frac{\varepsilon L_0^{D_\tau} (2 - D_f) \int_{r \frac{\varepsilon}{1-\varepsilon} \frac{D_f - 1}{D_f}}^{r \frac{\varepsilon}{1-\varepsilon} \frac{D_f - 1}{kD_f}} \frac{2R^{D_\tau + 1 - D_f}}{2R + 3\lambda} dR}{\left[1 - k^{2-D_f}\right] \left(r \frac{\varepsilon}{1-\varepsilon} \frac{D_f - 1}{kD_f}\right)^{2-D_f}} \quad (8.36)$$

where k is the ratio between the maximum and minimum pore radii.

8.4.3 Experimental Measurement of Vapor Diffusivity

We measured vapor diffusivity by the inverted cup test method (Fig. 8.15). The nylon 6 particles were dissolved in formic acid with 20 wt% concentration and they were continuously stirred for 24 hours at room temperature. A positive potential was employed to the polymer solution by connecting a copper wire to the metal tip. The imposed potential difference between the tip and the collector

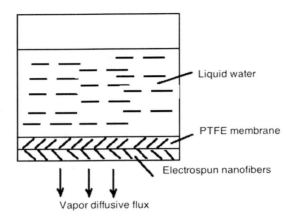

Figure 8.15 An inverted cup test setup for vapor diffusivty.

was 20–30 kV. A rotating metal drum covered with aluminum foil, placed 15 cm away from the tip, was used to collect the electrospun fiber assemblies. The ejection rate of the solution was set as 0.3 mL/h.

An FEI Sirion 200 field emission scanning electron microscope (SEM) was used to image the electrospun nanofibers. Then ImageJ was used to measure individual fiber radii in each SEM micrograph.

The porosity of the electrospun fiber web was determined using the following equation:

$$\varepsilon = 1 - \frac{\rho_{medium}}{\rho_{nylon}} \tag{8.37}$$

where ε is the porosity, ρ_{nylon} is the density of solid nylon 6, and ρ_{medium} is the density of the fibrous medium.

In Fig. 8.15, an inverted cup was filled with water in a conditioned room. The room had a controlled temperature of $20 \pm 0.5°C$ and a controlled relative humidity of $62 \pm 1\%$. To prevent the water in the cup from wetting and pressing on the sample, a breathable hydrophobic PTFE membrane covered the opening of the cup. Moisture vapor diffused from the liquid water in the cup to the air outside the cup across the PTFE and the sample. The cup assembly was then weighed hourly. Effective diffusivity can be calculated by

$$D_{eff} = \frac{h_i}{\frac{\Delta C}{J_0} - \frac{\Delta C}{J_i}} \tag{8.38}$$

where ΔC is the difference in vapor concentration, J_0 is the diffusion rate of a layer of the PTFE membrane, and J_i is the diffusion rate of the PTFE membrane and sample layers with total thickness h_i. We measured diffusion rates with 0, 1, 2, and 3 layers of samples and averaged the effective diffusivity using Eq. 8.40. Here, the bulk diffusion coefficient of moisture vapor in air, D_b is $2.45 \times 10^{-5} \mathrm{m}^2/\mathrm{s}$, the density of saturated vapor ρ_v in air is about $17.3 \mathrm{m}^3$ [97], and the mean free path of vapor molecules, λ is around 0.1 μm [98].

8.4.4 What Can Be Obtained from the Diffusion Model?

In this part, we compare our model of effective vapor diffusivity with experimental results. Then, the influence of microstructures on diffusion behaviors is extensively analyzed.

On the basis of Eq. 8.35, the area fractal dimension D_f for layered fibrous media is given by [99]

$$D_f = 2 - \frac{\ln \varepsilon}{\ln \left(\frac{R_{min}}{R_{max}} \right)} \tag{8.39}$$

and the tortuosity fractal dimension is expressed as [100]

$$D_\tau = 1 + \frac{\ln \langle \tau \rangle}{\ln \frac{L_0}{\langle R \rangle}} \tag{8.40}$$

where, $\langle \tau \rangle$ is the average tortuosity of the fibrous layer. The average tortuosity is given by [101]

$$\langle \tau \rangle = \left(\frac{0.89}{\varepsilon - 0.11} \right)^{0.785} \tag{8.41}$$

Diffusivity predictions of nylon 6 electrospun nanofibrous membranes are compared with the experimental results of vapor diffusivities. Two types of conventional microfiber nonwovens are also added for comparison. The fiber radius of the electrospun membranes is around 50 nm and the fiber radius of the conventional fibrous samples is 15 μm. Both Knudsen diffusion and bulk diffusion co-exist in electrospun nanofibrous layers due to the wide pore size distribution. Yet only bulk diffusion occurs in the microfiber nonwoven webs because their pore size is much larger than λ. For a sample of electrospun web with a porosity of 0.9, its maximum pore radius measured was 5 μm. The pore radius was close to the predicted value of 2.1 μm using the formula $R_{\max} = 4r\sqrt{\varepsilon/\pi}/(1 - \sqrt{\varepsilon})$ [102]. Here, navigation and determination of the minimum pore radius $R_{\min}$ in such a random fibrous mat is very difficult. We calculate $R_{\min}$ on the basis of Eq. 8.34 and find that the mean pore radius is a function of the minimum pore radius and the area fractal dimension. With the maximum pore radius 5 μm by measurement and 2.1 μm by prediction, the corresponding dimensionless effective diffusivities were calculated as 0.67 and 0.7, respectively. They are similar with each other. As such, a reasonable estimated ratio between the minimum and maximum radii, $k = 0.05$, was employed in this study. And the corresponding maximum pore radius is equal to 4.4 μm, between the predicted 2.1 μm and the measured 5 μm. In the meantime, the fractal theory holds as

$$\int_{-\infty}^{+\infty} f(R)\, dR = \int_{-\infty}^{+\infty} \frac{1}{N_t dN} = 99.72\% \approx 1 \qquad (8.42)$$

We compare the computed diffusivities with experimental data of both electrospun nanofibrous membranes and conventional nonwoven webs. A good agreement is evident as seen in Fig. 8.16. In Fig. 8.17, the dimensionless effective diffusivity is found to increase monotonously with an increase in porosity and fiber radius. The nanoscale (Knudsen) effect becomes significant when the fiber radius is comparable with λ. It is worthwhile to note that this trend is different from that of the pressure-driven flow, in which the nanoscale effect results in increased permeability due to slip flow at the fiber surface. Moreover, the effective diffusivity becomes independent of the fiber radius when the fiber radius is larger than 500 nm. From Fig. 8.16 and Fig. 8.17, we can conclude that the effective diffusivity of the electrospun nanofibrous membrane was smaller than the microfiber nowoven webs, but they still remain in the same magnitude. However, electrospun nanofibrous membranes are much thinner in thickness [8]. Therefore, light and thin electrospun protective clothing can be as breathable as conventional microfiber webs.

The effective diffusivities of electrospun nanofibrous mats of $\varepsilon = 0.6$ and $\varepsilon = 0.8$, respectively, are plotted against the fiber radius in Fig. 8.18. The figure shows that higher porosity results in higher diffusivity, as expected. Furthermore, we can see that a decrease

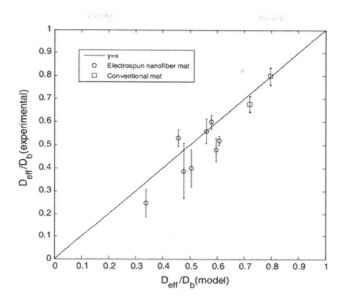

Figure 8.16 A comparison of effective diffusivities between the present model and the experimental results (with standard deviations) for electrospun nanofiber mats and conventional mats. With kind permission from Springer Science+Business Media: From Ref. [54].

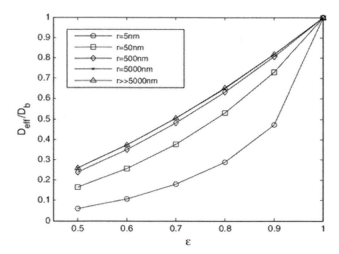

Figure 8.17 Effect of fiber radius on effective diffusivity versus porosity. With kind permission from Springer Science+Business Media: From Ref. [54].

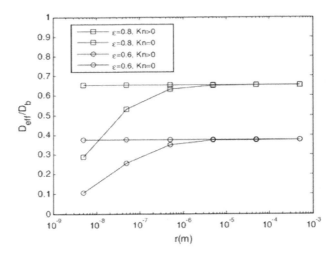

Figure 8.18 Effect of porosity on effective diffusivity versus fiber radius. With kind permission from Springer Science+Business Media: From Ref. [54].

in the fiber radius or an increased Knudsen number reduces the effective diffusivity. This effect is even more pronounced at lower porosity (e.g., $\varepsilon = 0.6$) than at higher porosity (e.g., $\varepsilon = 0.8$).

8.5 Summary and Future Work

8.5.1 Conclusive Summary

This chapter has briefly introduced electrospinning from production to application. The affecting factors on fiber morphology and fiber radii have been summarized. The application of electrospun nanofibers to filtration and protective clothing has been extensively discussed. The nanoscale effect of transport properties evolved in the two applications has received less attention than its fundamental position. Thus the development of theoretical analysis dealing with this problem will lead to much increased understanding of transport behaviors.

Unlike the continuum hypothesis for gas flow past coarse fibers, the slip velocity on the surface of nanofibers and microfibers is considered in the present model. Moreover, the random distribution of cells on the basis of orthogonal fibers enables more realistic characterizations of microstructures and so more accurate permeability predictions for a nanofiber layer. The fiber radius or Knudsen number is used to quantify the effect of slip flow in nanoscale and microscale regimes. It is found that the dimensionless permeabilities of both regular structures and random arrangements increase with decreased fiber radius or increased Knudsen number, because the slip flow velocity on the fiber surface becomes increasingly substantial compared to the bulk flow. When the fiber radius is smaller than 1 μm, it is necessary to take the slip flow into account. The slip effect is slightly more pronounced in fibrous systems with a higher FVF.

The fractal model of diffusion behavior of nanoscale and microscale fibrous media is validated by experimental data from the present measurement and literature. Electrospun nanofibrous membranes are found to be good breathable materials with a small diffusive resistance. It is found that gas diffusion is slowed down by Knudsen diffusion due to a fiber size that decreases to a nanoscale.

8.5.2 Future Perspective

On the basis of the progress achieved through the present study, the following further work is suggested:

- Apply nanoscale transport models to engineering problems such as protective clothing and filtration. Design optimal fibrous structures of electrospun nanofiber mats with required or maximum/minimum permeability, diffusivity, or production expense. Structural parameters, including porosity (or FVF), thickness, fiber size, fiber distribution, scale hierarchy, surface roughness, layer distribution, edge effect, inclusion influence, and layer arrangement, can be optimized on the basis of the specific requirement.
- With analogy theory, apply the models of effective permeability and diffusivity to heat transfer, electrical conduction, elastic, etc. In addition, extend present models to investigate dynamic transport behaviors and transport properties in deformed electrospun nanofibrous constructs.

- Perform numerical simulations of coupled transport properties in complex fibrous composites from nanoscale to macroscale on the basis of present models. Then develop easy-to-use software to describe the complex transport phenomena.
- Explore the mechanism of generation of electrospun nanofiber mats, which enables one to better characterize fibrous structures and thus transport behaviors.

Acknowledgments

This work was supported by a Discovery Project from the Australia Research Council.

References

1. Huang, Z. M., Zhang, Y. Z., Kotaki, M., and Ramakrishna, S. A review on polymer nanofibers by electrospinning and their applications in nanocomposites, *Compos. Sci. Technol.*, **63**, 2003, 2223–2253.
2. Wang, C.-s., and Otani, Y. Removal of nanoparticles from gas streams by fibrous filters: a review, *Ind. Eng. Chem. Res.*, **52**, 2013, 5–17.
3. Pant, H. R., Bajgai, M. P., Nam, K. T., Seo, Y. A., Pandeya, D. R., Hong, S. T., and Kim, H. Y. Electrospun nylon-6 spider-net like nanofiber mat containing TiO_2 nanoparticles: a multifunctional nanocomposite textile material, *J. Hazard. Mater.*, **185**, 2011, 124–130.
4. Yoshimoto, H., Shin, Y. M., Terai, H., and Vacanti, J. P. A biodegradable nanofiber scaffold by electrospinning and its potential for bone tissue engineering, *Biomaterials*, **24**, 2003, 2077–2082.
5. Wu, H. J., Fan, J. T., Qin, X. H., and Zhang, G. Thermal radiative properties of electrospun superfine fibrous PVA films, *Mater. Lett.*, **62**, 2008, 828–831.
6. Thavasi, V., Singh, G., and Ramakrishna, S. Electrospun nanofibers in energy and environmental applications, *Energ Environ. Sci.*, **1**, 2008, 205–221.
7. Wu, J., Wang, N., Zhao, Y., and Jiang, L. Electrospinning of multilevel structured functional micro-/nanofibers and their applications, *J. Mater. Chem. A*, **1**, 2013, 7290–7305.

8. Gibson, P., Schreuder-Gibson, H., and Rivin, D. Transport properties of porous membranes based on electrospun nanofibers, *Colloids Surf. A*, **187**, 2001, 469–481.
9. Brown, R. C. *Air Filtration: An Integrated Approach to the Theory and Application of Fibrous Filters*, Pergamon Press, Oxford, 1993.
10. Wendorff, J. H., Agarwal, S., and Greiner, A. *Electrospinning: Materials, Processing, and Applications*, Wiley-VCH, Weinheim, 2012.
11. Rayleigh, L. On the equilibrium of liquid conducting masses charged with electricity, *Philos. Mag.*, **14**, 1882, 184–186.
12. Zeleny, J. The electrical discharge from liquid points, and a hydrostatic method of measuring the electric intensity at their surfaces, *Phys. Rev.*, **3**, 1914, 69–91.
13. Taylor, G. Electrically driven jets, *Proc. R. Soc. London A*, **313**, 1969, 453–475.
14. Srinivasan, G., and Reneker, D. H. Structure and morphology of small-diameter electrospun aramid fibers, *Polym. Int.*, **36**, 1995, 195–201.
15. Chong, E. J., Phan, T. T., Lim, I. J., Zhang, Y. Z., Bay, B. H., Ramakrishna, S., and Lim, C. T. Evaluation of electrospun PCL/gelatin nanofibrous scaffold for wound healing and layered dermal reconstitution, *Acta Biomater.*, **3**, 2007, 321–330.
16. Deitzel, J. M., Kleinmeyer, J., Harris, D., and Tan, N.C.B. The effect of processing variables on the morphology of electrospun nanofibers and textiles, *Polymer*, **42**, 2001, 261–272.
17. Ki, C. S., Baek, D. H., Gang, K. D., Lee, K. H., Um, I. C., and Park, Y. H. Characterization of gelatin nanofiber prepared from gelatin-formic acid solution, *Polymer*, **46**, 2005, 5094–5102.
18. Sukigara, S., Gandhi, M., Ayutsede, J., Micklus, M., and Ko, F. Regeneration of Bombyx mori silk by electrospinning: part 1; processing parameters and geometric properties, *Polymer*, **44**, 2003, 5721–5727.
19. Haghi, A. K., and Akbari, M. Trends in electrospinning of natural nanofibers, *Phys. Status Solidi A*, **204**, 2007, 1830–1834.
20. Hohman, M. M., Shin, M., Rutledge, G., and Brenner, M. P. Electrospinning and electrically forced jets. II. Applications, *Phys. Fluids*, **13**, 2001, 2221–2236.
21. Demir, M. M., Yilgor, I., Yilgor, E., and Erman, B. Electrospinning of polyurethane fibers, *Polymer*, **43**, 2002, 3303–3309.
22. Yuan, X. Y., Zhang, Y. Y., Dong, C. H., and Sheng, J. Morphology of ultrafine polysulfone fibers prepared by electrospinning, *Polym. Int.*, **53**, 2004, 1704–1710.

23. Bhardwaj, N., and Kundu, S. C. Electrospinning: a fascinating fiber fabrication technique, *Biotechnol. Adv.*, **28**, 2010, 325–347.
24. Li, D., Wang, Y. L., and Xia, Y. N. Electrospinning nanofibers as uniaxially aligned arrays and layer-by-layer stacked films, *Adv. Mater.*, **16**, 2004, 361–366.
25. Xu, C. Y., Inai, R., Kotaki, M., and Ramakrishna, S. Aligned biodegradable nanofibrous structure: a potential scaffold for blood vessel engineering, *Biomaterials*, **25**, 2004, 877–886.
26. Reneker, D. H., and Chun, I. Nanometre diameter fibres of polymer, produced by electrospinning, *Nanotechnology*, **7**, 1996, 216–223.
27. Yang, Y., Jia, Z., Li, Q., Hou, L., Liu, J., Wang, L., Guan, Z., and Zahn, M. A shield ring enhanced equilateral hexagon distributed multi-needle electrospinning spinneret, *IEEE Trans. Dielectr. Electr. In.*, **17**, 2010, 1592–1601.
28. Niu, H. T., and Lin, T. Fiber generators in needleless electrospinning, *J. Nanomater.*, **2012**, 2012, 725950.
29. He, J.-H., Liu, Y., Xu, L., Yu, J.-Y., and Sun, G. BioMimic fabrication of electrospun nanofibers with high-throughput, *Chaos Soliton Fract.*, **37**, 2008, 643–651.
30. Ajayan, P. M., Schadler, L. S., and Braun, P. V. *Nanocomposite Science and Technology*, Wiley-VCH, Weinheim, 2003.
31. Gibson, P. W., Schreuder-Gibson, H. L., and Rivin, D. Electrospun fiber mats: transport properties, *AIChE J.*, **45**, 1999, 190–195.
32. Kirsh, V. A. The effect of van der Waals' forces on aerosol filtration with fibrous filters, *Colloid J.*, **62**, 2000, 714–720.
33. Wang, Q., Maze, B., Tafreshi, H. V., and Pourdeyhimi, B. A note on permeability simulation of multifilament woven fabrics, *Chem. Eng. Sci.*, **61**, 2006, 8085–8088.
34. Lee, S., and Obendorf, S. K. Use of electrospun nanofiber web for protective textile materials as barriers to liquid penetration, *Text. Res. J.*, **77**, 2007, 696–702.
35. Kim, J. S., and Reneker, D. H. Mechanical properties of composites using ultrafine electrospun fibers, *Polym. Compos.*, **20**, 1999, 124–131.
36. Darcy, H. *Les fontaines publiques de la ville de Dijon*, Dalmont, Paris, 1856.
37. Smith, W. F., and Hashemi, J. *Foundations of Materials Science and Engineering*, McGraw-Hill Higher Education, 2006.
38. Smith, W. F. *Foundations of Materials Science and Engineering*, McGraw-Hill, 2004.

39. Kuwabara, S. The forces experienced by randomly distributed parellel circular cylinders or spheres in a viscous flow at small reynolds numbers, *J. Phys. Soc. Jpn.*, **14**, 1959, 527–532.
40. Happel, J. Viscous flow relative to arrays of cylinders, *AIChE J.*, **5**, 1959, 174–177.
41. Lee, K. W., and Liu, B.Y.H. Theoretical-study of aerosol filtration by fibrous filters, *Aerosol Sci. Technol.*, **1**, 1982, 147–161.
42. Dhaniyala, S., and Liu, B. Y. H. Theoretical modeling of filtration by nonuniform fibrous filters, *Aerosol Sci. Technol.*, **34**, 2001, 170–178.
43. Hosseini, S. A., and Tafreshi, H. V. 3-D simulation of particle filtration in electrospun nanofibrous filters, *Powder Technol.*, **201**, 2010, 153–160.
44. Hosseini, S. A., and Tafreshi, H. V. Modeling particle filtration in disordered 2-D domains: a comparison with cell models, *Sep. Purif. Technol.*, **74**, 2010, 160–169.
45. Zhang, S., Shim, W. S., and Kim, J. Design of ultra-fine nonwovens via electrospinning of Nylon 6: spinning parameters and filtration efficiency, *Mater. Design*, **30**, 2009, 3659–3666.
46. Zhang, Y. Z., Ouyang, H. W., Lim, C. T., Ramakrishna, S., and Huang, Z. M. Electrospinning of gelatin fibers and gelatin/PCL composite fibrous scaffolds, *J. Biomed. Mater. Res., Part B*, **72B**, 2005, 156–165.
47. Vasita, R., and Katti, D. S. Nanofibers and their applications in tissue engineering, *Int. J. Nanomed.*, **1**, 2006, 15–30.
48. Baji, A., Mai, Y.-W., Wong, S.-C., Abtahi, M., and Chen, P. Electrospinning of polymer nanofibers: effects on oriented morphology, structures and tensile properties, *Compos. Sci. Technol.*, **70**, 2010, 703–718.
49. Gibson, P. W., and Charmchi, M. Modeling convection/diffusion processes in porous textiles with inclusion of humidity-dependent air permeability, *Int. Commun. Heat Mass*, **24**, 1997, 709–724.
50. Gibson, P., Rivin, D., Kendrick, C., and Schreuder-Gibson, H. Humidity-dependent air permeability of textile materials, *Text. Res. J.*, **69**, 1999, 311–317.
51. Gibson, P., and Charmchi, M. The use of volume-averaging techniques to predict temperature transients due to water vapor sorption in hygroscopic porous polymer materials, *J. Appl. Polym. Sci.*, **64**, 1997, 493–505.
52. Gebart, B. R. Permeability of unidirectional reinforcements for RTM, *J. Compos. Mater.*, **26**, 1992, 1100–1133.

53. Tamayol, A., and Bahrami, M. Analytical determination of viscous permeability of fibrous porous media, *Int. J. Heat Mass Transfer*, **52**, 2009, 2407–2414.
54. Shou, D. H., Fan, J. T., Mei, M. F., and Ding, F. An analytical model for gas diffusion though nanoscale and microscale fibrous media, *Microfluid. Nanofluid.*, **16**(1–2), 2014, 381–389.
55. Hosseini, S. A., and Tafreshi, H. V. Modeling permeability of 3-D nanofiber media in slip flow regime, *Chem. Eng. Sci.*, **65**, 2010, 2249–2254.
56. Ziarani, A. S., and Aguilera, R. Knudsen's permeability correction for tight porous media, *Transport Porous. Med.*, **91**, 2012, 239–260.
57. Huang, J. H., and Qian, X. M. A new test method for measuring the water vapour permeability of fabrics, *Meas. Sci. Technol.*, **18**, 2007, 3043–3047.
58. LaManna, J. M., and Kandlikar, S. G. Determination of effective water vapor diffusion coefficient in pemfc gas diffusion layers, *Int. J. Hydrogen Energy*, **36**, 2011, 5021–5029.
59. Chen, Y. S., Fan, J. T., Qian, X., and Zhang, W. Effect of garment fit on thermal insulation and evaporative resistance, *Text. Res. J.*, **74**, 2004, 742–748.
60. Fan, J. T., and Chen, Y. S. Measurement of clothing thermal insulation and moisture vapour resistance using a novel perspiring fabric thermal manikin, *Meas. Sci. Technol.*, **13**, 2002, 1115–1123.
61. Flueckiger, R., Freunberger, S. A., Kramer, D., Wokaun, A., Scherer, G. G., and Buechi, F. N. Anisotropic, effective diffusivity of porous gas diffusion layer materials for PEFC, *Electrochim. Acta*, **54**, 2008, 551–559.
62. Mu, D., Liu, Z. S., Huang, C., and Djilali, N. Determination of the effective diffusion coefficient in porous media including Knudsen effects, *Microfluid. Nanofluid.*, **4**, 2008, 257–260.
63. Clifford, S. M., and Hillel, D. Knudsen diffusion: the effect of small pore-size and low gas-pressure on gaseous transport in soil, *Soil Sci.*, **141**, 1986, 289–297.
64. Bosanquet, C. H. *British TA Report BR-507*, 1944.
65. Zalc, J. M., Reyes, S. C., and Iglesia, E. The effects of diffusion mechanism and void structure on transport rates and tortuosity factors in complex porous structures, *Chem. Eng. Sci.*, **59**, 2004, 2947–2960.
66. Gilron, J., and Soffer, A. Knudsen diffusion in microporous carbon membranes with molecular sieving character, *J. Membr. Sci.*, **209**, 2002, 339–352.

67. Sangani, A. S., and Acrivos, A. Slow flow past periodic arrays of cylinders with application to heat-transfer, *Int. J. Multiphase Flow*, **8**, 1982, 193–206.
68. Drummond, J. E., and Tahir, M. I. Laminar viscous-flow through regular arrays of parallel solid cylinders, *Int. J. Multiphase Flow*, **10**, 1984, 515–540.
69. Phelan, F. R., and Wise, G. Analysis of transverse flow in aligned fibrous porous media, *Compos. Part A*, **27**, 1996, 25–34.
70. Shou, D. H., Ye, L., Tang, Y. H., Fan, J. T., and Ding, F. Transverse permeability determination of dual-scale fibrous materials, *Int. J. Heat Mass Transfer*, **58**, 2013, 532–539.
71. Shou, D. H., Fan, J. T., and Ding, F. Hydraulic permeability of fibrous porous media, *Int. J. Heat Mass Transfer*, **54**, 2011, 4009–4018.
72. Mattern, K. J., and Deen, W. M. "Mixing rules" for estimating the hydraulic permeability of fiber mixtures, *AIChE J.*, **54**, 2008, 32–41.
73. Jackson, G. W., and James, D. F. The permeability of fibrous porous-media, *Can. J. Chem. Eng.*, **64**, 1986, 364–374.
74. Tamayol, A. T. A., and Bahrami, M. In-plane gas permeability of proton exchange membrane fuel cell gas diffusion layers, *J. Power Sources*, **196**, 2011, 3559–3564.
75. Tahir, M. A., and Tafreshi, H. V. Influence of fiber orientation on the transverse permeability of fibrous media, *Phys. Fluids*, **21**, 2009, 083604.
76. Ferenc, J. S., and Neda, Z. On the size distribution of Poisson Voronoi cells, *Physica A*, **385**, 2007, 518–526.
77. Ogorodnikov, B. I. Pressure-drop across FP fiber filters under gas slip-flow and in transition regime, *Colloid J. USSR*, **38**, 1976, 168–172.
78. Tomadakis, M. M., and Sotirchos, S. V. Ordinary, transition, and knudsen regime diffusion in random capillary structures, *Chem. Eng. Sci.*, **48**, 1993, 3323–3333.
79. Shou, D. H., Fan, J. T., and Ding, F. Effective diffusivity of gas diffusion layer in proton exchange membrane fuel cells, *J. Power Sources*, **225**, 2013, 179–186.
80. Tomadakis, M. M., and Sotirchos, S. V. Effective diffusivities and conductivities of random dispersions of nonoverlapping and partially overlapping unidirectional fibers, *J. Chem. Phys.*, **99**, 1993, 9820–9827.
81. Sahimi, M. *Flow and Transport in Porous Media and Fractured Rock*, VCH, Weinheim, 1995.

82. Blunt, M. J., Jackson, M. D., Piri, M., and Valvatne, P. H. Detailed physics, predictive capabilities and macroscopic consequences for pore-network models of multiphase flow, *Adv. Water Resour.*, **25**, 2002, 1069–1089.
83. Liang, Z., Ioannidis, M. A., and Chatzis, I. Geometric and topological analysis of three-dimensional porous media: pore space partitioning based on morphological skeletonization, *J. Colloid. Interface Sci.*, **221**, 2000, 13–24.
84. Houst, Y. F., and Wittmann, F. H. Influence of porosity and water-content on the diffusivity of CO_2 and O_2 through hydrated cement paste, *Cem. Concr. Res.*, **24**, 1994, 1165–1176.
85. Mandelbrot, B. B. *The Fractal Geometry of Nature*, W. H. Freeman, New York, 1982.
86. Shou, D. H., Fan, J. T., and Ding, F. A difference-fractal model for the permeability of fibrous porous media, *Phys. Lett. A*, **374**, 2010, 1201–1204.
87. Zhu, Q. Y., Xie, M. H., Yang, J., Chen, Y. Q., and Liao, K. Analytical determination of permeability of porous fibrous media with consideration of electrokinetic phenomena, *Int. J. Heat Mass Transfer*, **55**, 2012, 1716–1723.
88. Yu, B. M., and Lee, L. J. A fractal in-plane permeability model for fabrics, *Polym. Compos.*, **23**, 2002, 201–221.
89. Yu, B. M., and Liu, W. Fractal analysis of permeabilities for porous media, *AIChE J.*, **50**, 2004, 46–57.
90. Yu, B. M. Analysis of flow in fractal porous media, *Appl. Mech. Rev.* **61**, 2008, 050801.
91. Welty, J. R., Wicks, C. E., and Wilson, R. E. *Fundamentals of Momentum, Heat, and Mass Transfer*, John Wiley and Sons, New York, 1984.
92. Xu, P., and Yu, B. M. Developing a new form of permeability and Kozeny-Carman constant for homogeneous porous media by means of fractal geometry, *Adv. Water Resour.*, **31**, 2008, 74–81.
93. Xiao, B. Q., Fan, J. T., and Ding, F. Prediction of relative permeability of unsaturated porous media based on fractal theory and monte carlo simulation, *Energy Fuel*, **26**, 2012, 6971–6978.
94. Papadopoulos, G. K., Theodorou, D. N., Vasenkov, S., and Karger, J. Mesoscopic simulations of the diffusivity of ethane in beds of NaX zeolite crystals: comparison with pulsed field gradient NMR measurements, *J. Chem. Phys.*, **126**, 2007, 094702.

95. Tomadakis, M. M., and Robertson, T. J. Survival and relaxation time, pore size distribution moments, and viscous permeability in random unidirectional fiber structures, *J. Chem. Phys.*, **122**, 2005, 094711.
96. Tomadakis, M. M., and Robertson, T. J. Pore size distribution, survival probability, and relaxation time in random and ordered arrays of fibers, *J. Chem. Phys.*, **119**, 2003, 1741–1749.
97. Bolz, R., and Tuve, G. *Handbook of Tables for Applied Engineering Science*, 2nd ed., CRC Press, Cleveland, 1976.
98. Phattaranawik, J., Jiraratananon, R., and Fane, A. G. Effect of pore size distribution and air flux on mass transport in direct contact membrane distillation, *J. Membr. Sci.*, **215**, 2003, 75–85.
99. Yu, B. M., and Li, J. H. Some fractal characters of porous media, *Fractals*, **9**, 2001, 365–372.
100. Yu, B. M. Fractal character for tortuous streamtubes in porous media, *Chin. Phys. Lett.*, **22**, 2005, 158–160.
101. Tomadakis, M. M., and Robertson, T. J. Viscous permeability of random fiber structures: comparison of electrical and diffusional estimates with experimental and analytical results, *J. Compos. Mater.*, **39**, 2005, 163–188.
102. He, G., Zhao, Z., Ming, P., Abuliti, A., and Yin, C. A fractal model for predicting permeability and liquid water relative permeability in the gas diffusion layer (GDL) of PEMFCs, *J. Power Sources*, **163**, 2007, 846–852.

Biography

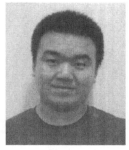

Dahua Shou was born in Longquan, China. He received his PhD degree in 2013 from the Hong Kong Polytechnic University. His PhD research was focused on modeling gas and vapor transport in nano- and microfibrous materials. During this time he received an attachment program scholarship to study composite materials at the University of Sydney.

Dr. Shou is now working as a postdoctoral research associate at the Centre for Advanced Materials Technology (CAMT), University of Sydney. His current research interests are smart composite materials and structures, transport in porous media, and nanofibers.

Dr. Shou is a member of the Australian Nanotechnology Network. He has published 16 first-author journal papers and has served as a referee for over 10 journals as of December 2013.

Chapter 9

An Introduction to Blender 2.69 for Scientific Illustrations

Iwan Kelaiah

Australian Centre for Fields Robotics, University of Sydney,
Sydney, NSW 2006, Australia
iwan.kelaiah@gmail.com

As the saying goes, "A picture is worth a thousand words." A picture illustrates more than the shape of an object. It also informs us about the object's size, its relation to other objects, interactions, characteristics, colors, etc. Scientific publications use illustrations to convey condensed information, including abstract and difficult concepts.

This chapter introduces Blender 2.69—a free and open source 3D modeling, animation, and rendering package—to create scientific illustrations [1]. The participants in the book workshop have been introduced to Blender to produce many of the illustrations in the color pages of this book. In this introduction an image of a simple human hepatitis B virus (HBV) has been used to illustrate the use and capability of Blender. Blender also offers tools to create production-quality movies and is being used by academia in creating 3D objects, including virtual environments and virtual actors for research [2–5].

Nanomaterials: Science and Applications
Edited by Deborah Kane, Adam Micolich, and Peter Roger
Copyright © 2016 Pan Stanford Publishing Pte. Ltd.
ISBN 978-981-4669-72-6 (Hardcover), 978-981-4669-73-3 (eBook)
www.panstanford.com

This chapter does not attempt to cover Blender functionalities in detail. Many books have been written showcasing these, such as using Blender Game Engine (BGE) to create real-time applications [6], realistic lighting, materials and textures [7–9], advanced 3D modeling, animation and rendering [10, 11], and postprocess special effects and compositing [12]. Rather, this chapter presents a brief introduction to Blender 2.69 by creating a scientific illustration of human HBVs, presented especially for those with little experience of Blender.

It is best to read this chapter while running Blender on a computer. It is suggested to read through a section prior to attempting the tasks in that section. The next objective will be clear at the end of each section. This chapter is divided into eight sections. The first section explains how to set up Blender. Section 9.2 introduces Blender's user interface (UI). Section 9.3 explains the hotkeys of Blender and some transformation exercises using keyboard shortcuts. Section 9.4 shows the steps to create a 3D model of HBV from a 3D cube. Scene preparation for rendering, including lighting and shading, is presented in Section 9.5. Section 9.6 demonstrates how to render and save 3D illustrations. Finally, Section 9.7 is the conclusion.

9.1 Setting Up Blender 2.69

9.1.1 *Getting the Latest Version of Blender*

At the time of writing, the latest version of Blender was 2.69. It can be obtained from http://www.blender.org/download/. The download page offers packages for various platforms: Windows, Mac OSX, and GNU/Linux operating system. Blender developers recommend the following hardware specifications:

- 64-bit quad core CPU with 8 GB RAM
- Full HD display with 24-bit color
- Three-button mouse
- OpenGL-compatible graphics card with 1 GB RAM

For bigger projects that demand movie production-grade outputs, the following hardware specifications are recommended:

- 64-bit eight core CPU with 16 GB RAM
- Two full HD displays with 24-bit color
- Three-button mouse and graphics tablet
- Dual OpenGL-compatible graphics cards with 3 GB RAM

9.1.2 Installing and Running Blender 2.69

Installing and running Blender is as simple as downloading an appropriate package for your platform, unpacking the compressed file, and running the executable file. A self-extracting installer is also provided for Windows. For portable Windows installations, extract the compressed file onto a USB drive and launch it by double-clicking blender.exe. For Mac OSX users, download the .zip file from Mac OSX tab on the download page, extract it, and launch Blender by double-clicking blender.app.

GNU/Linux users have two choices to install Blender, using a package manager or downloading the source code provided on the download page. Blender can be compiled by running the install_deps.sh script, with administrator access to install the required dependencies and compile them.

Figure 9.1 shows a screenshot of the default Blender user interface (UI) when installed correctly. Blender's UI on Mac OSX and GNU/Linux would appear similar but with a different window title bar. The default scene contains a cube, a render camera, and a point light. They are circled (by pink, blue, and yellow in the e-book) from left to right, respectively, in Fig. 9.1.

9.1.3 Setting Up User Preferences

This section shows the author's recommended settings for using Blender. The **User Preferences** menu is in the **File** > **User Preferences** menu, or simply use the keyboard shortcut by pressing **Ctrl + Alt + U**. It has seven tabs, but only **Interface**, **Input** and **Addons** tabs will be covered here. As users gain more proficiency

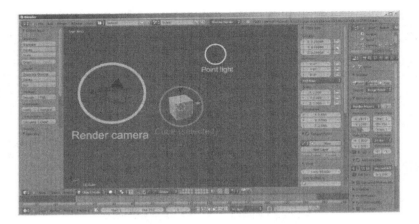

Figure 9.1 The default Blender UI.

in Blender, they can experiment with various settings to increase productivity.

Under the **Interface** tab, as shown in Fig. 9.2, enable the **Zoom To Mouse Position** and **Rotate Around Selection** options. **Zoom To Mouse Position** enables users to point the mouse cursor to specify the location for zoom rather than zooming at the centre of the screen. Further, **Rotate Around Selection** allows the user to dolly/orbit around a selected object. This is particularly useful when working with a number of objects where users would like to inspect each object by orbiting around it. Commonly, the object must be selected first using **[RMB]** (the right mouse button) and focused by using the [**Numpad .(dot)**] key.

Under the **Input** tab, as shown in Fig. 9.2, enable **Continuous Grab**. This option allows users to perform transformation tools (translate, rotate, and scaling) using the mouse beyond Blender's window. Transformation using mouse movement will not be interrupted when the cursor reaches Blender's window.

Under the **Addons** tab, as shown in Fig. 9.2, enable **3D View: Dynamic Spacebar Menu** by clicking the checkbox on the top-right corner of the menu. This is very handy as it allows users to access commonly used menus in Blender by pressing the **[Spacebar]** key in the 3D viewport window.

User Interface | 339

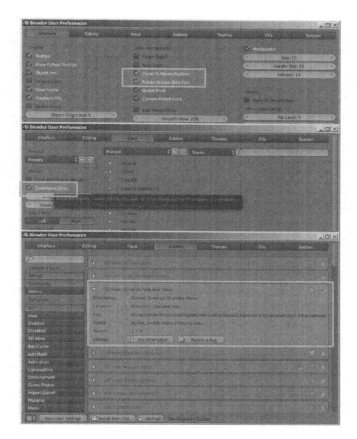

Figure 9.2 Suggested settings for **Interface**, **Input**, and **Addons** tabs in the **User Preference** menu.

Lastly, the new settings can be saved permanently by clicking **File > Save Startup File** or pressing **[Ctrl + u]**. If it is necessary to restore the default factory settings, go to **File > Load Factory Settings**.

9.2 User Interface

Blender's UI is a rectangular, nonoverlapping windowing system, as shown in Fig. 9.3. Each window is resizable and can be maximized

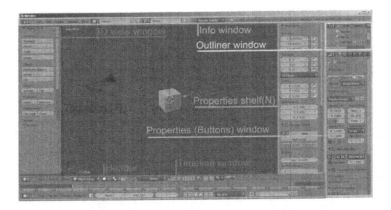

Figure 9.3 Blender's nonoverlapping windowing system.

using the [**Ctrl** + ↑] keys. By default, there are five windows visible on the UI: Information (appears as the top menu bar), 3D View, Timeline, Outliner, and Properties. These windows are marked distinctly in Fig. 9.3. The 3D View window has additional shelves: tool and property shelves that can be enabled/disabled by using [**t**] or [**n**] keys. Tool shelves contain tools for transformation and 3D modeling processes such as rotate, translate, delete, remove double faces, and enable smooth shading. The Properties shelf contains details of the selected object, such as position and orientation, name, and the perspective camera settings (not the render camera).

3D modeling and animation takes place in the 3D View window. The Outliner window shows the list of objects in a scene. It is like a shipping manifest of the scene. The name of an object can be set from the properties shelf—[**n**], under the **Item** submenu. If objects are created without specifying a name, the Outliner window might display the default names of the object, along with an incremental number. For example, creating three items beginning with three cubes, without specifying any name, would appear in the Outliner window as cube, cube.001, and cube.002. Thus, it will become difficult to identify objects of interest in a complex scene.

Each window contains a header that provides additional functionalities depending on the window type. With the 3D View window, the header is located at the bottom of the window, that is, it

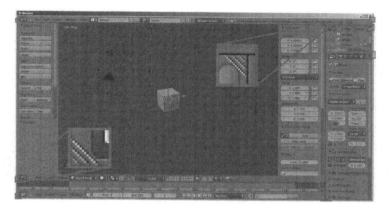

Figure 9.4 Each window has two draggable regions at the top-right and bottom-left corners.

is a footer. Underneath the 3D View window, there is an Animation window. This helps animators to inspect animation quickly across the length of the timeframe. The Animation window is beyond the scope of this chapter. Please refer to books on Blender animation and compositing to see how animators use this window [10, 12].

9.2.1 Splitting Windows

Each window can be resized by dragging its border and can be split to create more windows. Splitting windows is as simple as dragging the top-right or bottom-left corner region of each window marked by three diagonal lines (Fig. 9.4).

Splitting windows is crucial as tasks become complex. For example, it is easy to set up lights and materials for rendering a scene by having two 3D views, one for inspecting results by enabling interactive rendering and the other to set up Lights, Properties, and Node windows simultaneously. Hence, changes in the position of the light will be reflected immediately in the other window that shows render results. Interactive rendering and light setup will be covered in the next section. Blender allows users to split out as many windows as required.

To create or split a new window to the right of an existing window, drag the top-right corner region of the existing window to

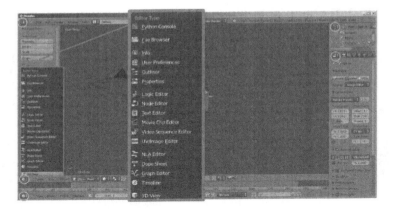

Figure 9.5 Each header has a window-type icon, as circled (5 circles, light blue in e-book).

the left. If a new window is needed to the left of an existing window, simply drag the bottom-left corner region to the right. The same rule applies to create a new window on the top or bottom of an existing window.

9.2.2 Customising Window Types

Each window type contains different information that allows users to do different tasks. As shown in Fig. 9.5, each header has a window-type icon marked by circles (light blue in e-book). These icons can be clicked to bring a list of window types. Currently, there are 17 window types in Blender:

- Python Console brings up the Python console and allows users to write Python script to automate tasks.
- File Browser brings up a file browser.
- Info Window provides scene information, and it appears at the top toolbar by default.
- User Preferences brings up user preferences options.
- Outliner allows users to manage and find objects in a scene.
- Properties Editor displays attributes of the selected object, such as constraint, material, texture, and modifier stack.

- Logic Editor provides options to set up the behavior of objects in Blender Game Engine.
- Node Editor brings up a workspace to compose nodes for texturing materials and compositing.
- Text Editor enables the writing of notes and documentation.
- Movie Clip Editor gives tools for motion tracking.
- Video Sequence Editor provides advanced tools to manipulate video streams. It is particularly useful for compositing and camera tracking to combine computer graphics and real footage.
- Image/UV Editor provides advanced 2D texture editing tools for texture mapping 3D objects and image editing along U and V axes.
- Nonlinear Animation (NLA) Editor is a higher abstraction or higher layer for managing animations. It provides tools to combine actions in a nonlinear way.
- Dope Sheet gives an overview of all animations in a scene.
- Graph Editor allows users to visualize and manage the animation keys of an object as graphs.
- Timeline shows controls for playing back and scrubbing animation.
- 3D view shows the content of a scene in 3D; this is the window where most users do 3D modeling.

The 3D modeling task in this chapter is simple. It does not require animations, complex UV unwrapping, or compositing with motion-tracked video streams of live footage. Hence, only Node Editor, 3D View, and Properties Editor window types will be used in this chapter.

9.2.3 Properties Window

In the previous versions of Blender, the Properties window was known as the Buttons window. The header of the Properties window changed depending on the selected object in the scene. If a 3D object containing vertices is selected, the header of the Properties window shows 12 buttons (Fig. 9.6). The first four buttons—Render, Render Layer, Scene, and World—show up panels, and their settings apply

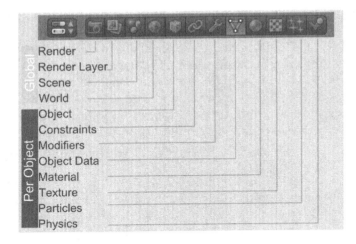

Figure 9.6 Schematic of the header of the Properties window.

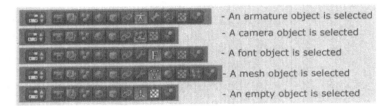

Figure 9.7 Some examples of the header of the Properties window with different Object Data icons selected.

globally in the current scene. The rest of the buttons bring up panels and settings that only apply to the selected object. Each button brings up differing panels to set the properties of the scene in or for the selected object.

Figure 9.7 shows some examples of differing Object Data button icons, depending on the object selected in the scene. Users are able to tell what objects are currently selected in the scene by the icons on the Properties window header.

The Object Data button resembles three vertices connected by two edges. When a light object is selected, its icon resembles a picture of the sun. It turns to an F when a 3D font is selected. If a camera object is selected, its icon resembles a camera. If an armature object is selected, additional buttons will appear to set up joints for the character for animation. The Object Data icon turns into a chevron if an empty is selected. An empty is basically an object that has no visual appearance when rendered. Its sole purpose is to help scene management.

9.3 Using Hotkeys in Blender

Blender has a lot of functionalities and users can access them by clicking appropriate buttons on the UI. As proficiency in Blender increases, more keyboard shortcuts will be used instead of mouse movements. Consider a scenario of enabling a translation tool by using only a mouse operation. This involves the following steps: (1) The tool shelf must be opened by pressing **[t]** if it is closed, (2) the mouse cursor must be moved to the top of tool shelf, and lastly (3) the Translate button should be clicked. On the other hand, the **[g]** key enables the translation tool in one action. Thus, it is good practice to learn the hotkeys in Blender to work efficiently.

Table 9.1 shows the list of hotkeys commonly used in Blender. Some exercises are provided below to help readers familiarize themselves with these hotkeys prior to attempting 3D modeling. More hotkeys will be provided, as needed, throughout this chapter.

9.3.1 Exercise: Orientation in 3D Space, Switching Orthogonal/Perspective View, and Rendering

(1) Start a new scene by pressing **[Ctrl + n]**.
(2) Select the cube object at the origin with **RMB**.
(3) Drag the **MMB** to the right to dolly around the object horizontally 360 degrees.
(4) Zoom out until the cube appears very small in the middle of the screen by using the mouse wheel.
(5) Press **[Num .]** to focus on the cube.
(6) Pan the camera so that the cube object touches the right side of the monitor by using **[Shift]** and dragging the **MMB**.
(7) Pan the camera so that the cube object touches the left side of the screen.

Table 9.1 Commonly used keyboard shortcuts in Blender. Those marked with an asterisk (*) require the user's mouse cursor to hover on top of the 3D View window

Key / Mouse actions	Function
LMB click on 3D View window	Set the position of the 3D cursor.
RMB click on any 3D object	Select an object.
MMB drag on 3D View window	Dolly/Orbit the 3D View window.
[Ctrl + MMB]*	Zoom the 3D View window.
[Shift + MMB]*	Pan the 3D View window.
[g]*	Translate tool. Type **[g]**, **[x]** to constrain movement along the global *x* axis, **[g]**, **[y]** to constrain movement along the global *y* axis, and **[g]**, **[z]** to constrain movement along the global *z* axis. For greater accuracy, a value can be added after specifying the constraining axis. For example, typing **[g]**, **[-]**, **[5]** and pressing the **[Enter]** key will move the object along the global *z* axis −5 units.
[r]*	Rotate tool. It has similar features to other transformation keys—**[g]**, **[r]**, and **[s]**.
[s]*	Scale tool. It has similar features to other transformation keys—**[g]**, **[r]**, and **[s]**.
[Tab]*	On a selected object, toggle between the object and the edit mode.
[Num 7]/[Num 1]/[Num 3]*	Switch the 3D view into top/front/right orthogonal view.
[Num .]*	Focus current view on the selected object.
[a]*	Toggle select all or none.
[b]*	Rectangle the object selection mode.
[c]*	Paint the selection mode; radius can be modified by using the mouse wheel. Press **RMB** to exit the paint selection mode.
[Shift +c]*	Reset the 3D cursor by placing it at the origin (0, 0, 0) and 3D view to capture all objects in the scene.
[Shift +d]*	Duplicate the selected object(s).
[z]*	Toggle the 3D View window between the shaded and the wireframe mode.
[Ctrl +s]	Save the current scene to a file.
[Num 0]*	Align the perspective view with an active render camera.
[Ctrl +Alt +Num 0]*	Align the active render camera to the current view in the 3D View window.
[F12]	Render the current scene onto the UV/Image Editor window. Press the **[Esc]** key to return to the 3D View window. Alternatively, click UV/Image Editor icons on the header to switch to other window types.

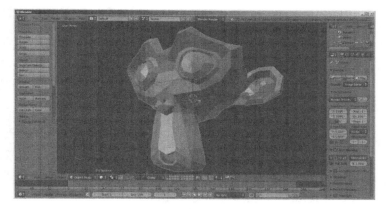

Figure 9.8 One of the primitive 3D objects in Blender—a monkey head called Suzanne.

(8) Switch to the right orthogonal view with the **[Num 3]** key.
(9) Switch to the front orthogonal view with the **[Num 1]** key.
(10) Switch to the top orthogonal view with the **[Num 7]** key.
(11) Drag the **MMB** to reposition 3D view, as shown in Fig. 9.8.
(12) Align the render camera to the current perspective view by pressing **[Ctrl + Alt + Num 0]**.
(13) Press **[F12]** to render the results in the UV/Image Editor window. Click the UV/Image Editor icon on the left-most side of the header to switch back to the 3D View window, or simply press **[Esc]**.

9.3.2 *Exercise: Object Creation, Deletion, and Transformation*

(1) Start a new scene by pressing **[Ctrl +n]**. The default scene contains a cube, a render camera, and a lamp object.
(2) Select the cube by aiming the mouse cursor on top of it and clicking **RMB**.
(3) Delete the existing cube by pressing the **[x]** key.
(4) Create a monkey primitive object by pressing **[Spacebar]** and clicking **Add Object Menu > Add Mesh > Monkey** or type **[a]**, **[a]**, and **[m]**.

(5) Scale the monkey head half its size by typing **[s]**, **[0]**, **[.]**, **[5]** and press **[Enter]**.
(6) If the 3D cursor is not at the origin, press **[Shift + c]** to reset it. Create another monkey head by pressing **[Spacebar]** and clicking **Add Object Menu** > **Add Mesh** > **Monkey** or type **[a]**, **[a]**, and **[m]**.
(7) Select the second monkey head.
(8) Move it one unit along the global z axis by typing **[g]**, **[z]**, **[1]** and press **[Enter]**.
(9) Rotate it along the global z axis 45 degrees by typing **[r]**, **[z]**, **[4]**, **[5]** and press **[Enter]**.
(10) Deselect all objects by using the **[a]** key.

9.3.3 Exercise: Object Editing, Transformation, and Rendering

(1) Start a new scene.
(2) Select all objects by pressing **[a]** or **[a]** twice if an object is already selected in the scene.
(3) Delete selected objects by using **[x]**, including the default lamp and render camera objects.
(4) Create a monkey primitive object.
(5) Get a good close look at the nose, as shown in Fig. 9.9.

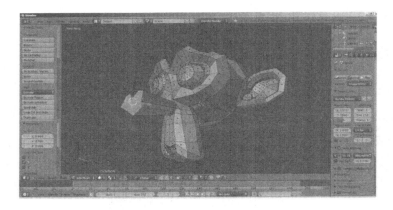

Figure 9.9 Editing the shape of the nose in the edit mode.

(6) Press the **[Tab]** key to get into the edit mode. Now, in the edit mode you can change the appearance by modifying the vertices, edges or polygons.
(7) We make the nose bigger by modifying the polygons. Press the **[Ctrl +Tab]** keys. This displays the selection mode. The default selection mode is the vertices selection mode.
(8) Select option number 3, **Faces**.
(9) All faces are selected by default. Clear all selections by pressing the **[a]** key.
(10) Select four polygons at the tip of the nose by holding down **[Shift] + RMB**.
(11) Scale these polygons twice the size and move them -0.5 units along the global y axis to achieve the effect, as shown in Fig. 9.9. Use the **[s]** key for scaling. These keystrokes can be used to translate those face polygons -0.5 units along the global y axis: **[g]**, **[y]**, **[-]**, **[0]**, **[.]**, **[5]**, and **[Enter]**.
(12) Clear all selections.
(13) Switch to the front orthogonal view by typing **[Num 7]**.
(14) Enable the wireframe display mode of the 3D View window by pressing the **[z]** key.
(15) Press **[b]** to use the rectangle selection mode or **[c]** to enable the paint selection mode. Press **RMB** to quit the paint selection mode, when finished. Select the polygons that make up the left half of the monkey head, as shown in Fig. 9.10.

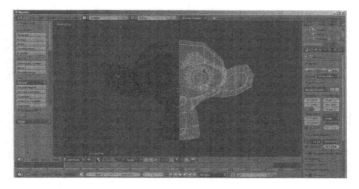

Figure 9.10 The polygons that make up the left half of the monkey head are selected in the front orthogonal view.

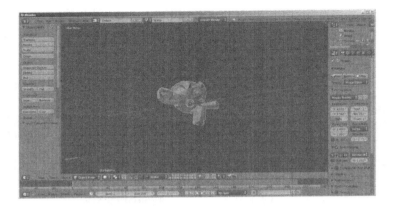

Figure 9.11 The outcome of the exercise in Section 9.3.3.

(16) Once these polygons are selected, press **RMB** to quit the paint selection mode. Press **[x]** and choose **Faces** to delete those polygons.
(17) Return to the shaded display mode of the 3D View window by pressing the **[z]** key.
(18) Press the **[Tab]** key to leave the edit mode. It is a good idea not to create a new object in the edit mode. New objects created in the edit mode will always be part of the object that you are currently editing. Always leave the edit mode when editing is done.
(19) Orient your 3D view to display the result, as shown in Fig. 9.11.
(20) Save this scene by pressing **[Ctrl + s]** keys. Specify a new filename instead of using the default filename (untitled.blend) in the File window and click the Save button.

9.4 3D Modeling

This section describes the necessary steps to create 3D models for simple scientific visualization. This section provides fewer common hotkeys, for example, *switch of wireframe mode* rather than *switch to wireframe mode by using* **[z]**. Please refer to Table 9.1 for a list of commonly used hotkeys.

9.4.1 *Planning*

Planning is paramount in every discipline. In some cases, a slight miscalculation could mean the end of a project and any future funding. In mission- and life-critical systems, poor planning can lead to loss of lives. Jumping into 3D modeling and animation without good planning potentially leads to time wasting and undesirable results [7]. Some questions demand answers before 3D models are created for any kind of illustration with any 3D modeling package. These include:

- The layout of the illustration for publication:
- What is its size? Will it be printed on A4 paper or A3?
- What is the orientation? Will it be in portrait or landscape?
- The content of the illustration:
- What will be portrayed? What will be in it? How will you arrange the objects in the scene?
- How much detail is needed?
- Do you require some postprocessing effects, such as motion blur, chromatic aberrations, or sepia tone?

Spend time researching the scene or objects that must be created. Use Google, YouTube, scholarly databases, and other resources to become familiar with 3D objects of interest (Fig. 9.12). Download images, videos, articles, presentations, and other types of information and examine how others present their 3D scientific illustrations. The above list is not exhaustive. There is more information needed when dealing with complex 3D animations than simple 3D illustrations, including objects of interest, paths of

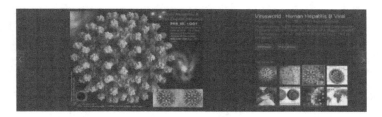

Figure 9.12 The Google search engine can be used to find image references to assist in creating 3D models of interest, in this case HBVs.

the cameras, timing, and stop positions. Be aware that producing your own illustrations means you will be differentiating these from the work of others and you will avoid any violation of copyright. Referring to the work of others serves as a stimulus and examples.

Brief research into the characteristics of a hepatitis B virus (HBV) reveals the shape of an HBV (Fig. 9.12) and its size is about 42–47 nm [13]. At this stage, the physical appearance is more important than its size. Chiefly, there is no other object in the scene. If the sketch contained red blood cells, the size of an HBV would be about 177 times smaller than the size of a red blood cell.

Sketches help us to plan where the objects will be in the scene, the colors that will be used for each object, and the required visual details and to visualize how an illustration will appear in the publication. For a small project, sketches do not have to be of high quality. However, larger-scale projects require better-quality sketches (e.g., character designs, virtual cities, etc.). For simplicity, Fig. 9.13 is a reference schematic that is used to place HBV objects in the scene. The illustration in this chapter has omitted medium-size surface protein information.

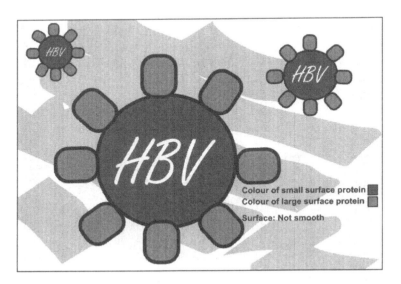

Figure 9.13 A simple sketch to show the placements of HBVs.

9.4.2 Creating a 3D Model of a Hepatitis B Virus

3D modeling is all about problem solving. What would be the best starting point when creating a complex HBV shape? If the shape is complex, break it down into manageable portions and address one shape or component at a time. Once the basic shape is formed, details can be added, as required. Never start 3D modeling with a complex shape. Begin with a simple shape and add details, as needed. At this stage, the concern is to become familiar with Blender by creating a simple visualization of an HBV instead of creating a fully accurate, protein-by-protein model of it.

Identifying the basic shapes that make up an object helps us to identify the primitives. Primitives are basic mesh shapes or objects where 3D modeling begins. Blender provides a number of primitives such as plane, cube, circle, UV sphere, icosphere, cylinder, cone, grid, monkey head, and torus. There are other add-ons for extra primitives, such as gemstones and gears. A UV sphere is composed of n segments and m rings. An icosphere is composed of triangles. Consider a scenario of creating an apple. An apple resembles a sphere. Hence, the right primitive to begin with is a sphere. It is incorrect to say that we cannot start creating an apple by using monkey head or plane primitives. We can but with increased difficulty.

An HBV resembles a sphere with many cylinders protruding out of it. In other words, any kind of sphere, and plenty of cylinders, would make an HBV. Making a 3D HBV can be as simple as creating a 3D sphere in the scene and placing as many cylinders as required. This is a valid decision. However, let us start more simply with a cube—six polygons primitive—instead of a sphere that contains 256 polygons (32 segments and 16 rings). This might sound confusing, as we have identified the basic primitives for an HBV as a sphere and cylinders, not a cube and cylinders. A cube can be transformed into a sphere-like object (although not a perfect sphere) by performing multiple subdivisions.

The strategy is to start as simply as possible and slowly add details. First, start with a cube and add a subdivision to obtain a sphere-like object. Having a perfect sphere is not a critical requirement. Second, cylinder shapes can be added or shaped by extruding polygons of the cube object. Surface imperfection will be added last. The following table (Table 9.2) shows the steps in creating a 3D HBV from a cube.

9.4.3 Placing Objects in the Scene

Figure 9.13 shows a schematic of the planned scene. Press **[NUM 0]** to see the scene through the render camera. The rendering process takes into account what the activated render camera sees but not

Table 9.2 Steps in creating a 3D HBV from a cube

Step no.	Description
1	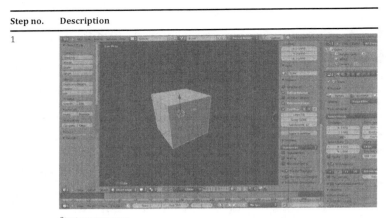 Start a new scene.
2	Apply a Subdivision Surface modifier by clicking the spanner icon in the Properties window, and then click **Add Modifiers** > **Subdivision Surface**.

3D Modeling | 355

Step no.	Description
3	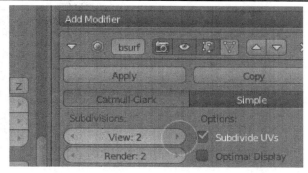 Set the subdivision view and render values to 2. A subdivision adds polygons for adding details.
4	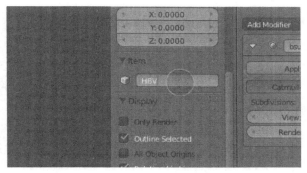 Set the name of the modified cube to "HBV" under **Item** on the Properties shelf—**[n]**.
5	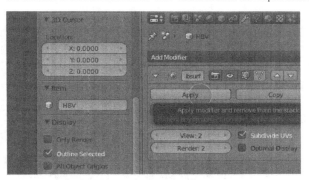 Return to the modifier options in the Properties window and click the **Apply** button to apply the subdivision permanently.

(Contd.)

Table 9.2 (*Contd.*)

Step no.	Description
6	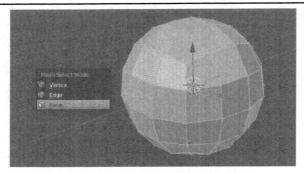 Enter the edit mode using the **[Tab]** key and change the selection mode to **Faces**. All the faces *must* be selected before moving to the next step.
7	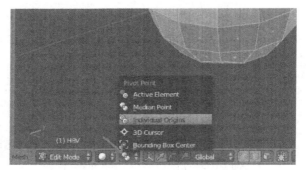 Change the pivot point to **Individual Origins**. This step is important as each face will be edited simultaneously on its own origin, not the object's origin.
8	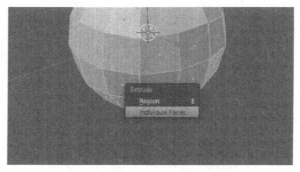 Press **[Alt +e]** to bring up the extrusion menu and choose **Individual Faces**. New faces will be created directly on top of the selected faces.

Step no.	Description
9	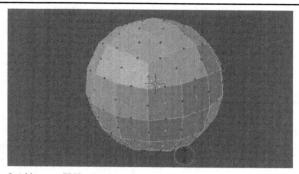 Quickly press **RMB** to terminate extrusion.
10	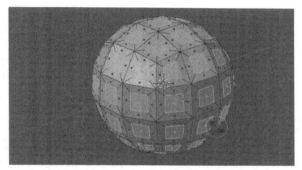 Scale each face approximately to half of its size by using **[s]** and moving the mouse cursor. Click the **LMB** or press **[Enter]** to confirm.
11	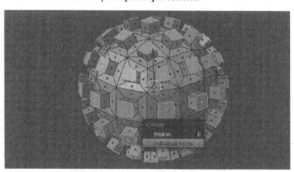 Perform small extrusions on those scaled faces by pressing **[Alt +e]** and select **Individual Faces**.

(*Contd.*)

Table 9.2 (*Contd.*)

Step no.	Description
12	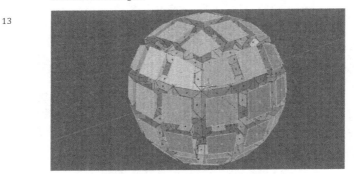 Perform another small extrusion on those faces by pressing [Alt +e] and select **Individual Faces** again.
13	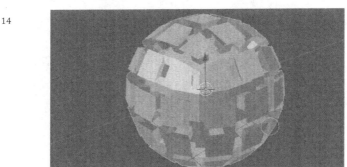 While those faces are still selected, scale them up about twice the original size.
14	Switch to the object mode. At this stage, the cube is now transformed into a low-polygon version of an HBV.

3D Modeling | 359

Step no.	Description
15	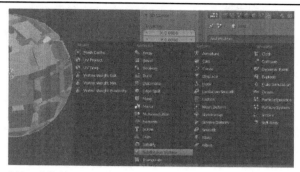 Add a subdivision modifier, as explained in Step 2.
16	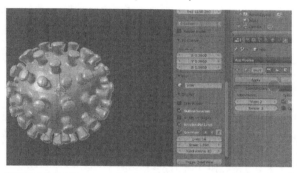 Set the subdivision view value and the render value to 2. Now the cube more closely resembles an HBV.
17	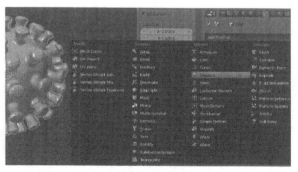 Add imperfections on the surface by adding another modifier—**Add Modifier** > **Displace**.

(*Contd.*)

Table 9.2 (*Contd.*)

Step no.	Description
18	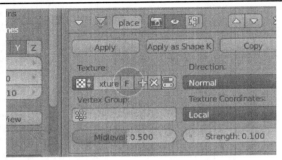
	Set the strength value to 0.1 for now and create a new noise texture by clicking the **+New** button under the Texture heading in the current Displace modifier. The HBV object appears more irregular at this stage than before.
19	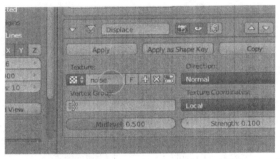
	The new texture material will have "Texture" as the default name. Change it to something more descriptive, like "Noise Texture" or "Noise."
20	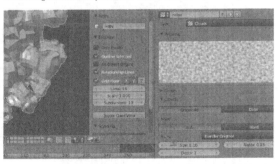
	Set the properties of the new texture for creating geometrical noise by clicking the texture icon on the header of the Properties window. The icon looks like a checkered red-white pattern. By default, the texture type is Clouds.

Step no.	Description
21	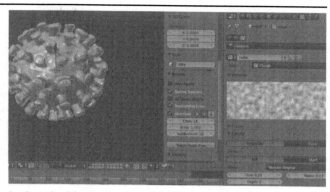 Set the scale of the Clouds noise to 0.1. This gives a less uniform surface on the HBV object than before.
22	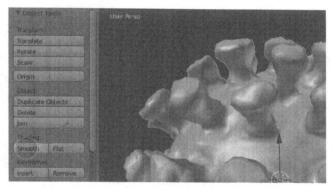 Head to the tool shelf—[t]—and change the shading type to Smooth. Thus, Blender averages out the light calculation between faces and gives a smoother HBV appearance than before.

(Contd.)

Table 9.2 (*Contd.*)

Step no.	Description
23	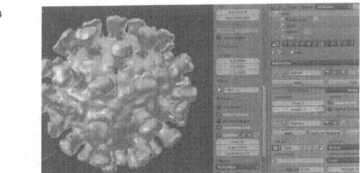 Return to the Modifier menu (spanner icon) in the Properties window. Increase the subdivision visual value to 3 and reduce the displacement strength to 0.085.
24	Set the value of the subdivision render to 3, matching the view value. It tells Blender to render the object at subdivision level 3. You may finalize and remove these modifiers from the stack by pressing the **Apply** button of each modifier.

Cycles, Light, and Materials | 363

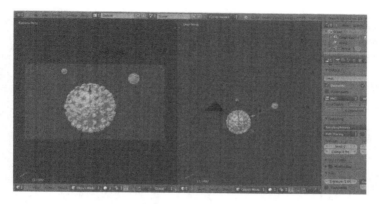

Figure 9.14 The task of arranging objects and visualizing their placement in render output is simpler by having two 3D View windows side by side rather than one.

the current transformation of the perspective view. There are two ways to make the scene look like the proposed sketch. First, leave the render camera as it is. Duplicate the HBV object by using **[Shift + d]** and transform it to match the sketch. Repeat this twice, as there are two HBVs in the background. Second, transform both the camera and the objects to obtain a scene, as illustrated in the sketch. To make the task easier, create another new 3D View window. Set one 3D view to look through the active render camera by hovering the mouse cursor on the designated 3D View window and pressing **[NUM 0]**. Use the other 3D View window for arranging objects in the scene, as shown in Fig. 9.14. Object transformations in the perspective view of one 3D View window will be reflected in other 3D View windows. Splitting windows in Blender was covered in Section 9.2.1.

9.5 Cycles, Light, and Materials

9.5.1 Using Cycles Render

Cycles Render is a new rendering engine added for the Blender 2.6x series. It is a ray-tracing render engine supporting interactive rendering, new texture workflow, new shading node system, and graphics processing unit (GPU) acceleration. Cycles can be enabled

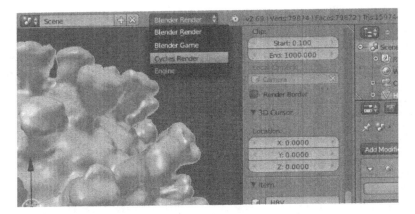

Figure 9.15 Cycles Render is not enabled by default. It must be enabled manually.

by clicking the default renderer **Blender Render**, on the top menu bar, and clicking **Cycles Render** (Fig. 9.15). Additionally, enable GPU rendering if a Nvidia graphics card(s) is available. This option is located in **File > User Preferences > System**, and look for the **Compute Device** option and select **CUDA**. Ensure that the latest driver for Nvidia CUDA is installed.

Rendering is the process of computing vertex information deformations, physics, lighting, and surface information in a 3D space onto a 2D image. Commonly, a rendering process is not interactive. The **Render** button must be pressed every time changes occur in order to inspect the 2D image output. Cycles Render is a fast, interactive renderer that gives render outputs quickly (subject to PC configuration and GPU capability). Hence, if a material is altered, Cycles computes quickly how that material would interact with other objects in the scene, such as reflection, ambient occlusion, and refraction. The next section shows how to use Cycles interactive rendering in 3D View windows.

9.5.2 Lighting and Background Color

For simplicity, this chapter shows how to create a three-point light setup only (Fig. 9.16). Three-point light is the standard in

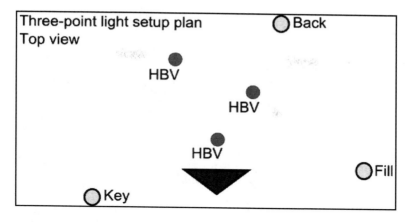

Figure 9.16 Three-point light setup for the HBV scene.

photography and cinematography as it creates a pleasant and natural look [11]. Three-point light, as the name implies, is a setup requiring three light sources: key, fill, and back lights. Key light is the primary light source in the scene. The fill light softens the shadows of the key light. The back light separates the objects of interest from the background. The following table (Table 9.3) shows the steps in adding three light sources to create a three-point light setup in Blender.

9.5.3 Shading

In this short section, the node system of creating materials will be introduced. Materials may contain textures or images that give a surface definition, for example, streaks or patterns on a wood material. Multiple nodes, with differing functions, can be chained together to create complex materials that define the surface appearance of an object in Blender. It is like a visual scripting way of creating surface information in Blender. It can be used to create lifelike textures and materials, such as metals, glasses, water, and eroded metals [9]. Before setting up materials in Blender, a sufficiently large workspace must be prepared for putting nodes together. This can be done by increasing the size of the Timeline window and switching its window type to Node (Fig. 9.17).

Table 9.3 Steps in adding three light sources to create a three-point light setup in Blender

Step no.	Description
1	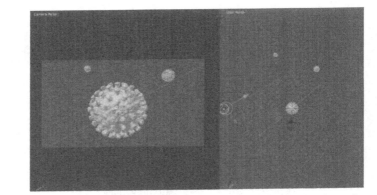 Split a new 3D window and set one 3D View window to look at the scene through the render camera. Make sure that Cycles Render is enabled from Blender's top toolbar (Fig. 9.15).
2	Use the other 3D View window to move the default lamp to the left of the render camera, on the same xy plane as the HBV closest to the camera.

Cycles, Light, and Materials | 367

Step no.	Description
3	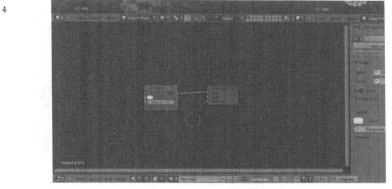
	While the lamp is selected, open up the property shelf of the 3D View window and set the default lamp name to "key light."
4	Add another point light by pressing **[Spacebar]** and selecting **Add Object Menu > Add Lamp > Point**.

(Contd.)

Table 9.3 (Contd.)

Step no.	Description
5	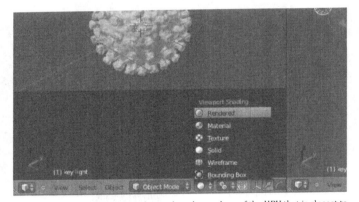
	Position the new point light to the right of the render camera about the same xy plane. Change its default name, "Point," to "fill light" via the properties shelf—[n].
6	Add another light and position it lower than the xy plane of the HBV that is closest to the camera. Place it roughly between the two HBVs further from the render camera. Change its name to "back light."

Step no.	Description
7	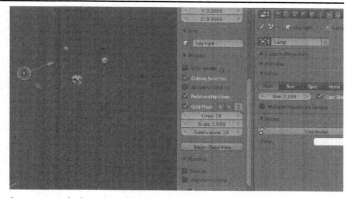 Set viewport shading of the 3D View window that looks through the active render camera to **Rendered**. This enables Cycles interactive rendering in the 3D View window. Users can move objects, and the results will be rendered instantly.
8	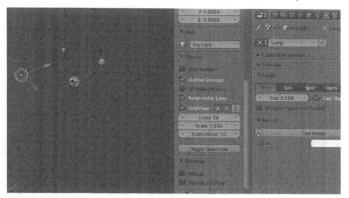 Select the key light from the 3D View window. Go to the Properties window on the right-hand side of the screen and click the light icon. Click **Use Node** to use the node system in setting up the light.

(Contd.)

Table 9.3 (*Contd.*)

Step no.	Description
9	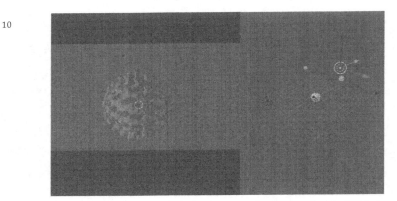
	New variables will appear in the light panel: surface, color, and strength. Change the strength of the key light to 500. The result will be instantly rendered on the other 3D view with the **Rendered** shading mode.
10	
	Repeat Step 9 for the fill and the back light sources. Set the strength of the fill light to 350 and the back light to 150.

Step no.	Description
11	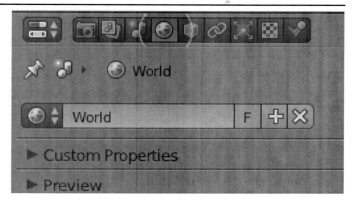 Set the background color to soft pink, as shown in the sketch proposed earlier (Fig. 9.13). The World panel must be opened by clicking the **World** button, the fourth icon on the header from the left, in the Properties window.
12	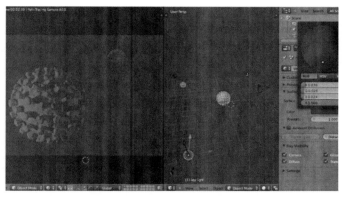 Set the background color by clicking the color field. This brings up a color selector. Set the values of R, G, and B to 0.07, 0.026, and 0.024, respectively.

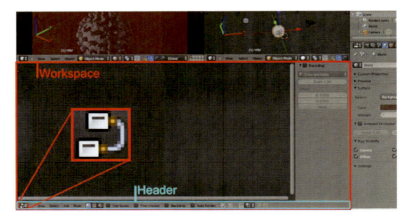

Figure 9.17 A node workspace prepared by increasing the size of the Timeline window upward and switching its window type to the Node window type. The icon looks like two squares connected by a blue line. The node workspace area is marked by a red rectangle and its header blue (e-book).

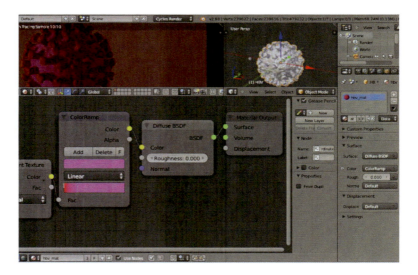

Figure 9.18 Node recipe for producing red color on the small surface protein and purple on the large surface protein on the basis of height of the surface from the center of the HBV object.

The material for the HBV will be created on the basis of the sketch as shown in Fig. 9.13. The color of the small surface protein of the HBV is purple, and the long surface protein is red. One way of accomplishing this is to set up nodes to tell Blender to color the surface of that object on the basis of the height of the surface. Four nodes can be used to accomplish this task (Fig. 9.18):

- Material Output node: What we see on the screen
- Diffuse BSDF (bidirectional scattering distribution function) node: Surface properties that give a surface appearance like plastic or rubber, and it takes color input from the Color Ramp node
- Color Ramp node: Used to adjust surface color based on distance of the surface from the center of the object
- Texture Coordinate node

The following table (Table 9.4) shows the steps in putting nodes together for the material of the HBV object and applying it to all the HBV objects in the scene.

Table 9.4 Steps in putting nodes together for the material of the HBV object and applying it to all the HBV objects in the scene

Step no.	Description
1	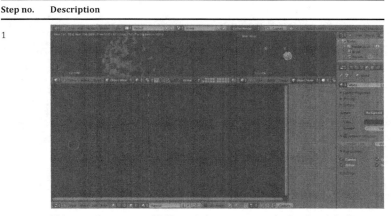 Make sure there are two 3D View windows, one set to the **Rendered** shading type. Additionally, set a sufficiently large Node window for composing nodes.

Table 9.4 (Contd.)

Step no.	Description
2	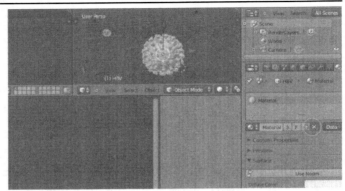 Select the HBV closest to the camera and click the **Material** button, fourth from the right of the header, in the Properties window. By default, it has been assigned as "Material." Unseat this material from the HBV object by pressing the **X** button.
3	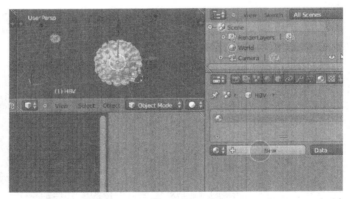 Once the default material is unset, a **New** button will appear to create a new material.

Step no.	Description
4	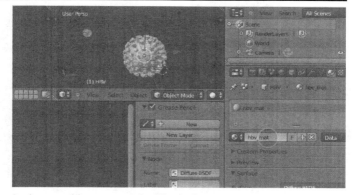 Set the name of the new material to "hbv_mat."
5	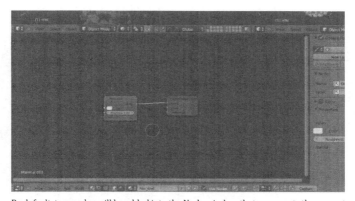 By default, two nodes will be added into the Node window that represents the current material. If these do not appear, click the **Material** button on the Node window's header and select hbv_mat from the pull-down/pull-up menu.

(Contd.)

Table 9.4 (*Contd.*)

Step no.	Description
6	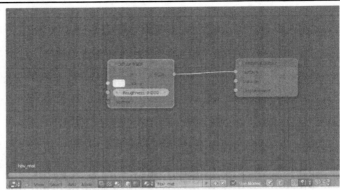

If the nodes appear small, use the mouse wheel or press [Ctrl] + [MMB] to zoom in and out of the Node workspace. Drag the MMB to pan the workspace around. Currently, the Diffuse BSDF node is connected to the Material Output node.

| 7 | 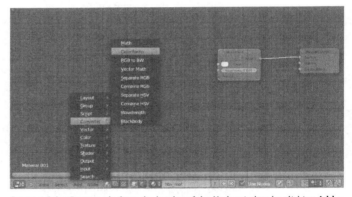 |

Create a Color Ramp node from the header of the Node window by clicking **Add** > **Converter** > **ColorRamp**.

Step no.	Description
8	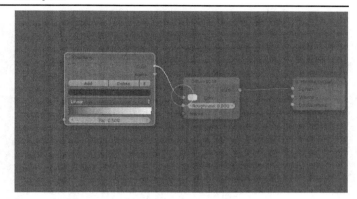 Connect the Color output of the Color Ramp node to the Color input of the Diffuse BSDF node.
9	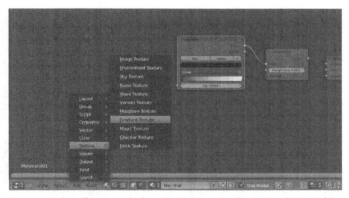 Create a Gradient Texture node from the Node window header by clicking **Add** > **Texture** > **Gradient Texture**.

(Contd.)

Table 9.4 (Contd.)

Step no.	Description
10	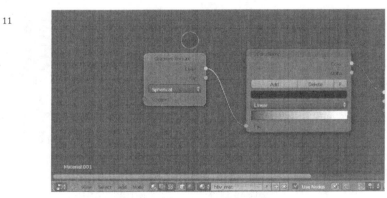 Connect the Color output of the Gradient Texture node to the Factor input of the Color Ramp node.
11	Set the Gradient Texture node's property to "Spherical."

Step no.	Description
12	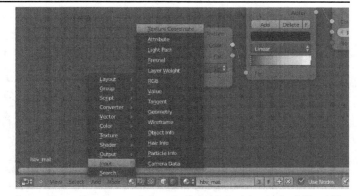 Create a Texture Coordinate node from the Node window's header by clicking **Add > Input > Texture > Coordinate**.
13	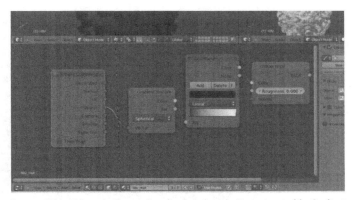 Connect "Object" from the Texture Coordinate node to the Vector input of the Gradient Texture node. Immediately, the 3D View window that renders interactively gives an interesting result: a gray HBV with a large surface protein in black.

(Contd.)

Table 9.4 (Contd.)

Step no.	Description
14	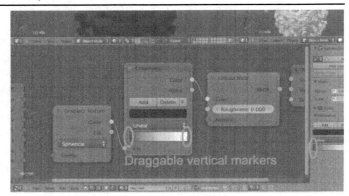

Now that the nodes are in place, changing the color of the HBV material is easy. By default, the Color Ramp node provides a gradient from black to white. Black seems to be allocated at the tip of the HBV. The Color Ramp node also allows us to add and delete more colors into the current gradient. For now, only two colors are needed. Each color—black and white—that makes up the gradient has a vertical bar marker that can be dragged to the left/right across the gradient color (marked in green circles).

15	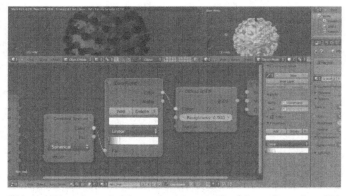

Click the **LMB** on the vertical line on the rightmost side of the gradient color, which represents white. Drag it to the left until the black color only is on the stumps.

Step no.	Description
16	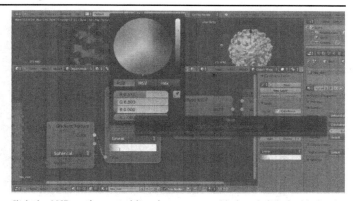 Click the **LMB** on the vertical line that represents black and click the black-color region on top of the Linear option to bring up the color chooser. Use the following R, G, and B values: 0.573, 0.003, and 0.0.
17	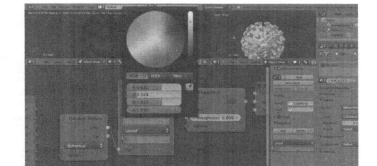 Use the following R, G, and B values: 0.622, 0.128, and 0.633. Replace the white color on the ramp. The material for the HBV is now complete.

(Contd.)

Table 9.4 (*Contd.*)

Step no.	Description
18	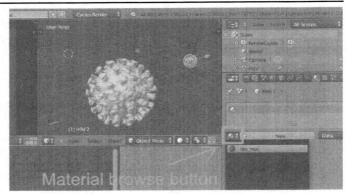 Select one of the HBV objects with no material and click the **Material** button in Properties window. Blender allows us to link existing material to the selected HBV object by clicking the browse button and selecting the existing hbv_mat.
19	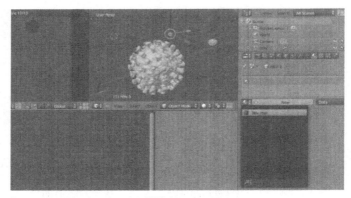 Repeat Step 18 for the other plain HBV object.

Step no.	Description
20	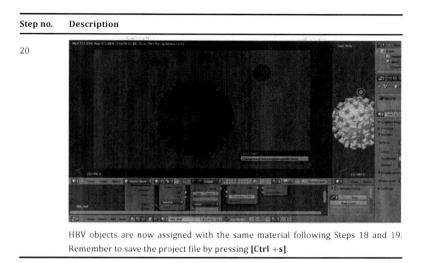 HBV objects are now assigned with the same material following Steps 18 and 19. Remember to save the project file by pressing [Ctrl +s].

9.6 Render Setup and Saving Results

Rendering to a 2D image in Blender is as simple as pressing **[F12]**. However, this does not always give the desired output. The size of the rendered image and its quality must be known before clicking the **Render** button. Render settings can be accessed from the Properties window and clicking the **Render** button (the first button on the header from the left). This reveals additional options to adjust the size, performance, and quality of rendering. In brief, there are three submenus discussed here: Dimensions, Sampling, and Light Paths.

The size of the rendering output can be adjusted from the Dimensions submenu (Fig. 9.19). The quality of the render can be altered from Sampling and Light Paths submenus, as marked by yellow (middle) and red (bottom) rectangles. The image in the UV/Image window, as shown in Fig. 9.19 was rendered at a 50% size of 1920 × 1080, with the default **Final** preset for Sampling and the default **Full Global Illumination** preset for Light Paths. Also, high sampling was used to produces a high-quality output. The

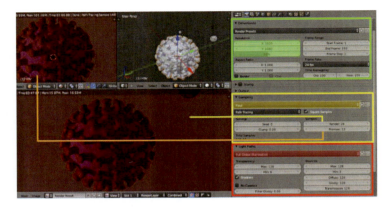

Figure 9.19 Settings to adjust size (green, top) and quality (yellow, middle; and red, bottom) of render output.

interactive rendering in the 3D View window used half of the final render sampling value to improve interactivity.

9.6.1 *Setting Render Size and Quality*

The Dimensions submenu has parameters for setting image dimensions. For an A4 size at 96 dots per inch (dpi), the optimal render size is 1123 × 794 pixels. If 600 dpi quality is required for A4-size printing, the optimal size is 7016 × 4961 pixels. The larger the pixel size, the longer it takes for rendering.

Under the Sampling submenu, there are options to control the number of samples for ray tracing. There are two presets, Preview and Final. Increasing samples is often necessary if there are acoustic objects in the scene, such as oceans or glasses. The number of samplings for preview is generally lower than the final render itself for performance reasons. The Preview quality is what the interactive render shows in the 3D View windows. Under Light Paths, there are presets to control how rays bounce on the surface and inside a material: **Direct Light**, **Full Global Illumination**, and **Limited Global Illumination**. Again, in the presence of glassy materials, normally a good render would require a higher number of rays to bounce on the surface and within the materials. Better-quality images take more time to complete than lower-quality ones.

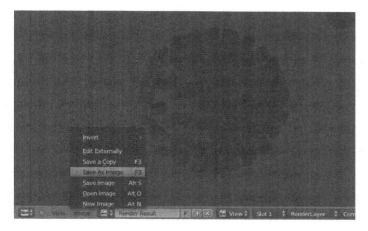

Figure 9.20 Render results can be saved into an image file from the Image >Save As Image menu of the UV/Image Editor window or by pressing [F3].

There is no hard-and-fast rule for setting the values for Sampling and Light Paths. It takes time to tweak and to find the best balance between an acceptable quality for a given resolution size and render time. Given a scene that does not contain light caustics or glassy materials, setting the number of rays to 1000 and increasing the number of diffuse reflection bounces to 500 might have little quality improvement with a longer render time in comparison to ray samples of 100 and a bounce value of 50. It is best to do tests at 25% or 50% render size for evaluation before committing the time and computing resources to do a full-size render. If the resolution is low without much detail, using lower-quality settings might be acceptable.

9.6.2 *Saving Images*

After rendering is finished, the result can be saved to a local or network hard drive by pressing **[F3]**. Alternatively, if the UV/Image Editor window is open, click **Image > Save As Image** on the header (Fig. 9.20).

By default images will be saved as PNG images. This can be changed by clicking the **PNG** button in the **Save as Image** panel on the left bar to bring up various formats Blender exports to

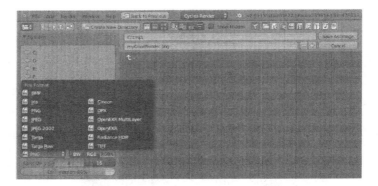

Figure 9.21 The image file format can be specified from the File window prior to saving the render result. This window appears after pressing [F3].

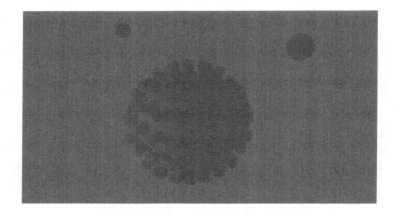

Figure 9.22 Final result of the HBV scene.

(Fig. 9.21). Click the **Save As Image** button next to the folder field to save the image to disk.

The successfully created 3D model of the HBV scene, as rendered, is shown in Fig. 9.22. This render took approximately 45 seconds to complete at 1920×1080 resolution by enabling the CUDA option (Section 9.5.1), with a 4-core i7 2nd generation CPU, 10 GB RAM, and 1 GB NVIDIA GT 640 M. It is possible to further explore and/or modify the scene, such as to create a dramatic effect, as shown in Fig. 9.23, using the tools of Blender.

Figure 9.23 Author's render of the HBV scene with the subdivision modifier set to 6 for rendering, three-point light, postprocessing effect, and mixing Diffuse BSDM with Velvet BSDM nodes.

9.7 Conclusion

This chapter has introduced the basics of Blender for scientific visualization by creating a scene containing HBV objects (Fig. 9.22). Blender is free and available for popular computing platforms: Windows, MacOSX, and GNU/Linux. Blender is not only a 3D modeling suite, but it also enables users to create complex materials and rendered images. It also includes many tools that are not covered in this chapter, which allow users to create real-time applications, camera tracking, video compositing, and posteffect productions. Blender has many functionalities that can be accessed from its UI. However, learning Blender's keyboard shortcuts is important to be able to create illustrations in a time-efficient manner. Solely relying on mouse movements and clicks to find a particular functionality hinders productivity and may increase the risk of repetitive strain injury.

The 3D modeling process should begin with a plan and a model with appropriate simplifications but should not be overly simplified. Always begin with low-polygon primitives and gradually increase the polygon count, as needed, for details. Setting up material and light follows logically after 3D modeling and composing objects in the scene. Lastly, the rendering stage must be carefully planned. It takes time to balance the image size, the quality, and an acceptable result. It is best to do render tests at a lower resolution quickly prior to committing to a higher resolution that would take more time and computing resources.

This chapter has touched lightly on what Blender 2.96 offers. Blender's online documentation lists complete functionalities, along with some tips and examples [14]. Scientists can use these tools to create illustrations that will significantly enhance the ease of uptake and impact of the research being reported.

References

1. Blender Foundation. *Blender*, http://www.blender.org (last accessed January 2014).
2. Kelaiah, I. *The Visual Complexity of Instructional Animations in Training Simulations to Promote Learning*, Macquarie University, Sydney, Australia, 2012, 468. Available at Macquarie University Library Automated Retrieval Collection Thesis (QA76.9.P75 K45).
3. Bigoin, N., Porte, J., Kartiko, I. and Kavakli, M. Effects of depth cues on simulator sickness, *Proc. 1st Int. Conf. Immersive Telecommun.: IMMERSCOM 2007*, 2007, 1–4.
4. Kavakli, M., Szilas, N., Porte, J. and Kartiko, I. *Architectural Design of Multi-Agent Systems: Technologies and Techniques*, Lin H, ed., Information Science Reference, 2007, 356–376.
5. Richards, D., Jacobson, M. J., Taylor, M., Newstead, A., Taylor, C., Porte, J., Kelaiah, I. and Hanna, N. Learning to be scientists via a virtual field trip (demonstration), *Proc. 11th Int. Conf. Auton. Agents Multiagent Syst.*, Richland, SC, International Foundation for Autonomous Agents and Multiagent Systems, 2012, doi:http://dl.acm.org/citation.cfm?id=2343896.2344062.
6. Bacone, V. K. *Blender Game Engine Beginner's Guide*, Packt, Birmingham, UK, 2012.
7. Brito, A. *Blender 3D 2.49 Architecture, Buildings, and Scenery*, Packt, Birmingham, UK, 2010.
8. W. Powell, A. *Blender 2.5 Lighting and Rendering: Bring Your 3D World to Life with Lighting, Compositing, and Rendering*, Packt, Birmingham, UK, 2010.

9. Valenza, E. *Blender 2.6 Cycles, Materials and Textures Cookbook,* Packt, Birmingham, UK, 2013.
10. Mullen, T. *Mastering Blender,* Wiley, Indianapolis, 2012.
11. Simonds, B. *Blender Master Class: A Hands-On Guide to Modeling, Sculpting, Materials, and Rendering,* No Starch Press, San Francisco, 2012.
12. Wickes, R. D. *Foundation Blender Compositing,* friendsofED, Berkeley, CA, 2009.
13. Datta, S., Chatterjee, S., Veer, V. and Chakravarty, R. Molecular biology of the hepatitis B virus for clinicians, *J. Clin. Exp. Hepatol.*, **2**(4), 2012, 353–365. doi:http://www.sciencedirect.com/science/article/pii/S0973688312000801.
14. Blender Community. *Blender 2.6 Online Documentation,* 2014, http://wiki.blender.org/index.php/Doc:2.6/Manual.

Index

Abraxane 5, 10
AFM, *see* atomic force microscope
AID peptide 38–39, 41–42, 44–45, 47
AID-TAT 39, 42–43, 46
AlGaN/GaN heterostructure 148–149, 161, 168
AlGaN/GaN sensor 152, 163–164, 166–167
AlGaN/GaN surfaces 151, 161
ammonia 128, 254
amorphous semiconductor model 175, 179–181, 186, 188–189, 195
anatase 250–251
anatase TiO_2 257
antibodies 18, 22, 80, 85, 88, 149
atom transfer radical polymerization (ATRP) 72–73, 75–76
atomic force microscope (AFM) 115–116, 138
ATRP, *see* atom transfer radical polymerization

biocompatibility 18, 72, 78–79, 86, 93, 147, 156, 158–159
bioelectronics 176, 197
biosensors 149, 165, 168
Brownian diffusion 299–300
Brownian motion 139–140
bulk semiconductor 205–206

calcium dosing 166–167
cancer 10, 19, 22, 32, 47
cancer cells 22, 85, 88
cantilever beams 110–112, 130, 138–139
cantilever–grating separation 123, 133–134
capacitance 117, 153, 155, 247
  chemical 247
cardiac myocytes 38, 42–43, 47
CBD, *see* chemical bath deposition
CCD, *see* charge-coupled device
CdSe 209, 212, 215, 218, 242
CdSe QDs 204, 207, 209–210, 212–214, 219–221, 225–226
cell mortality 158–160
cell-penetrating peptides (CPPs) 17, 19, 39
cellular uptake 18–19, 36, 40, 42
charge-coupled device (CCD) 211
charge transfer resistance 244, 247
chemical bath deposition (CBD) 241
chemical sensors 149
chemical vapor deposition (CVD) 203
chemotherapeutics 9, 94
chemotherapy 90–95
clathrin 12, 14
co-structure-directing agents (CSDAs) 68, 70

colloidal synthesis 203, 206
comproportionation reaction 176, 178, 193–194, 197–198
computed tomography (CT) 23, 25
conduction band 204, 206, 235, 237, 239, 261
continuum mechanics 290, 297–298
controlled release 10, 18–19
convective flow resistance 295, 304–305
CPPs, see cell-penetrating peptides
creatine kinase 46
CSDAs, see co-structure-directing agents
CT, see computed tomography
CVD, see chemical vapor deposition

Darcy's law 296, 305, 308
deflection noise density (DND) 133–136
delivery, nanoparticle-mediated 42, 45
delivery vehicles, nanoparticle 3, 47
dendrimers 4, 6–7, 9
DHI, see 5,6-dihydroxyindole
DHICA, see 5,6-dihydroxyindole-2-carboxylic acid
diffusivity 325
  effective 308, 316, 319–324
5,6-dihydroxyindole (DHI) 179
5,6-dihydroxyindole-2-carboxylic acid (DHICA) 179
DLS, see dynamic light scattering
DMPC, see dynamic moisture permeation cell
DND, see deflection noise density
docetaxel 83–84
drug delivery 2, 4, 9, 11, 18–19, 22–24, 32, 35–36, 69, 91
drug delivery vehicles 3, 6, 9–10
drug testing 162–167

DSSCs
  see dye-sensitized solar cells
  efficiency of 263, 265
  high-efficiency 258, 265, 268–270
dye-sensitized solar cells (DSSCs) 231–258, 262–264, 266–267, 269–271
dynamic light scattering (DLS) 40–41, 211, 213, 215
dynamic moisture permeation cell (DMPC) 304–305

EIS, see electrochemical impedance spectroscopy
electrochemical impedance spectroscopy (EIS) 244, 247, 261, 267
electron diffusion coefficient 265
electron paramagnetic resonance (EPR) 19, 193–194
electron transport 238, 247, 256, 264–265, 270
electrospinning 290–294, 324
electrospun fiber mats 304–305
electrospun nanofiber filters 301, 303
electrospun nanofiber mats 291, 295, 301–302, 304–308, 323, 325–326
electrospun nanofiber webs 295, 297
electrospun nanofibers 289–298, 300–302, 304, 306, 308, 310, 312, 314, 316, 318, 320, 322, 324, 326
electrospun nanofibrous membrane 321–322, 325
electrostatic actuation 126, 129
encapsulation 6, 9, 11, 36, 151, 156–157
endocytosis, clathrin-mediated 14–15

EPR, *see* electron paramagnetic resonance
eumelanin 179

fast-Fourier transform (FFT) 216–217, 251
FDTD, *see* finite-difference time domain
FETs, *see* field-effect transistors
FFT, *see* fast-Fourier transform
fiber volume fraction (FVF) 299–301, 311–312, 314, 325
fibrous filters 296, 298–299, 301, 307
fibrous porous media 296, 317
field-effect transistors (FETs) 149–150, 153, 176
finite-difference time domain (FDTD) 121, 134
free-radical density 193, 195
FVF, *see* fiber volume fraction

gadolinium-labeled magnetite nanoparticles (GMNPs) 30–31
gas diffusion layer (GDL) 308
gas flow in nanofibrous media 309–313
GDL, *see* gas diffusion layer
gel permission chromatography (GPC) 78
gene delivery 62
GMNPs, *see* gadolinium-labeled magnetite nanoparticles
GPC, *see* gel permission chromatography
graphene 204, 207–208, 218–226, 244
graphene sheets 180, 203–204, 207–208, 218–219, 221–223, 225
graphene surface 222, 225

Hank's balanced salt solution (HBSS) 163, 165
HBSS, *see* Hank's balanced salt solution
HBV, *see* hepatitis B virus
HCAEC, *see* human coronary artery endothelial cells
HeLa cells 15–16, 86–87
HEMTs, *see* high-electron-mobility transistors
hepatitis B virus (HBV) 335–336, 351–355, 358–359, 363, 366, 368, 373–374, 380–381
high-electron-mobility transistors (HEMTs) 148
high-resolution transmission electron microscopy (HRTEM) 203, 216, 221
HRTEM, *see* high-resolution transmission electron microscopy
human coronary artery endothelial cells (HCAEC) 165
hydrogen 113–114, 195
hydronium 193–194, 197
N-hydroxysuccinimide 80, 265, 269–270

interrogating grating 119, 122, 126, 134, 139
ion-sensitive field-effect transistors (ISFETs) 150–153
ischemia-reperfusion injury 37, 46–47
ISFETs, *see* ion-sensitive field-effect transistors

Johnson noise 134, 137

Knudsen diffusion 298, 316, 321, 325

lactate dehydrogenase (LDH) 46
lauryl sulfonate betaine (LSB) 63, 68
LDH, see lactate dehydrogenase
LEDs, see light-emitting diodes
light-emitting diodes (LEDs) 148
light harvesting 232, 252, 255, 262, 265, 269
light-harvesting efficiency 234, 266–267, 269–270
light scattering 255, 266, 268–269
  dynamic 40–41, 211
liposomes 4, 6–9, 21
living radical polymerization (LRP) 72–74, 95
localized surface plasmon resonance (LSPR) 254
LRP, see living radical polymerization
LSB, see lauryl sulfonate betaine
LSPR, see localized surface plasmon resonance

macromolecules 11, 13, 79
macrophages 13, 15, 21
macropinocytosis 12, 14–15
magnetic field 28, 30, 85, 93, 192
magnetic resonance imaging (MRI) 23, 25, 27–30, 44–45, 89–90, 93–94
magnetite 30, 40, 42, 208
MDD, see minimum detectable deflection
melanin 175–198
  conductivity of 183
  dry 182–183, 196
  hydrated 193–194
  water content of 183–185, 187
melanin charge transport 181–183
melanin dark conductivity 186–187
melanin polymers 180

MEMS, see microelectromechanical systems
MEMS beams 111, 114, 116
MEMS cantilever 110, 117, 128, 138, 140
MEMS devices 112, 116–118, 127–128, 130, 140
MEMS sensors 109, 113–115, 118
MEMS structures 109, 111, 126, 129
mesoporous silica nanoparticles (MSNs) 75, 78–79, 91
metal organic chemical vapor deposition (MOCVD) 206
micelles 4–8, 67
microcantilevers 111, 115, 120–121, 127, 130–133, 136, 138
microelectromechanical systems (MEMS) 107–109, 111–112, 116–118
microfibers 290, 297, 304, 310, 321, 324
micromachined beams 118–119
minimum detectable deflection (MDD) 133–135, 137
MOCVD, see metal organic chemical vapor deposition
MRI, see magnetic resonance imaging
MSNs, see mesoporous silica nanoparticles
multifunctional nanoparticle system 18, 35
muon mobility 190, 192–193
muon spin resonance 183, 190–191, 193, 195
muons, positive 190–191
myocytes 42–44

nanobeams 116–117
nanocapsules 4, 6, 10

nanofibers 290, 294, 296–297, 308, 310, 315, 324
nanofibrous media 309, 311, 313, 315, 317, 319, 321, 323
nanoparticle endocytosis 14–15
nanoparticle surface charge 15
nanoparticle surface coating 13, 21
nanoparticle synthesis 3, 33
nanoparticle toxicity 32, 34
nanoparticle uptake 13–14, 16
nanoparticles
   AID-tethered 43–44, 46
   anionic 16
   biodegradable polymeric 4, 10
   cationic 16
   gold 25, 27
   hydrogel 15
   iron oxide 25, 30
   multifunctional 17–19, 23
   multifunctional PGMA 45, 47
   multifunctional polymeric 36, 45
   octafunctional 19
   PEI-functionalized 41–42
   PGMA 37, 39–40, 45, 47
   polymeric 10–11, 36
   silica 66, 70, 72, 75, 77–80
   mesoporous 75
   yolk–shell 61–62
nanostructured photoanodes 234, 248–249, 251, 253, 255, 257, 259, 261, 270
nanotoxicology 33–34
neurons 32, 150, 178
nitroxide-mediated radical polymerization (NMP) 73, 75, 77
NMP, see nitroxide-mediated radical polymerization
NMR, see nuclear magnetic resonance
nonphagocytic pathways 12, 14

nuclear magnetic resonance (NMR) 28, 211

OBD, see optical beam deflection
octadecene (ODE) 218–219, 224–225
OCVD, see open-circuit voltage decay
ODE, see octadecene
OECT, see organic electrochemical transistor
open-circuit voltage decay (OCVD) 247, 269
optical beam deflection (OBD) 115–116
organic dyes 80, 234, 241
organic electrochemical transistor (OECT) 176, 178, 194, 196
orthogonal fibers 310, 312–313, 325

pair distribution function (PDF) 211, 214
palladium 113
patch-clamp technique 150
Pauw geometry 186–188
PDF, see pair distribution function
PECVD, see plasma-enhanced chemical vapor deposition
PEDOT 176–178, 196
PEI, see poly(ethyleneimine)
PEI functionalization 40–41
PEI-functionalized nanoparticle surface 41
peptides 1, 18–19, 27, 37–39, 41–44, 47, 80
   therapeutic 2, 35, 37, 39, 42
PET, see positron emission tomography
PGMA, see poly(glycidyl methacrylate)
phagocytosis 12–13

photoanodes 231, 234–235, 237–238, 249–250, 252, 256, 265–266, 268–269
photodynamic therapy 7–8
photoelectrodes 267, 269–270
photothermal therapy 62, 82, 88, 91–93, 95
photovoltage 239–240, 246, 261–262
photovoltaics 232
plasma-enhanced chemical vapor deposition (PECVD) 128
poly(ethyleneimine) (PEI) 16, 36–37, 40, 86, 93
poly(glycidyl methacrylate) (PGMA) 2, 35–37, 39, 41, 43, 45, 47
polystyrene 15, 72
positron emission tomography (PET) 23, 25
powder X-ray diffraction (PXRD) 203, 211–213, 215–216, 220, 222
power conversion efficiency 245, 266
protective clothing 289–290, 295–296, 298–299, 301, 303–305, 307–308, 322, 324–325
proteins
  fluorescent 32
  small surface 372–373
protons 89, 190–192, 194, 240
PXRD, see powder X-ray diffraction

QDs, see quantum dots
quantum confinement 204–206, 225
quantum dots (QDs) 2–3, 18, 31–32, 203–215, 217–223, 225–226, 239, 241–242

RAFT, see reversible addition-fragmentation chain transfer
RAFT polymerization 73, 75
readout technique 107, 114–115, 118, 133, 137–140
red blood cells 352
reversible addition-fragmentation chain transfer (RAFT) 72, 75–76

scanning electron micrograph (SEM) 130, 161, 257, 320
SEM, see scanning electron micrograph
semiconductors 181–182, 214, 237–239
  amorphous 179, 181–182, 189
semiquinones 193–194, 197
SERS, see surface-enhanced Raman scattering
SFEs, see single-fiber efficiency
silane chemistry 72, 80
silica 65, 70–71, 74–75, 80, 82, 86–87, 112, 121–122, 158
  epitaxial 122, 126–127
silica nanorattles 84, 91–92
single-fiber efficiency (SFEs) 299–301
siRNA 16, 19, 86–87
solar cells 208, 231, 245–246
SPR, see surface plasmon resonance
surface-enhanced Raman scattering (SERS) 94
surface-initiated ATRP technique 76–77
surface plasmon resonance (SPR) 112
surface-protected etching method 65–66
synergetic chemo-/radiotherapy 94

TAT, *see trans*-activator of transcription
TAT-mediated delivery 42, 45, 47
TAT peptide 17, 39
TEM, *see* transmission electron microscopy
thin films 175, 178, 196, 237, 255
TiO_2 66, 70, 237–238, 251, 255–257, 259, 268
TiO_2 beads, mesoporous 252–254
trans-activator of transcription (TAT) 17–18, 39, 44, 46
transmission electron microscopy (TEM) 40, 161, 211
tumor vasculature 19–20, 22
tumors 8, 19–22, 27, 84, 90, 92, 94

vapor diffusion 289–290, 296, 298, 315, 317
vapor diffusion in nanofibrous media 315–323
vasoactive intestinal peptide (VIP) 9

VIP, *see* vasoactive intestinal peptide

water vapor diffusion resistance 304, 306–307

yolk–shell-structured nanoparticles (YSNs) 61–72, 74, 76, 78, 80, 82, 84–88, 90–96
YSNs, *see* yolk–shell-structured nanoparticles
YSNs for biomedicine applications 82–93

ZB, *see* zinc blende
ZB–CdSe 213, 216–217
zinc blende (ZB) 209, 211–214, 221
zinc-blende structures 209
ZnO nanowires 258–259, 265–267

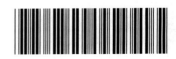